Measuring Health

Measuring Health:
A Review of Subjective Health, Well-Being and Quality of Life Measurement Scales

FOURTH EDITION

Ann Bowling

Open University Press

Open University Press
McGraw-Hill Education
8th Floor
338 Euston Road
London
NW1 3BH

email: enquiries@openup.co.uk
world wide web: www.mheducation.co.uk

and Two Penn Plaza, New York, NY 10121-2289, USA

First published 1991
Second edition published 1997
Third edition published 2004
First published in this fourth edition 2017

A catalogue record of this book is available from the British Library

ISBN-13: 978-0-33-526194-9
ISBN-10: 0-33-526194-9
eISBN: 978-0-33-526195-6

Library of Congress Cataloging-in-Publication Data
CIP data applied for

Typeset by Transforma Pvt. Ltd., Chennai, India

Printed and bound by Bell & Bain Ltd, Glasgow.

Praise page

"The world of measurement scales, which ones to use and for what purpose, is a complex one even for experienced qualitative researchers. It is easy for less experienced researchers to lose their way. Ann Bowling's book provides an up to date and coherent guide and assessment of measurement tools which is comprehensible and well organized."

Virginia Berridge, Professor of History and Director, Centre for History in
Public Health, London School of Hygiene and Tropical Medicine, UK

"In her latest edition of Measuring Health: A Review of Subjective Health, Well-Being and Quality of Life Measurement Scales, *Professor Ann Bowling has, once again, provided us with an essential for our bookshelves. It is a vital resource for anyone investigating health and well-being – whether novice student researcher or experienced academic.*

Written in an accessible, easy to use style, we are initially taken through the importance of measuring and understanding lay people's experiences of their physical and social health. The mechanics and challenges of measurement of subjective health are then described. Later chapters include handy definitions of relevant concepts and detailed descriptions of specific scales – both familiar and relatively new ones – including psychometric testing and use. This text is packed with useful information and can be used both as a resource for an overall understanding of measuring health and well-being or for selecting specific patient-based health scales for research projects."

Dr Nan Greenwood, Reader in Health and Social Care Service Research,
St George's University of London and Kingston University, UK

Contents

Preface to the fourth edition

Since the publication of the previous editions of this book, interest in patient-based evaluation of health and service outcomes has continued to increase. This fourth edition has been based on systematically conducted internet searches of new and established measurement scales. It would not be feasible in a book of this size to include reference to all published studies utilizing a specific scale. The studies which have been referenced include those that have provided pertinent information on the psychometric properties of an instrument. Also, while many new measures have been developed, few have undergone extensive psychometric testing.

New measures have been included where an emerging body of evidence supports their use (e.g. on well-being and quality of life – QoL). New inclusions are: the additional World Health Organization WHOQOL group quality of life measures (WHOQOL-BREF and WHOQOL-OLD); the Older People's Quality of Life questionnaire (OPQOL and OPQOL-Brief); the Warwick-Edinburgh Well-being Scale (WEWBS); the Adult Social Care Outcomes Toolkit for assessing social care-related QoL (ASCOT); and the Short-Form McGill Pain Questionnaire (SF-MPQ). An expanded, headed section on the Functional Independence Measure (FIM) and Functional Assessment Measure (FAM) has also been included.

Some measures have been removed from this edition, such as the Symptoms of Anxiety and Depression Scale (SAD). This is because, while it was a popular tool in the UK for use with older populations, it is no longer used as a stand-alone instrument. It is used mainly in the USA along with the SCL-90 subscale on anxiety (the DSSI/SAD) (Bedford et al. 1976; Bedford and Deary 1997). Also removed is the Geriatric Mental State, due to the retirement of its developer and as no current sources or contacts for support have yet been found (Copeland et al. 1976).

The Family Relationship Index (Moos and Moos 1981) has been removed due to lack of recent evidence of its psychometric properties. The Cornell Medical Index (CMI) (Brodman et al. 1949) has been removed due to its withdrawal from use by its owners at Cornell University Medical College (now the Weill Medical College of Cornell University), on the grounds that it is outdated and no longer suitable for clinical research. Cornell retains the copyright to enable it to reinitiate the CMI if revision and revalidation are carried out (Brodman et al. 1986; Weill Cornell Medical Library 2003). The Crichton Royal Behaviour Rating Scale (CRBRS) has been removed due to less published use (Robinson 1968; Wilkin and Jolley 1979), as has Evans and Cope's (1994) Quality of Life Questionnaire (QLQ). The short mental status scales have also been removed: the Mental

Status Questionnaire (MSQ) and its modified version (Kahn *et al.* 1960a, 1960b; Pfeiffer 1975) and the Abbreviated Mental Test Score (AMTS) (Hodkinson 1972) in order to give Chapter 5 more focus.

While this volume includes a wide selection of popularly used generic and domain-specific measurement scales, there are inevitable omissions in a book of this size. Notably, classic scales of stress, adjustment and coping ability have been omitted (see Kasl and Cooper 1987; Maes *et al.* 1987; Cooper and Kasl 1995; Schwarzer and Schwarzer 1996). Overviews of research methods and terminology can be found in Bowling (2014b), Bowling and Ebrahim (2005) and Earl-Slater (2002).

Copyright permissions were re-sought to reproduce the items from the scales in this volume, and the author is grateful to the scale developers and distributors for their consent. Some scales are too long to reproduce in full here, and others are strictly copyrighted and only available commercially (which prevents reproduction in full or of more than a small number of items). It was, as before, decided to aim for consistency and only reproduce a selection of scale items as examples, except where scales are very brief.

Potential users are advised to consult the authors or distributors of scales before use, in order to avoid copyright infringement. Informed use also assists authors of scales to compile bibliographies of users and results, and handbooks; computerized scoring templates or user guides may be available.

An updated selection of useful addresses has been included in scale boxes in order to assist readers. Where a contact address has not been given for a particular scale, it is usually because there is no current contact for that scale, and readers should consult the references to the scale, as well as conduct electronic searches, for further details. It may also be because the scale has been reproduced in full in one of the key publications listed in the references (e.g. many of the older social support scales have been reproduced in this way).

The current addresses of scale developers and distributors are not always easy to trace, and scale developers sometimes change which publishers hold the copyright and licences for use. Some measures that have long been free to use are later available only with payment of a fee (unfunded academic research is sometimes exempt from charges). I would again like to repeat an early plea made by Wilkin *et al.* (1992) that authors should be encouraged to publish their scales in full in key journal publications or, where copyright, length or commercial reasons prevent this, to, at minimum, publish the address of the scale distributor. Care is also needed to ensure the version accessed is the most up to date available.

Finally, as before, section summaries recommending a 'best buy' have not been included as each scale has its strengths and weaknesses, most scales are being continually developed or tested, and ultimately the choice of which scale to use is dependent on the aims of the study, its population type and the judgement of the investigators. Also, some scales have not been subjected to the fullest psychometric testing; it should be noted that testing is an ongoing process and can take many years.

Acknowledgements

I would like to thank Richard Townrow and Karen Harris at Open University Press for all their hard work and patience, and also Jon Ingoldby, for copy-editing the manuscript so efficiently.

List of abbreviations

ABS	Affect-Balance Scale
ADDQoL	Audit of Diabetes Dependent Quality of Life
ADL	activities of daily living
AIMS	Arthritis Impact Measurement Scales
AKPS	Australian-modified Karnofsky Performance Status
AMTS	Abbreviated Mental Test Score
APA	American Psychiatric Association
ASCOT	Adult Social Care Outcomes Toolkit
ASSIS	Arizona Social Support Interview Schedule
AUC	area under the curve
BDI	Beck Depression Inventory
CAL	chronic airflow limitation
CAMDEX	Cambridge Examination for Mental Disorders of the Elderly
CAPE	Clifton Assessment Procedures for the Elderly
CARE	Comprehensive Assessment and Referral Evaluation
CASP-19	Control, Autonomy, Self-realisation and Pleasure 19-item questionnaire
CES-D	Center for Epidemiologic Studies Depression Scale
CMI	Cornell Medical Index
CRBRS	Crichton Royal Behaviour Rating Scale
CSEI	Coopersmith Self-esteem Inventory
DIS	Diagnostic Interview Schedule
DSM	*Diagnostic and Statistical Manual*
D–TFS	Delighted–Terrible Faces Scale
ECOG PS	Eastern Cooperative Oncology Group Performance Status
EQ-5D	EuroQol
ERSS	Edinburgh Rehabilitation Status Scale
FAI	Functional Assessment Inventory
FIM/FAM	Functional Independence Measure and Functional Assessment Measure
FLP	Functional Limitations Profile
FRI	Family Relationship Index
GDS	Geriatric Depression Scale
GHQ	General Health Questionnaire
GHRI	General Health Rating Index
GHS	General Household Survey
GMS	Geriatric Mental State
GWBS	(Psychological) General Well-Being Schedule

HADS	Hospital Anxiety and Depression Scale
HANES	Health and Nutritional Examination Survey
HAQ	(Stanford Arthritis Center) Health Assessment Questionnaire
HIS	Health Insurance Study (RAND)
HSQ-12	Health Status Questionnaire-12
HUI3	Health Utilities Index mark 3
IADL	instrumental activities of daily living
ICD	International Classification of Diseases
ICF	International Classification of Functioning, Disability and Health
IQOLA	International Quality of Life Assessment
IRT	item response theory
ISEL	Interpersonal Support Evaluation List
ISSB	Inventory of Socially Supportive Behaviours
ISSI	Interview Schedule for Social Interaction
KPI	Karnofsky Performance Index
LASA	Linear Analogue Self-Assessment
LEIPAD	LEIden and PADua quality of life questionnaire
LHS	London Handicap Scale
LSIA	Life Satisfaction Index A
LSIB	Life Satisfaction Index B
LSIZ	Life Satisfaction Index Z
LSNS	Lubben Social Network Scale
MACTAR	McMaster-Toronto Arthritis and Rheumatism
MADRS	Montgomery-Asberg Depression Rating Scale
MCS-36	Mental Component Summary Score
MHIQ	McMaster Health Index Questionnaire
MOS	Medical Outcomes Study (RAND)
MOT	Medical Outcomes (Study) Trust
MPQ	McGill Pain Questionnaire
MSE	Mental State Examination
MSQ	Mental Status Questionnaire
NHP	Nottingham Health Profile
OARS	Older Americans' Resources and Services Schedule
OMFAQ	OARS Multi-Dimensional Functional Assessment Questionnaire
ONS	Office for National Statistics
OPQOL	Older People's Quality of Life questionnaire
OPQOL-Brief	Older People's Quality of Life questionnaire – brief
PCA	principal components analysis
PCS-36	Physical Component Summary Score
PGCMS	Philadelphia Geriatric Center Morale Scale
PGI	Patient Generated Index
PEWBI	Psychological General Well-Being Index
PGWBS	Psychological General Well-Being Schedule
PWB	Scales of Psychological Well-Being

QALYs	quality-adjusted life years
QL Index	(Spitzer's) Quality of Life Index
QLQ	Quality of Life Questionnaire
QoL	quality of life
QWBS	Quality of Well-Being Scale
RA	rheumatoid arthritis
RADS	Reynolds Adolescent Depression Scale
RCT	randomized controlled trial
ROC	receiver operating characteristic
SAS	Statistical Analysis Systems
SCRQoL	social care-related QoL
SEIQoL	Schedule for the Evaluation of Individual Quality of Life
SF-MPQ	Short McGill Pain Questionnaire
SF-6D	Short Form-6D
SF-8	Short Form-8
SF-12	Short Form-12
SF-36	Short Form-36
SIP	Sickness Impact Profile
SNS	Social Network Scale
SOC	Sense of Coherence Scale
SS-A	Social Support Appraisals Scale
SS-B	Social Support Behaviours Scale
STAI	State–Trait Anxiety Inventory
STAI-Y	State–Trait Anxiety Inventory – Form Y
SWLS	Satisfaction with Life Scale
TAPS	Team for the Assessment of Psychiatric Services
TSCS	Tennessee Self-Concept Scale
UCLA	University of California at Los Angeles
VAS	Visual Analogue Scale
WEMWBS	Warwick Edinburgh Mental Well-Being Scale
WHO	World Health Organization
WHOQOL	World Health Organization Quality of Life
WONCA	World Organization of Family Doctors
ZSDS	Zung's Self-Rating Depression Scale

CHAPTER 1

CONCEPTS OF FUNCTIONING, HEALTH, WELL-BEING AND QUALITY OF LIFE

CHAPTER COVERAGE

MEASUREMENT

Researchers in health and social care are increasingly focused on the measurement of the outcomes of service interventions, based on patients' or clients' perspectives. The conceptualization and methods of measurement of outcomes is still controversial, although there is general recognition that meaningful measures of people's broader health status and quality of life should be used.

In social care, the measurement of the effectiveness of services was relatively limited for many years, but there is now an increasing emphasis on service monitoring, objectives, measuring people's needs, met needs and outcomes based on clients' perspectives – rather than just, for example, measuring their levels of functioning.

In health care, outcome assessment has a longer tradition. Clinical indicators traditionally reflect a 'disease' model – a medical conception of pathological abnormality which is indicated by signs and symptoms. But a person's 'ill health' is indicated by feelings of pain and discomfort or perceptions of change in usual functioning and feeling. Illnesses can be the result of pathological abnormality, but not necessarily so. A person can feel ill without medical science being able to detect disease.

Broader measures of health status need to take both concepts into account. What matters is how the patient feels, rather than how professionals think they feel. Symptom response or survival rates are no longer enough. For example, where people are treated for chronic or life-threatening conditions, the therapy has to be evaluated in terms of whether it is more or less likely to lead to an outcome of a life worth living in social and psychological, as well as physical, terms.

Moreover, there are multiple influences upon patient outcome, and these require a broad model of health to incorporate them. The non-biological factors which can affect recovery and outcome include patient psychology, motivation, coping strategies, access to health care, social support networks, values and cultural beliefs, health behaviours, self-management style, adherence to therapy, and socio-economic status. Many of these concepts have been long recognized in research on health behaviour (Becker 1974), and require recognition in other studies which aim to understand the factors influencing service outcomes.

MEASURING HEALTH OUTCOME

In order to measure health outcomes a measure of health status is required which needs to be based on a concept of health. The limitations of the widely used negative definition of health as the absence of disease, and the unspecific World Health Organization's (1948a, 1948b) definition of health as total physical, mental and social well-being, have long been recognized. In the absence of satisfactory definitions of health, the question is: how should the outcome of interventions and services be measured?

One commonly used source of information about the functioning of health services is routinely collected data about processes and outcomes – *health service use* information. For example, the USA relies heavily on health insurance data for information about service use, and the UK relies on routinely collected information from the National Health Service about deaths and discharges from hospital by the patients' diagnosis, surgical interventions performed, socio-demographic details, and geographical area. All routinely collected data about usage are subject to problems of inaccuracy. Also, indicators of service use reflect the policies and practices of service providers, their resources and priorities, and provide no information about the impact of treatment on a person's life. Service-use rates also reflect people's 'illness behaviour' (the extent to which people perceive, react to, and act upon their symptoms of ill health), which varies by their socio-demographic and cultural characteristics (there is a long history of sociological research on illness behaviour, including work by Mechanic 1962, 1978; Kasl and Cobb 1966; Cockerham 1995). It is now recognized that routine data needs to be supplemented with patient-based information to be of value in outcome assessments.

As stated earlier, the traditional indices of outcomes of health care are negative in their focus. The main clinical outcome measures are mortality rates (length of survival), morbidity, complications, biochemical tests, physical condition, symptoms and, in the past, speed of return to work. Clinicians have traditionally judged the value of an intervention mainly in terms of the five-year survival period. While important, many health care interventions will have little or no impact on mortality rates (e.g. chronic conditions).

In recognition of this, since the 1980s there has been an exponential increase in the additional use of indicators of broader health status and health-related quality of life (Garratt *et al.* 2002; for range see Bowling 2001). But many measures of health status, broader health status and health-related quality of life take health and life quality as a starting point and measure deviations away from it, rather than also encompassing gradations of healthiness and good quality of life. A perspective which captures the positive end of the spectrum is required to create a balance and a less skewed viewpoint. In contrast to the emphasis on negative health, Merrell and Reed (1949), in a classic early paper, proposed a graded scale of health from positive to negative health. On such a scale people would be classified from those who are in top-notch condition with abundant energy, through to people who are well, to fairly well, down to people who are feeling rather poorly, and finally to the definitely ill. The word 'health' rather than 'illness' was chosen deliberately to emphasize the positive side of this scale. Despite the existence of single item ranking scales asking people to rate their health from 'Excellent' to 'Very poor', the development of a broader health status scale along such a continuum is still awaited.

Standardized items or measures of subjective health status are increasingly included in population health surveys, in evaluations and clinical trials of service interventions. These are measures which ask people to rate their own health status and the impact of their health on various aspects of their lives. They are often referred to as patient-based measures. Detailed information about self-perceived health and its effects can be collected from large numbers of people using self-report questionnaires. They can be administered to the target group of interest by post, telephone, computers, in clinical settings, or in face-to-face home interviews (although caution may be needed in interpretation, as different methods of questionnaire administration can result in different findings – Bowling 2005a). The group of interest may be a patient or client group or a sample of the general population, depending on the aims of the study. Survey information about health and illness at population level is collected routinely by several governments (e.g. government-sponsored interview surveys in the USA since 1956, in Britain since 1971 and in Finland since 1964).

As concepts are often used interchangeably in the literature on patient-based health and quality of life outcomes research, there is a general lack of consensus over their definition and measurement. The following sections examine the main concepts that are widely used and which arguably make up broader health status, and, ultimately, health-related and generic quality of life.

THE CONCEPT OF FUNCTIONAL ABILITY

Functional status, in its broadest sense, is the degree to which someone is able to perform social roles free of physical or mental health-related limitations. One of the oldest, and most common, broader methods of assessing outcome of health and social care is in terms of people's physical functioning, especially their performance of tasks of daily living. Such measures are regarded as more meaningful to people's lives than objective biochemical measures, or measures of timed 'get up and go' and walk speed tests, balance, lower limb strength and grip strength. Even short measures of physical function can be predictive of loss of independence, mortality and nursing home admissions (Guralnik *et al.* 1994).

There are several models of disability (see review by Putnam 2002). Social models of disability attempt to explain what disability is and how it is experienced; it is held that disability is a function of the interaction between a person and the demands of their environment. The original World Health Organization social model of disability recognized that the terms 'impairment', 'disability' and 'handicap' are often erroneously used interchangeably. The increasing use of the concept of functional dependency has recently added to the confusion. The World Health Organization's (WHO 1980) early *International Classification of Impairments, Disabilities and Handicaps* provided a consistent, if over-simple, terminology and classification system (since revised to present a more complex, positive model, see later). It defined the terms 'impairment', 'disability' and 'handicap' and linked them together conceptually:

Disease or Disorder $\longrightarrow$ Impairment $\longrightarrow$ Disability $\longrightarrow$ Handicap

e.g.:

Blindness $\longrightarrow$ Vision $\longrightarrow$ Seeing $\longrightarrow$ Orientation

Rheumatism $\longrightarrow$ Skeletal $\longrightarrow$ Walking $\longrightarrow$ Mobility

Impairment was defined as '. . . any loss or abnormality of psychological, physiological or anatomical structure or function'. It represents deviation from some norm in the individual's biomedical status. While impairment is concerned with biological function, disability is concerned with activities expected of the person or the body. Disability was defined as '. . . any restriction or lack (resulting from an impairment) of ability to perform an activity in the manner or within the range considered normal for a human being'. Functional handicap thus represents the social consequences of impairments or disabilities. It is a social phenomenon and a relative concept. The attitudes and values of the non-handicapped play a major part in defining a handicap. It was defined as a disadvantage for a given individual, resulting from an impairment or a disability, that limits or prevents the fulfilment of a role that is normal (depending on age, sex and social and cultural factors) for that individual. More detailed classifications have since been proposed (e.g. Nagi 1965, 1991).

A related concept is dependency – on other people or service providers. Impairment and disability may or may not lead to dependency in the same way they lead to handicap. As with the concept of handicap, functional 'dependency' is a social consequence – societal attitudes decide on its definition and existence. Wilkin (1987) defined dependency as 'a state in which an individual is reliant upon other(s) for assistance in meeting recognized needs'. In summary, impairment and disability may lead to dependency in the same way they lead to handicap. However, they cannot be equated with dependency, nor is there a necessary relationship. On the basis of the previous definitions, functional status can be defined as the degree to which an individual is able to perform socially allocated roles free of physically (or mentally in the case of mental illness) related limitations.

The WHO classifications above constituted useful working definitions of impairment, disability and handicap. A working definition, as distinct from an operational definition, must be precise enough to suggest the content of the indicators but must not be so precise that it cannot be generalized to a variety of contexts. Operational definitions, in contrast, are usually specific to a particular measurement instrument and even to a particular type of study. They define the specific behaviours and the ways in which they are to be classified. Most operational definitions in this area concentrate upon activities of daily living, often subdivided into domestic and self-care activities. Thus the operational definition of dependency is failure to perform certain specified activities independently to a predefined standard.

The WHO (1998) has since updated and revised its classification to produce a more complex model in a move away from a 'consequence of disease' classification, to a more positive classification of 'Impairments (of structure), Activities (previously called disabilities), and Participation (previously called handicaps)', and a 'components of health' classification, known as the International Classification of Functioning, Disability and Health (ICF) (WHO 2001). In the latter, the aim was to provide a unified and standard language and framework for the description of health and health-related states. Functioning was described as an umbrella term for all body functions, activities and participation in life situations, and disability as an umbrella term for impairments, activity limitations or restrictions on participation. The first part of the ICF contains two main lists: 'body functions and structures' – for example, specific mental functions (such as memory) and structures of the nervous system (e.g. the spinal cord), and 'activities and participation' (e.g. mobility and community recreation). The second part incorporates environmental factors (e.g. support and relationships or services, systems and policies). The WHO conceived a person's functioning and disability as a dynamic interplay between health and environment and personal factors. There is no formal definition of disability within their revised model; it is the umbrella term for any impairment of body structure or function, limitation of activities, or restriction in participation. It provides a framework of human functioning on a continuum, rather than just at the extreme points, and it complements the WHO's (2004) *International Classification of Diseases* – 10th Revision (ICD) which classifies diagnosis and type of condition.

There is, then, a clear distinction between functioning and general health status. Functioning is directly related to the ability to perform one's roles and participate in life. As such, functional status is just one component of health – it is a measure of the effects of disease.

THE CONCEPT OF POSITIVE HEALTH

It was pointed out earlier that, in medicine, health is usually referred to negatively as the absence of disease, illness and sickness. A narrow focus solely on objective data has been criticized in terms of its inability to capture factors pertinent to health status, to the way people feel, and the context in which they live (Patrick 2003). Although social scientists view health as a continuum along which people progress and regress, and despite Merrell and Reed's early (1949) proposal for a graded scale of health from positive to negative health, current measures of health status still take health as a baseline and then measure deviations away from this. They measure ill health because it is easier to measure departures from health rather than to find indices of health itself. Health has been operationalized (e.g. definition to enable proxy measurement) in most patient-based research in terms of self-reported (mental and physical) health status and broader health status (which includes the ability to continue with everyday social role functioning). But developed scales still tend to measure the negative, rather than the positive ends of continua.

Of course, when studying severely ill populations, the most effective strategy may be to employ measures of negative health status. However, only approximately 15 per cent of a general population in a western society will have chronic physical limitations, and some 10–20 per cent will have substantial psychiatric impairment (Stewart *et al.* 1978; Ware *et al.* 1979). Large numbers of very old people have also reported in surveys that they are relatively healthy, although this might partly reflect the survival of the fittest (Nybo *et al.* 2001). Thus reliance on a negative definition of health provides little information about the health of the remaining 80–90 per cent of general populations.

In its 1946 constitution (WHO 1948a, 1948b), the WHO adopted a positive definition of health and specified that 'Health is a state of complete physical, mental and social well-being and not merely the absence of disease and infirmity.' However, no conceptual or operational definitions were attempted. Despite the controversy provoked by this utopian definition, it led to a greater focus on a broader, more positive concept of health, rather than a narrow, negative (disease-based) focus (Seedhouse 1986). The WHO's concept of health in social, psychological and physical terms has become accepted to the extent that a measure of health status that fails to incorporate one of these dimensions is likely to receive negative evaluation. Since the 1980s, as a result of the increasing focus on health promotion worldwide (WHO 1985, 2002), the search for positive health definitions and indicators has intensified.

However, a positive conception of health is still difficult to measure because of the lack of agreement over its definition. Without an operational definition it is not possible to determine if and when a state of health has been achieved by a population. While clinical judgements focus upon the absence of disease, classic sociological research has reported that lay people may hold a variety of concepts of health such as the ability to carry out normal everyday tasks, feeling strong, good, fit and so on (Cox *et al.* 1987, 1993).

There is broad agreement that the concept of positive health is more than the mere absence of disease or disability and implies 'completeness' and 'full functioning' or 'efficiency' of mind and body and social adjustment. Beyond this there is no one accepted definition. Positive health could be described as the ability to cope with stressful situations, the maintenance of a strong social support system, integration in the community, high morale and life satisfaction, psychological well-being, and even levels of physical fitness as well as physical health (Lamb *et al.* 1988). It is composed of distinct components that must be measured and interpreted separately.

The concept of health, even when defined broadly, and with a positive slant, for example in terms of the ability to continue with everyday social role functioning, is theoretically distinct from health-related quality of life. Although health is valued highly by people, it is just one of several valued components of life (Bowling *et al.* 2003; Bowling 2005b); by definition, health status and health-related quality of life are only part of overall quality of life. Broader quality of life, and health-related quality of life, are more comprehensive than health status per se, and include aspects of the environment and living circumstances that may or may not be affected by health (Patrick 2003).

THE CONCEPT OF SOCIAL HEALTH

Donald *et al.* (1978) aimed to measure 'social health' in the Rand Health Insurance Study. Social health was viewed as a dimension of individual well-being distinct from both physical and mental health. They conceptualized social health both as a component of health-status outcomes (as a dependent variable) and, following Caplan (1974) and Cassel (1976):

> in terms of social support systems that might intervene and modify the effect of the environment and life stress events on physical and mental health (as an intervening variable). Measurement of social health focuses on the individual and is defined in terms of interpersonal interactions (e.g. visits with friends) and social participation (e.g. membership in clubs). Both objective and subjective constructs (e.g. number of friends and a rating of how well one is getting along, respectively) are included in this definition.
>
> (Donald *et al.* 1978)

Social functioning, then, is the ability to interact effectively with others, and with the social environment, including social role performance and participation in social groups, networks, activities and engaging in satisfying personal relationships. It is an essential dimension of quality of life (Bowling 2005b). It can be influenced by opportunities available – features of the social and community setting – which are not always within an individual's control.

Others have also conceptualized social health as a separate component of health status, defining it in terms of the degree to which people function adequately as members of the community (Renne 1974; Greenblatt 1975). Lerner (1973) noted that health status may be a function of non-health factors external to the individual, such as the environment, the community and significant social groups, and recommended that social well-being measures focus on constructs such as role-related coping, family health and social participation. He hypothesized that socially healthy persons would be more able to cope successfully with day-to-day challenges arising from performance of major social roles; would live in families that are more stable, integrated and cohesive; would be more likely to participate in community activities; and would be more likely to conform to societal norms. Lack of social support, via influences on mood, or via heightened levels of social stress and lack of a 'buffer' to stress (the support), has also been implicated in poor outcome of depression (George *et al.* 1989). It has been hypothesized to increase health risks by social influences: influencing opportunities for companionship, social activities and participation, maintenance of self-efficacy beliefs, access to help, material goods and services, shared norms and health behaviours (Berkman and Glass 2000).

Kaplan (1975) outlined a broad range of types of social support, including workplace support; family support, social activity and friendships; existence of a confidant(e); financial adequacy, personal achievements, philosophy and sexual satisfaction. Berkman and Glass (2000) also included definitions of network characteristics: size (number of members); density (connectiveness of members); boundedness (structural characteristics such as work, neighbourhood); homogeneity (similarity between members); and network ties (frequency of contact, types of support/transactions, duration known each other, reciprocity between members).

Most investigators of social health in these areas have focused on individual social network and support systems rather than on community resources and integration. But human ecology theory also holds that the quality of life of humans and the quality of their environment are interdependent, and the former cannot be considered apart from the whole ecosystem (Rettig and Leichtentritt 1999). Cultures, the environment, societal resources and facilities can all contribute to health.

Social cohesion and social capital are collective, ecological dimensions of society, distinct from the concepts of social networks and social support which are measured at the level of the individual. Social cohesion refers to the connectedness and solidarity between groups of people (Kawachi and Berkman 2000).

As Durkheim (1895, 1897) recognized long ago, society is not simply the sum of individuals, and well-being is influenced by society as a whole. Therefore, in order to understand individuals we must study them in the context of external, societal as well as internal, personal forces. Brissett *et al.* (2000), taking Durkheim's (1897) classic research on suicide risk and lack of social ties, focused more specifically on measures of participation in a range of social relationships (social integration), citing evidence that people who are more socially integrated live longer and have better health outcomes (from number of types of relationships, frequency of activities, perceived integration, to more complex combinations of these to form an index). However, there is also much inconsistent evidence in relation to the influence of social capital on health (Choi *et al.* 2014).

Social capital is a subset of the concept of social cohesion and integration, and refers to the extent to which communities offer members opportunities, through active involvement in social activities, voluntary work, group membership, leisure and recreation facilities, political activism and educational facilities, to increase their personal resources (i.e. their social capital) (Coleman 1984; Putnam 1995; Brissette *et al.* 2000). It is a stock of tangible or less tangible resources (Kawachi and Berkman 2000). It can also be defined as those features of social structures which act as resources for individuals and facilitate collective action, such as high levels of interpersonal trust and mutual aid (Kawachi and Berkman 2000). Social capital needs to be incorporated into a model of social health, and included in broader studies of health and quality of life.

The concept of social health is a dimension of both broader health and of quality of life. Having social relationships, being involved in social activities, and living in safe neighbourhoods with good facilities have all been nominated by the public as giving their life quality; conversely, their absence has been said to take quality away from their lives (Bowling *et al.* 2003).

THE CONCEPT OF SUBJECTIVE WELL-BEING

In 1946, the constitution of the WHO (1948a, 1948b) recognized the importance of broader well-being to health. Its definition of health was 'a state of complete physical, mental and social well-being and not merely the absence of disease or infirmity'. The implication of this was that measurement of broader health should include well-being. General well-being is a dynamic, multi-faceted concept, and includes subjective, social, physical and psychological dimensions. The specific concept of subjective well-being emerged in the 1950s in attempts to move beyond reliance on objective indicators of life quality in the monitoring of social change (e.g. income, crime, housing quality), and towards more subjective measurement, in order to more meaningfully reflect people's lives and experiences. This became the tradition of social indicators research (Noll 2004).

In contrast to objective indicators, subjective indicators are those which involve some evaluation of one's circumstances in life (e.g. of well-being and quality of life). Subjective well-being is more than the absence of physical and mental health problems or psychological morbidity and 'ill-being', such as anxiety and depression; it has a positive dimension. Measurement of well-being usually involves subjective self-assessments of life satisfaction and/or morale (involving cognitive components in their evaluation), positive emotions such as happiness, involving an affective or emotional component (hedonic), reflecting the influence of early Greek and nineteenth-century utilitarian philosophy (Andrews and McKennel 1980; Bowling 2005b), and whether their life is meaningful, or functioning with optimal effectiveness in individual and social life (the eudaimonic perspective) (Deci and Ryan 2008).

Psychological models of well-being are distinct but related, and emphasize existential challenges of life: personal growth, control, autonomy, self-efficacy or self-mastery (Larson 1978; Keyes *et al.* 2002). The distinction is discussed further in Chapter 7. However, few investigators have distinguished between these concepts and they are commonly used interchangeably.

The dimensions of well-being have been measured with what social scientists have called 'subjective indicators', on the grounds that it is unlikely that human happiness and satisfaction can be understood without asking people about their feelings. Subjective or experiential social indicators are based on the model of subjective well-being as defined by people's 'hedonic feelings or cognitive satisfactions' (Diener and Suh 1997). People are routinely engaged in evaluating themselves in relation to the life domains they consider to be of relevance, and important, to themselves. Subjective indicators formalize these natural tendencies. Veenhoven (1991) has argued that making an overall judgement about one's life implies a cognitive, intellectual activity and requires the assessment of past experiences and estimation of future experiences: 'Both require a marshalling of facts into a convenient number of cognitive categories. It also demands an evaluation of priorities and relative values' (Veenhoven 1991). Life assessment is also bipolar, consisting of the independent dimensions of positive and also negative affect. The difficulty for research lies in capturing the relevant and important areas to most people. While biases inevitably threaten all subjective measures (Veenhoven 2002), researchers have risen to the challenge with exhaustive, now classic, investigations of the validity of measures of reported well-being (Andrews and Crandall 1976).

Reasons for discontent with subjective indicators have been described, and counterargued, by Veenhoven (2002) and include the difficulties of comparing people because of varying standards for comparison, shifting standards over time (e.g. when living standards improve, standards for comparison might rise and lead to increasing dissatisfaction); also the partly unconscious and implicit criteria which underlie subjective appraisals (e.g. people may be able to state how satisfied they are, but be less certain why). Subjective measures have also been controversial in mental health research because of the subjectivity of individuals' self-assessments – which might be distorted by mental health symptoms (Katschnig 2005).While random errors are not always problematic, Veenhoven (2002) admits that social desirability bias can inflate certain self-ratings of circumstances and happiness; and interviewing biases, question sequence and response format can lead to systematic distortion of data (see Schwartz and Strack 1999). These criticisms apply to all social research with human participants, including the measurement of health status. As Veenhoven (2002) pointed out, despite criticism over the biases inherent in measuring subjective perceptions, subjective indicators are still needed in the setting of policy goals based on what people need and want, and in evaluations of outcome in terms of public support. Objective indicators alone do not provide sufficient information.

Lay perceptions of subjective concepts are important to understand, if policy evaluation is to include social relevance. Lay perceptions of well-being, as well as of successful ageing, active ageing and quality of life have been elicited, in separate national population surveys of adults and/or older adults, and considerable overlap between lay definitions of concepts was reported. For example, physical health and functioning, social relationships, social roles and activities, mental and cognitive functioning, and psychological resources (including positive thinking, outlook) were the most common lay definitions of active ageing, successful ageing, quality of life and well-being (Bowling et al. 2003; Bowling and Dieppe 2005; Bowling 2006, 2008, 2009a, 2011). These results support the use of broader definitions of each concept. The question of how well-being should be defined, and its components distinguished and measured, remains to be resolved (see overview by Dodge et al. 2012). An ongoing confusion in well-being research is its overlap with concepts and measurement of quality of life.

THE CONCEPT OF QUALITY OF LIFE

In general terms quality can be defined as a grade of 'goodness'. Quality of life (QoL) encompasses how an individual perceives the 'goodness' of multiple aspects of their life.

There is wide recognition of this subjective and multi-dimensional nature. Models of QoL have been heavily influenced by the early social science literature on well-being and satisfaction with life (Andrews and Withey 1976; Campbell *et al.* 1976). But broader QoL is more than well-being.

Measurement of QoL is relevant to the evaluation of outcomes of health and social care interventions and in relation to conditions which can affect a person's whole life. While broader QoL is about the goodness of life, in relation to health it is about the goodness of those aspects of life affected by health. Health-related QoL is one dimension of broader QoL. The former is an evaluation of domains of life affected by one's health. A wide range of domains of health-related QoL have been identified, including emotional well-being (e.g. measured with indicators of life satisfaction and self-esteem), psychological ill-being (e.g. measured with indicators of anxiety and depression), physical well-being (e.g. measured with measures of physical health status and physical functioning) and social well-being (e.g. measured with indicators of social network structure and support, community integration, functioning in social roles). Some investigators also prefer to measure areas of QoL that are specific to diseases and health conditions. This may increase the sensitivity of measurement but also prevents comparisons being made across conditions. Definitions of disease-specific QoL overlap with broader health status, and include physical, mental, social and role functioning, and health perceptions (Ware and Sherbourne 1992).

The wide range of definitions of QoL, health-related QoL, and their inconsistent structures, was reviewed by Farquhar (1995a), and the diverse contributions of sociology (functionalism) and psychology (subjective well-being) to the theoretical foundations of the concept were described by Patrick and Erickson (1993). QoL has been defined in macro (societal, objective) and micro (individual, subjective) terms. The former includes income, employment, housing, education, and other living and environmental circumstances. The latter includes perceptions of overall QoL, individuals' experiences and values. Some definitions overlap. For example, Shin and Johnson (1978) suggested that QoL consists of 'the possession of resources necessary to the satisfaction of individual needs, wants and desires, participation in activities enabling personal development and self-actualization and satisfactory comparison between oneself and others', all of which are dependent on previous experience and knowledge. Veenhoven (2000) also distinguished between *opportunities* (chances) for a good life and the good life (outcomes) itself. Each area of QoL can also have knock-on effects on the others. For example, having access to transport may promote independence and social participation, promote life and enhance perceived quality of life (Bowling *et al.* 2003), but the former are partly dependent on having health and adequate finances. These can also be influenced by local transport facilities, type of housing, community resources to facilitate social participation and social relationships.

QoL appears to be a complex collection of interacting objective and subjective dimensions (Lawton 1991), and most investigators focus on its multi-dimensionality. Beckie and Hayduk (1997) argued, however, that multi-dimensional definitions of QoL confound the dimensionality of the concept with the multiplicity of the causal sources of that concept. They argued that QoL could be considered as a unidimensional concept with multiple causes, and a unidimensional QoL rating, such as 'How do you feel about your life as a whole?' could be the consequence of global assessments of a range of diverse and complex factors. Thus it is logical for a unidimensional indicator of QoL (e.g. a self-rating global QoL uniscale) to be the dependent variable in analyses, and the predictor variables include the range of health, social and psychological variables. The predictor variables in a model of global quality of life self-evaluation would, by necessity, have to include a wide range of life domains if it were to mirror how those evaluations were made. In addition, these factors may interact, adding to the complexity of the evaluation. Beckie and Hayduk argued that if the QoL evaluation is greater than the sum of its parts, then this can be problematic for causal analyses, but that the diversity, multiplicity and complexity of sources of the concept warrants treating its measurement in terms of a global assessment. Thus it appears reasonable that QoL is influenced by causal variables, and the level of QoL manifests itself in indicator variables. But the traditional approach to its measurement has implicitly assumed only indicator variables. An appreciation of the distinction between these types of variable may lead to more careful definition of concepts and the selection of more appropriate measurement scales (Zissi et al. 1998; Fayers and Hand 2002).

In relation to this, the effects of personality on perceived well-being and QoL are controversial, partly because of the debate about causal versus mediating variables. Extroversion and neuroticism have been reported to account for a moderate amount of the variation in subjective well-being (the trait of extraversion is associated with positive affect and with well-being; emotionality is associated with negative affect and poor well-being) (Costa et al. 1987). Spiro and Bossè (2000), on the basis of their survey of over 2,000 adults in the Normative Aging Study, reported the same association with personality traits and well-being, and also with health-related QoL. However, these personality factors are highly stable traits, while subjective well-being has been shown to have only moderate stability over time (Headey et al. 1985).

Despite classic work on mediators in the 1980s, theoretical and empirical development has made little progress (Abbey and Andrews 1986). Following Abbey and Andrews (1986), Barry (1997) and Zissi et al. (1998) argued that there is a need for a model of QoL which focuses on the potential link between psychological factors (e.g. self-esteem or self-worth; self-efficacy, perceived control and self-mastery; and autonomy) and subjective evaluations of QoL. Their theoretical model, which was supported by their data on people with mental health problems, focused on how subjectively perceived QoL is mediated by several interrelated variables, including self-related constructs, and how these perceptions are influenced by cognitive mechanisms. Zissi et al. (1998) pointed to the confusion surrounding the many psychological concepts commonly used to denote QoL, with their potential roles as influences, constituents or mediators of perceived life quality. They argued that perceived quality of life is likely to be mediated by several interrelated variables, including self-related constructs (e.g. self-mastery and self-efficacy, morale and self-esteem, perceived control over life) and these perceptions are likely to be influenced by cognitive mechanisms (e.g. expectations of life, social values, beliefs, aspirations and social comparison standards). Although the model is attractive, there is still little empirical data to support or refute the distinction between psychological constructs as mediating or influencing variables in determining QoL.

The main theoretical models of QoL, as opposed to basic definitions, include needs-based approaches derived from Maslow's (1954, 1962) hierarchy of human needs (deficiency needs: hunger, thirst, loneliness, security; and growth needs: learning, mastery and self-actualization) (Higgs *et al.* 2003). Overlapping with this are social-psychological models which emphasize autonomy and control, self-sufficiency, internal control and self-assessed technical performance, and social competence (Abbey and Andrews 1986; Fry 2000); classic models based on subjective well-being, happiness, morale, life satisfaction (Andrews and Withey 1976; Larson 1978; Andrews 1986); social expectations or gap models based on the discrepancy between desired and actual circumstances (Calman 1984; Michalos 1986); and phenomenological models of the individual's unique perceptions of their circumstances (O'Boyle 1997a, 1997b), based on the concept that QoL is dependent on the individual who experiences it, and should be measured using their own value systems (Ziller 1974; Benner 1985; Rosenberg 1995). The literature reveals that QoL encompasses self-evaluations of psychological well-being, as well as a wide range of more tangible life domains, including physical health and functioning, social support and resources, independence, material and financial circumstances, community social capital and the external environment (Brown *et al.* 2004). Due to the proliferation of definitions of QoL many investigators now refer to the WHO definition (WHOQOL Group 1993; and see 1995), as it is all-encompassing, and captures the subjectivity and context of the individual:

> . . . an individual's perception of their position in life in the context of the culture and value systems in which they live and in relation to their goals, expectations, and standards and concerns. It is a broad-ranging concept affected in a complex way by the person's physical health, psychological state, level of independence, social relationships, and their relationships to salient features of their environment.

While acknowledging the importance of the individual's perceptions, there is empirical evidence that most people hold a set of common values in relation to what gives QoL and what make up the important things in life, although priorities vary by people's socio-demographic characteristic. Research shows that most people define their QoL in terms of having a positive psychological outlook and emotional well-being, having good physical and mental health and the physical ability to do the things they want to do, having good relationships with friends and family, participating in social activities and recreation, living in a safe neighbourhood with good facilities and services, and having enough money and being independent (Bowling 1995; Farquhar 1995b; Bowling and Windsor 2001; Bowling *et al.* 2003; Bowling and Gabriel 2004; Bowling 2005b).

CHAPTER 2

THEORY OF MEASUREMENT

CHAPTER COVERAGE

CHOICE OF HEALTH INDICATOR

When deciding which measure to use, investigators need to assess whether a disease-specific or generic, broad-ranging instrument is required; the type of scoring that the instrument is based on (the complexity of the scoring; whether scores can be easily analysed in relation to other variables); the reliability, validity, sensitivity and factor structure of the scale; the appropriateness of the instrument for, and its acceptability to, the study population. It is also important to decide whether the study requires measurement on a nominal-, ordinal-, interval- or ratio-scale level; these terms are explained below.

MEASUREMENT THEORY

Descriptions can be placed on a nominal or an ordinal, interval or ratio scale. The requisite level of measurement depends on the intended applications of the indicator and on the question that the researcher is attempting to answer.

With a *nominal* scale, numbers or other symbols are used simply to classify a characteristic or item. This is measurement at its weakest level. For example, functional disability states and perceived health are defined by descriptions and thus a nominal or classification scale is constructed. For the purpose of the comparative evaluation of the outcome of intervention A in comparison with the outcome of intervention B, a nominal scale may be sufficient (e.g. 'died' or 'survived'). Hypotheses can be tested regarding the distribution of cases among categories by using the nonparametric test, $x2$, and also Fisher's exact probability test. The most common measure of association (correlation) for nominal data is the contingency coefficient.

An *ordinal* (or ranking) scale is applicable where objects in one category of a scale are not simply different from objects in other categories of that scale, but they stand in some kind of relation to them. For example, typical relations may be higher than, more preferred, more difficult (in effect, greater than). This is an ordinal scale. Many disability and health status measures are strictly of this type.

The most appropriate statistic for describing the central tendency of scores in an ordinal scale is the median, since the median is not affected by changes of any scores above or below it, as long as the number of scores above and below remain the same. Hypotheses can be tested using nonparametric statistics such as correlation coefficients based on rankings (e.g. Spearman r or the Kendall r). An ordinal scale is sufficient only for answering basic questions such as 'How does X compare with Y?'

An *interval* scale is obtained when a scale has all the characteristics of an ordinal scale, and when, in addition, the distances between any two numbers on the scale are of known size. Measurement considerably stronger than ordinality has thus been achieved. An interval scale is characterized by a common and constant unit of measurement which assigns a real number, but the zero point and unit of measurement are arbitrary (e.g. temperature – where two scales are commonly used as the zero point – differs on each and is arbitrary).

The interval scale is a truly quantitative scale and all the common parametric statistics (means, standard deviations, Pearson correlations, etc.) are applicable as are the common statistical tests of significance (t test, F test, etc.). Parametric tests should be used as nonparametric methods would not usually take advantage of all information contained in the research data. Interval scales are appropriate if the question is 'How different is X to Y?'

The *ratio* scale exists when a scale has all the characteristics of an interval scale and in addition has a true zero point as its origin. The ratio of any two scale points is independent of the unit of measurement. Weight is one example. Any statistical test is usable when ratio measurement has been achieved. Ratio scales are needed if the question is: 'Proportionately how different is X to Y?'

The most rigorous methods of data analysis require quantitative data. Whenever possible, measures which yield interval or ratio data should be used, although this is often difficult in social science. Measures of functional disability and health status never strictly reach a ratio or interval scale of measurement. However, methods of data transformation do exist which permit even nominal data to be made quantitative for purposes of analysis.

MEASUREMENT PROBLEMS

Measurement problems are rife when attempting to measure health outcomes. Indicators may work well or badly and are usually assessed by tests of validity and reliability.

Authors of the various measures often make claims for reliability and validity based on achieved coefficients, often without any reference to acceptable levels. Suggestions for acceptable levels for reliability and validity correlation coefficients range from 0.85 to 0.94, although often 0.50 is regarded as acceptable (Ware *et al.* 1980). A full discussion of the problems of achieving reliability and validity can be found in Streiner and Norman (2008). Main psychometric methods of assessment are summarized in Box 2.1.

Box 2.1 Summary of classic psychometrics in measurement scale development (summarized from Cano *et al.* 2012, Tables 1 and 8 and Bowling 2014b, Table 3.1)

Psychometric property	Criteria
Item generation and reduction	The generation of the item pool for inclusion within a measure should be derived from a sample of the target group; this item generation should be conducted alongside literature reviews and consultations with expert groups. The latter should not be used as a substitute for the target group. Then the pool of items is examined conceptually, and assessed again by the target group and experts. It is then reduced using standard psychometric approaches. Ideally, the resulting measure should be initially tested with the target group using cognitive interview techniques: the 'think aloud' method. This method asks people to verbalize their thought processes during completion, and enables examination of people's comprehension of the items and meaning of their responses. It aims to expose whether people interpret questions and responses differently to the researcher. Redundant items and those with weak measurement properties, floor and ceiling effects, as indicated by maximum endorsement frequencies (>80%) and high levels of missing data (>5%) can then be removed, and the resulting items grouped into scales using factor analysis, and then refined to form the intended measurement scale for testing for acceptability, reliability and validity, in a larger survey, before final refinement and final testing.
Acceptability	Assessed by data quality and targeting. Data quality: the completeness of item- and scale-level data, assessed by data completeness; criterion for missing data <5% (as above) (some use <10%, e.g. with sensitive topics). Targeting: the extent to which the range of the variable measured by a scale matches the range of that variable in the study sample; assessed by maximum endorsement frequencies <80% (as above), aggregate endorsement frequencies >10%, skewness statistic –1 to +1, proximity of scale mean score to scale mid-point (closer matches = better), acceptable distribution of scores (closer to 100% indicates better targeting).

Scaling assumptions	Assessed by the extent to which it is legitimate to sum a set of items, without weighting or standardization, to produce a single total score. Criterion is satisfied when items have adequate corrected-item total correlations ≥0.30, and grouping of items in subscales is correct. Assessed by principal components analysis (factor loadings >0.30, cross-loadings <0.20), item convergent and discriminant validity (item-own scale correlations >0.30, magnitude >2 standard errors than other scales).
Reliability	The extent to which scale scores are not associated with random error.
Internal consistency reliability	Precision of the scale based on the homogeneity (inter-correlations) of items at one point in time. Assessed by testing whether the items are inter-correlated, using tests of internal consistency (e.g. Cronbach's coefficient alpha ≥0.70; some use ≥0.80), mean item-item correlations (homogeneity coefficient) ≥0.30, and item-total correlations ≥0.30.
Test-retest reproducibility and inter-interviewer reliability	Agreement between respondent's scores at two short time intervals, expected to be stable; it estimates the stability of scales. Scale-level intra-class correlation coefficients ≥0.80, item-level intra-class correlation coefficients ≥0.50, should be achieved. Inter-interviewer reliability: reproducibility of the scale when administered to same respondents by different interviewers.
Validity	The extent to which a scale measures the construct that it purports to measure.
Face validity	An estimate of whether a test appears to measure a certain criterion.
Content-related validity	The ability of the measure to reflect what is predicted by the conceptual framework for the measure – this can include tests for discriminant, convergent and known-groups validity (see separate listings below).
Validity (within scale)	Evidence that a scale measures a single construct, and that scale items can be combined to form a summary score. Assessed using internal consistency reliability (Cronbach's alpha ≥0.70, again ≥0.80 is used by some) and factor analysis (factor loadings >0.30, cross-loadings <0.20).
Validity (correlations between scales)	Correlations between scales: moderate correlations (0.30–0.70) expected.
Discriminant validity	Evidence that a scale is not correlated with other measures of different constructs, hypothesized as not expected to be correlated with the scale.
Known-groups validity testing/ hypothesis tests	Ability of a scale to detect hypothesized differences between known subgroups.

Validity

Validity is concerned with whether the indicator actually does measure the underlying attribute or not. One of the most problematic aspects of assessing validity is the varying terminology. Textbooks have tended to focus on content validity, criterion validity and construct validity. Construct validity is differentiated into convergent and discriminant validity. However, all types of validity are addressing the same issue of the degree of confidence that can be placed on the inferences drawn from scale scores. These issues have been addressed more fully by Messick (1980) and Streiner and Norman (2008).

The assessment of validity involves assessment against a standard criterion. Because there is no 'gold standard' of health against which health status indices can be compared, the validation methods commonly used in the behavioural sciences are the assessment of content and construct validity (American Psychological Association 1974). The criteria of validity which should be met in general are as follows.

Content validity

Content validity refers to whether the components of the scale/item cover all aspects of the attribute to be measured, in a balanced way. At its most basic level, the content of the variable should match the name which it has been given. Each item should fall into at least one of the content areas being tapped. If it does not, then the item is not relevant to the scale's objectives, or the list of scale objectives is not comprehensive. The number of items in each area should also reflect its importance to the attribute. Content validity is more systematic than face validity, and judgements about these issues are usually made by a panel following literature reviews, focus groups and exploratory interviews with the target population. It is generally agreed that the content validity of subjective indicators should be judged by members of the target group being assessed (Patrick 2003).

Face validity

Face validity is more superficial than content validity. It is a subjective assessment by the investigators about whether the indicator, on the face of it, is a reasonable one and the items appear to be measuring the variables they claim to measure. The meaning and relevance of the indicator should appear self-evident.

Criterion validity

Criterion validity refers to whether the variable can be measured with accuracy. The traditional definition of criterion validity is the correlation of a scale with some other 'criterion' measure of the topic under study, ideally a 'gold standard'. Criterion validity is usually divided into two types: concurrent and predictive validity.

Concurrent validity

Concurrent validity is the independent corroboration that the instrument is measuring what it purports to measure against a criterion measure (e.g. the corroboration of a physical functioning scale with observable functioning). Thus, when a scale is tested against another scale measuring the same thing it is called concurrent validity, which refers to a scale's substitutability. Both scales are administered at the same time. It is most often used when attempting to develop a replacement scale which is simpler or less expensive to administer than an existing scale.

Predictive validity

Predictive validity refers to whether the measure can predict future differences in key variables in the expected direction (e.g. was the health status scale able to predict self-reported improvements in patients' health after treatment?). With this type of predictive validity, the criterion will be unavailable until some future end point.

Predictive validity has also been defined in terms of its discriminative ability (i.e. in tests of association, the percentage of respondents who have been correctly classified using the instrument). For example, if there are theoretically sound reasons to hypothesize that people in the lower socio-economic groups are more likely than people in higher socio-economic groups to report poor health status, then the health status of the two groupings can be compared as a check of predictive validity.

Construct validity

Construct validity is corroboration that the instrument is measuring the underlying concept it is intended to measure. This type of validity is relevant in more abstract areas such as psychology and sociology where the variable of interest cannot be directly observed. Unlike other types of validity testing, testing for construct validity involves assessing both theory and method simultaneously. It necessitates stating a conceptual definition of the construct to be measured, specifying its dimensions, hypothesizing its theoretical relationship with other variables, and then testing it. One problem is that, if the predictions made on the basis of theory are not confirmed, then the problem could be with the validity of the measure or the validity of the theory. This type of validity is generally divided into convergent and discriminant validity.

Convergent-discriminant validity

Convergent validity is the extent to which two measures which purport to be measuring the same topic correlate (that is, converge). The hypothesis to be tested is that the measure will correlate with variables which measure the same topic. It thus involves assessing the extent to which the scale is related to other variables and measures of the same construct to which it should be related. The interpretation is sometimes problematic with the measurement of similar concepts, as scale scores that correlate too highly may be measuring the same dimension. Some investigators have interpreted this definition technically incorrectly and have assumed that convergent validity has been obtained when a measure correlates highly with a measure on a different topic that it is expected to be associated with.

Conversely, discriminant validity (also known as divergent validity) requires that the construct should not correlate with dissimilar (discriminant) variables. Thus, the hypothesis to be tested is that the measure will not correlate with variables which measure a different, unrelated topic.

Convergent-discriminant validity is also referred to as multitrait-multimethod matrix validity (Campbell and Fiske 1959), which simply means that different methods of measuring the same construct should produce similar results (that is, correlate highly), and measures with different dimensions should produce different results (i.e. not correlate). The validation process thus involves calculation of the inter-correlations between measures.

Precision

This is the ability of an instrument to detect small changes in an attribute.

Responsiveness to change (sensitivity)

This is the ability of an instrument to be responsive (sensitive) to actual changes which occur over time. It is a measure of the association between the change in the observed score and the change in the true value of the construct. This involves correlating the instrument's scores with other measures which reflect any anticipated changes (e.g. in the case of a depression scale, it will need to be correlated with a standardized, structured psychiatric interview and any indicated changes in psychological status between the two methods of assessment compared).

Sensitivity

This refers to the proportion of cases (e.g. people with verified diagnoses of depression) that score as positive cases on an instrument (e.g. a scale of depression), and the ability of the gradation in the scale's scores to adequately reflect actual changes.

Specificity

This is a measure of the probability of the scale correctly identifying non-cases (e.g. people without depression) with the measure (e.g. of depression). It refers to the discriminative ability of the measure. Again, it also refers to the ability of the gradation in the scale's scores to adequately reflect actual changes.

ROC curves

The discriminant ability of a scale which uses continuous data can be investigated with receiver operating characteristic (ROC) curves. The ROC curve examines the degree of overlap of the distributions of scale scores for all cut-off points for defined groups; the curve itself is a plot of the true positive rate against the false positive rate for each point on the scale (sensitivity plotted against one minus specificity). The degree of overlap between the defined groups is measured by calculating the area under the curve (AUC), and its associated standard error (Hanley and McNeil 1982). The greater the total area under a plotted curve from all cut-off points, then the greater the instrument's responsiveness. A statistic of 0.5 indicates that prediction is no better than chance and 1.0 represents perfect accuracy.

FACTOR STRUCTURE

Principal components analysis and factor analysis are both from a family of techniques that aim to produce a smaller number of linear combinations of variables, accounting for most of their variability in correlation patterns, thus reducing a large number of interrelated observations to a smaller number of common dimensions (factors). Exploratory factor analysis is often used in the initial stages of analysis to explore inter-relationships between variables. Confirmatory factor analysis is used later on to test ('confirm') hypotheses about the structure underlying the variables.

There are technical differences in the processes of principal components analysis and factor analysis. Each has its followers, although researchers often use them interchangeably. Tabachnick and Fidell (1996) summarized the preference for their use as: factor analysis is preferred for a theoretical solution uncontaminated by unique and error variability; principal components analysis is preferred for an empirical summary of the data. Factor analysis can have a slight tendency to find a solution in fewer dimensions than principal components analysis (Blunch 2013).

In relation to the development of a measurement scale, the technique is used to identify and define a small number of separate dimensions that make up an instrument – that underlie a set of variables (the factor structure). It describes how the items in each dimension group together with sufficient consistency to each other. For example, if items relate to a single dimension, then the combination of items into a single measure is supported.

The selection of items in a measurement scale needs to consider the relevance of the items before discarding any of them following factor analyses. Juniper et al. (1997) compared two philosophically different methods for selecting items for a disease-specific quality of life (QoL) questionnaire: the impact method which selects items that are most frequently perceived as important by the target population and the psychometric method (factor analysis) which selects items primarily according to their relationships with one another. Based on research with 150 adult asthma patients, they reported that the impact method resulted in a 32-item instrument and the psychometric method led to a 36-item tool, with 20 items common to both. The psychometric approach had discarded the items relating to emotional function and environment, and included items mainly on fatigue instead. Thus the two approaches led to important differences. Again, Kane et al. (1998), in a comparative study of the USA and Europe, compared geriatric professionals' and lay people's ratings of the importance of 32 items measuring physical functioning. While the overall correlation between the groups was 0.82, in general lay people rated instrumental activities of daily living items more highly (e.g. (dis)ability to prepare meals, clean the house, shopping). The experts rated the most dysfunctional activities of daily living items higher than the lay people (e.g. (dis)ability to dress, feed self, get to/use toilet).

Modern psychometric item response theory

The classic psychometric method of principal components analysis, or factor analysis, requires item scores to be normally distributed and measured at interval level. It is commonly used with ordinal level data which risks biased or inconsistent results, and in these circumstances it should be used only as an approximate guide to factor structure. Modern psychometric item response theory (IRT) is a superior technique, but there are advantages and disadvantages of both approaches. Non-parametric IRT, or Mokken scaling modelling, can be used to evaluate the unidimensionality of the measure, as indicated by scalability (Mokken 1971; Sijtsma and Molenaar 2002). This is a monotone homogeneity model, which is a benchmark model within non-parametric item response theory. It assumes that all items in a test measure the same latent trait, that the relationship between the item score and the latent trait is monotone, and the test procedure is free of influences on test performance other than the latent trait (Sijtsma 2005). Mokken's monotone homogeneity model comprises an item selection phase, in which ordinal items measuring the same construct are clustered using an iterative (repeated) procedure, followed by tests of the monotonic relationship between each item and the resulting scale. The summed scores of a set of items conforming to this model stochastically orders respondents on a single dimension.

Reliability

An instrument will also require testing for reliability. A measure is judged to be reliable when it consistently produces the same results, particularly when applied to the same subjects at different time periods when there is no evidence of change. The methods of testing for reliability include multiple form, basic tests of internal consistency (e.g. split-half, item-item correlations and item-total correlations), test-retest, intra-rater and inter-rater agreement, and sensitivity to change. In addition, tests of internal consistency based on statistical models, for example using factor analysis are becoming widespread (Harman 1976).

Internal consistency

Internal consistency involves testing for homogeneity. This can take the form of correlations between the items in the scale, or within each scale domain, or between the two halves of the scale where the scale can be divided into two equivalent parts (split-half reliability); correlations between the items and the total score are also performed. Cronbach's alpha should be calculated (Cronbach 1951), which is based on the average correlation among the items and the number of items in the instrument (values range from 0 to 1). A low coefficient alpha (e.g. below 0.50) indicates that the item does not come from the same conceptual domain. More detailed information on the appropriate statistical methods to employ, and minimum acceptable values, are given in *Measuring Disease* (Bowling 2001).

As questions that deliberately tap different dimensions within a scale cannot be expected to necessarily have high item-item or item-total correlations, factor analysis should be used to identify the separate factors (e.g. domains) within the scale. Each item within a factor is judged to be worthy of retention in a scale if its eigenvalue (a measure of its power to explain variation between subjects) exceeds a certain value (usually 1.5).

Multiple-form reliability

This refers to the correlation between the subdomains of the scale.

Alternate forms reliability

Where measures have alternative formats – for example a version for interviewer administration and a version for self-administration, or a long and shorter version – they should be highly correlated.

Test-retest reliability

The test is administered to the same population on two occasions and the results are compared, usually by correlation. The main problem with this is that the first administration may affect responses on the second. There can be problems with interpretation of observed change, given the potential for observer errors with any scale, and the potential for genuine individual change between administrations which affects the estimate of reliability.

Intra-rater and inter-rater agreements

Intra-rater agreement is the reliability of the same rater's scores, of the same subjects, on different occasions. Inter-rater agreement is the concordance of scores achieved by different raters on the same occasion.

The achievement of standards of validity and reliability requires time and effort. It is a powerful reason for using existing scales.

TYPES OF INSTRUMENTS

Most instruments used in social science rely on self-reporting of feelings, attitudes and behaviour by people in an interview situation or in response to a self-administered questionnaire. Other measurement approaches include the use of records and the observation of behaviour. Each approach has its strengths and limitations. The optimal measurement strategy is to measure the same phenomenon using several different approaches (Webb *et al.* 1966).

SELF-REPORT MEASURES

Self-report measures are essential for much research because of the need to obtain subjective assessments of experiences (e.g. feelings about recovery, level of health and well-being). They have a broad appeal as they are often quick to administer and involve little interpretation by the investigator. Self-report measures may take a variety of forms.

Single-item measures

These are self-report questions which use a single question, rating or item to measure the concept of interest.

Battery

A series of self-report questions, ratings or items used to measure a concept. The responses are not summed or weighted. A battery is like a series of single-item measures, all tapping the same concept.

Scale

A series of self-report questions, ratings or items used to measure a concept. The response categories of the items are all in the same format, are summed and may be weighted.

Sometimes researchers do not wish to use a long scale, because their questionnaires are already fairly lengthy, and they prefer single-item questions. Generally, where questionnaire length permits, scales are preferred because they contain a larger number of items and are suitable for statistical calculations using summed and weighted scores. Single-item measures are least preferable because it is doubtful that one question can effectively tap a given phenomenon and it is also difficult to assess the adequacy of a single-item instrument.

SCALING ITEM RESPONSES

There is a wide variety of scaling methods for item responses. The finer the distinctions that can be made between subjects' responses, the greater the precision of the measure. For example, rather than asking a person to simply agree or disagree with a statement (which yields only two-response (nominal) categories), it is preferable to ask respondents to indicate their opinions along a continuum of agreement: for example, 'strongly disagree, disagree, no opinion, agree or strongly agree' (Likert 1952). Attitudinal and behavioural issues are not easily dichotomized; they often lie on a continuum. A question about any difficulty in washing oneself can elicit a range of responses from 'no difficulty', to 'slight', 'moderate' or 'severe' difficulty, to 'cannot do this at all'. Offering a wide range of choices is likely to reduce the potential for error due to confusion, although the continuum should not be too great, or meaningless responses will be elicited.

If the aim of the research is to elicit continuous rather than categorical responses, there are several techniques available. One approach is to ask respondents to indicate their replies on a visual analogue scale (e.g. a line of 100 mm), with descriptions such as 'very depressed' to 'not at all depressed' at each end. Respondents are asked to place a mark on the line corresponding to their state. There is little evidence that different methods (e.g. categorical response choices or a visual analogue scale) produce different responses and the choice of method is ultimately the investigator's preference.

A common method for developing scales is Thurstone's method. This involves asking respondents to rank statements relating to the variable of interest, which are typed onto cards, into hierarchical order, from the most to the least desirable. The details and scoring systems of this technique are described by Streiner and Norman (2008) and in most psychology and methodology textbooks.

In relation to functional status, many methods exist of scoring or assessing 'function' by scaling, whereby a set of items can be put in a hierarchy of severity. The notion is that patients who can perform a particular task will be able to perform all tasks more easily. Conversely, if they cannot perform a particular task, they will be unable to perform tasks rated as higher. Guttman's (1944) scaling of disability was one of the earliest attempts in this field. He ranked degrees of patient disability in respect of a number of activities, such as feeding, continence, ambulation, dressing and bathing. This method assumes that disabilities can be ordered. Provided that disability progressed steadily from one activity to another (i.e. patients first have difficulty in bathing, then in bathing and dressing, and so on until they are disabled in respect of all five activities), this method of scaling yields a single rating from 1 (no disability) to 6 (disabled on all five). For example, four disabilities always score worse than three, and a score of 6 would assume that all disability items 2–5 had been affirmed. Examples of well-known measures using this scaling method are the Index of Activities of Daily Living (ADL) and the Arthritis Impact Measurement Scales (AIMS). A more recent Guttman scaling instrument has been developed by Williams *et al.* (1976). The activities which make up the scale are not comprehensive in terms of describing activities of daily living. The instrument has the advantage of having two scales, one for men and one for women. Work on developing and refining the scale is continuing. Guttman scaling, although popular, has been criticized for its method of attributing equal weights to item responses. For example, with responses per item ranging from 1 to 6, the higher the score the greater the debility; it cannot be assumed that 6 is six times as bad as 1 (Skinner and Yett 1972).

WEIGHTING SCALE ITEMS

Many scales simply involve summing the item scores, each of which has been given an equal weight. This is the easiest solution to the scale scoring. There is a fundamental problem with this method: some items may be more important to the construct underlying the scale than others and should therefore contribute more to the total score. Summing also erroneously converts what is at best ordinal data into interval levels of measurement when applying statistical techniques. Statistical caution is required.

The problem with many scoring methods, particularly when equal weight for each item is applied, is that a given score can be arrived at in different ways. A person who is cheerful and lucid but unable to walk due to arthritis may achieve the same scale score as someone who is physically mobile but disoriented and withdrawn. While this may be useful for assessments of staff workload, it is not useful in assessing patient outcome in any detail. Scoring may exacerbate the instrument's distortion of the experiences of individuals. The problem may be avoided by treating all aspects of disability and health status as equal contributors to overall severity, and expressing the results for each item separately.

The disadvantage of this method is that multiple disabilities are not then evident and this type of breakdown can be cumbersome in analysis. The alternative is to assign different values (weights) to different scale items for scoring purposes. The normative scale relies on the classification of items into major or minor categories; for example, with disability items, 'being able to feed oneself' is given twice the weight of 'being able to dress oneself'. Principal component scaling relies on the internal evidence of the data being scaled, thus calculating the relative weights to be given to each item to construct a linear additive index. Numerous health index questionnaires fall into these categories. The main methods of weighting have been clearly and fully described by Streiner and Norman (2008). The most common uses a different number of items to measure the various aspects of the trait, proportional to its importance within the construct. The total for any subscale would be the number of items with a response of interest divided by the total number of items within the subscale. The subscale scores can be added together for the scale total. Thus, each subscale contributes equally to the scale's total score, even though each may consist of a different number of items.

In practice, however, it is frequently found that weighting items makes little difference to subjects' relative scores, despite the inherent logic of this technique. This is because people who score high on one scale variant often score high on others. Examples of this have been given by Streiner and Norman (2008). On the other hand, weighting items can increase the predictive ability of an index (Perloff and Persons 1988). Streiner and Norman (2008) concluded that when the scale contains at least 40 items, or when the items are fairly homogeneous, then differential weighting contributes little (except complexity in scoring).

UTILITY RATING SCALES

Finally, economists have devised a series of econometric scaling techniques in an attempt to assign a numerical value to a health state. These are known as utility ratings, the most well-known application of these being the quality-adjusted life year (QALY) (Chiange 1965; Rosser and Watts 1971; Kaplan and Bush 1982). A QALY is a year of full life quality. Poor health may reduce the quality of a year. In QALYs, improvements in the length and QoL are combined into one single index. Each life year is quality adjusted with a utility value, where 1 = full health. QALYs are measures of units of benefit from a medical intervention, aiming to reflect the change in survival with a weighting factor for QoL.

Different types of medical interventions are then compared by calculations of costs per gained QALY (Williams 1985). QALYs can be derived by several different methods (e.g. the Rosser Index of Disability, Rosser and Watts 1972), standard gamble, trade-off and rating scale techniques (Torrance et al. 1972, 1982; Torrance 1986, 1987). These will be only briefly referred to here; interested readers should consult specialist texts for their evaluation (e.g. Torrance 1986; Teeling Smith 1988).

The rating scale

The rating scale is suitable for measuring preferences for chronic or temporary health states. A typical rating scale consists of a line drawn on a page with clearly defined end points such as 'death/least desirable' at one end and 'healthy/most desirable' at the other. The remaining health states are then located on the line between these two in order of their preference, such that the intervals between them correspond to the differences in preference between the health states, as perceived by the respondent. This is the interval-scaling technique. The scale is measured from 0 assigned to the worst health state of the group and 1 assigned to the best. The person is asked to select the best and worst health states from the group and then locate the other states on the scale relative to each other, according to the interval-scaling principle.

The standard gamble

With this technique, people are asked to choose between a gamble, with a desirable outcome, with risk P, and a less desirable outcome, with risk 1-P, and a certain option of intermediate desirability. The person is asked what probability of getting the desirable or less desirable outcome will make him/her indifferent between the gamble and the certainty.

An example of the standard gamble is to take a person faced with the choice of remaining in a poor state of health versus taking a gamble on treatment that could fully restore health or result in death (e.g. surgery for angina). If the probability of restoring full health is varied there will be a point where the person is indifferent between his/her current poor state of health and taking the gamble of surgery. If the person perceives his/her poor health state as particularly undesirable, he/she will be more likely to accept a greater probability of death in order to escape it.

Equivalence

A similar technique is the 'equivalence technique' whereby respondents are asked to identify their point of indifference between keeping alive a group of people in a state of fairly good health and a larger group, whose size is determined by the respondent, of less well people.

Time trade-off

With this method, the technique is to vary the length of time in each health state with treatment choice. For example, the respondent is presented with two alternatives and asked to select the more preferred. Alternative 1 offers the respondent a particular health outcome for a specified length of time followed by death, and alternative 2 offers a different outcome for a different length of time. The time is varied until the respondent is indifferent between the two alternatives.

This technique then requires people to judge how long a period in one state of health could be 'traded' for a different period in another state of health. The assumption underlying this concept is that the better their state of health, the shorter period of life people would accept as a 'trade-off' for longer survival in a less desirable state.

All utility scales achieve interval scale level. Research has found that people find the trade-off techniques the easiest of the utility measures, the standard gamble has been found to be more difficult for people, and the rating scale the most difficult. One main criticism of these techniques is that disease sufferers probably assign more positive utilities to states of ill health than normal people in hypothetical disease states. Very elderly persons may feel that a frail and painful existence is just as valuable to them as someone else's apparently healthier state.

Such models suffer from several limitations. They have not been adequately tested for validity and reliability, and they rarely ask sufferers themselves to make ratings (Carr-Hill 1989; Carr-Hill and Morris 1991). Judgements are usually made by 'proxy' patients or 'experts' (e.g. doctors, nurses and medical students). They assume that people are rational when assessing QoL, and that individual value judgements are not interfering with their ratings. It is also difficult to quantify QoL, which is a multi-dimensional concept, in terms of one figure.

The following chapters present relatively concise reviews of generic health status measures, and measures of specific domains of broader health-related, including generic, QoL. A generic scale is useful when the investigator aims to make comparisons between conditions or population groups; a domain-specific scale should be used when the topic covered is of particular interest to the investigator. Some domain-specific scales overlap with disease-specific scales (e.g. scales of physical functioning and psychological well-being). Disease-specific scales are useful when the attributes of particular diseases or conditions require assessment, as they will usually be more relevant to the condition and more sensitive. Disease-specific scales were reviewed in *Measuring Disease* (Bowling 2001).

CHAPTER 3

MEASURING FUNCTIONAL ABILITY

CHAPTER COVERAGE

MEASUREMENT

There are a number of methodological techniques available for measuring function: direct physical tests of function, direct observation of behaviour and interviews with the person concerned or a third party. Each method has its limitations, as has been indicated. Direct observation is rarely used because it is so time consuming. Direct tests of functioning, such as range-of-limb movement, grip strength and walking time; or standards such as joint swelling, pain scores, morning stiffness, erythrocyte sedimentation rate and joint counts, while objective, may not necessarily give an accurate indication of ability or performance. Grip strength tests can confirm how much a patient can and will squeeze a bag on a particular day, but patients may be more concerned with subjective feelings and reductions in activities associated with daily living (ADL).

Most measures of functional disability are self-report methods. Respondents are asked to report limitations on their ADL. Sometimes researchers do not wish to use a long scale to measure functioning, usually because their questionnaires are already fairly lengthy, and opt to use single-item questions. A long-used question asks if respondents have any longstanding illness, disability or infirmity, and whether this limits their activities (Office of Population Censuses and Surveys 1987; Office for National Statistics 2002; Ayis et al. 2003). Like the popular single-item question asking people to self-rate their general health status, responses to this question can be influenced by psychological distress (Ayis et al. 2003). An updated, harmonized version amends this question, and removes the word 'disability' giving 'Do you have any physical or mental health conditions or illnesses lasting or expected to last for 12 months or more?' (Office for National Statistics 2015).

The main criticism of this type of measure is that responses may vary with people's expectations of health and illness and perceptions of limitations. Subjectivity is involved. People who are shortsighted might reply 'yes' or they might not define their condition as a 'longstanding illness, disability or infirmity' or as limiting. Also, people who are used to their conditions and the restrictions they impose may have adjusted to them and no longer define them as limiting. However, if a measure of perceived health status is required, rather than objective morbidity indicators, then this inherent subjectivity is the strength of the measure.

There are many measures of functional ability. Some measures focus on basic mobility (e.g. walking indoors/outdoors), although most also include self-care ADL (including ability to wash self, bathe, use the toilet, eat/drink) along with instrumental activities of daily living (IADL), which encompass the activities that are required for the maintenance of independence and optimum levels of functioning (e.g. do laundry, shop, housework, prepare meals/cook).

Only those measures which are most well tested for validity and reliability, of topical interest, frequently used, or potentially applicable in Europe as well as in the USA are presented in detail. Other scales which are less well tested, older, but which are popular or are frequently used, are also presented, but in less detail (e.g. the Index of Activities of Daily Living, Barthel Index and the Karnofsky Performance Index). While Deyo (1993) recommended that these older scales of functioning should be abandoned in favour of the more recently developed scales (e.g. the HAQ and AIMS), these older scales continue to be popular among many investigators, possibly because they are relatively brief and simple to score, comparisons with studies using the same measures over time can be made, and they are simply well known. Readers are referred to *Measuring Disease* (Bowling 2001) for measures used in a wider variety of generic and disease-specific contexts. There are also several available measures of broader health status which incorporate subscales of functional ability. These are discussed in Chapter 4 on broader measures of health status.

Measures of functional ability are frequently used in population surveys and evaluative studies because they are socially relevant and interpretable. However, self-care limitations are rare in a general population – less than 0.5 per cent are likely to report limitations in eating, dressing, bathing or using the toilet due to poor health. Thus in studies of the general population these items should be selected sparingly in contrast to studies of the severely ill or very elderly where self-care measures may be more appropriate. Broad measures of function are also likely to miss specific effects of disease, and generic measures should be supplemented with more highly focused measures of disease impact.

Most measures of functioning focus narrowly on mobility, self-care and instrumental tasks, often ignoring financial, emotional and social needs which may be equally or more important. Measures of physical functioning and activity limitations do not always provide assessments of functioning in everyday social roles, mental functioning, sexual functioning, pain and comfort. More meaningful aspects of household roles are also largely ignored: for example, the effect of the condition on the *time taken* to perform chores such as cooking, shopping, cleaning, errands, childcare and other roles. Assessments of patients' satisfaction and choice with regard to level of functioning are seldom made. For example, people may prefer to have a strip wash rather than to risk slipping while getting into the bath. On scales of functioning it is often assumed by investigators that respondents achieving a low score necessarily have a poorer quality of life than a patient with a higher score. Thus someone who is wheelchair-bound might have a low functional ability score, and thereby be assumed by investigators to have a poor quality of life (QoL), despite the fact he or she may be receiving good quality social support and rate their own QoL as good.

Most scales have been developed on the basis of professionals' (e.g. doctors') judgements about essential abilities for daily living. Berg *et al.* (1976) asked 150 health workers to assign weight from 0 to 10 for 50 listed abilities or functions; open-ended questions to elicit functions not listed were also used. Serious problems were documented in finding simple and meaningful terms to describe functional loss to many respondents. Respondents assigned the largest average values to ability to use one's mental abilities, to see, to think clearly, to love and be loved, to make decisions for oneself, to live at home, to walk, to maintain contact with family and friends, and to talk. Although the sample was limited to health workers, the results indicate a need to consider lay persons' judgements of essential functions and to include these in measures of health outcomes. Also there are often differing viewpoints of how people ought to be performing, for instance, on the part of clinicians and patients. The patient may want to walk without aids or limp, while the clinician may regard 'walking with aids and limp' as indicative of a satisfactory outcome.

The problem of measuring functional disability is compounded by conceptual difficulties and interactive factors. One of the major problems with using a functional index is that different people may react differently to apparently similar levels of physical impairment, depending on their expectations, priorities, goals, social support networks and so on. Functional disability, like dependency, is a multidimensional concept which may relate to physical, mental, cognitive, social, economic or environmental factors (Wilkin 1987). Thus it is an interactive concept – it is not a necessary consequence of impairment but perhaps, for example, of the siting of bathrooms, toilets and other facilities and the necessity for negotiating stairs. In terms of dependency, severity might be a function of the existence of aids or the frequency and timing of help. Perceptions of severity with both disability and dependency will also be influenced by previous history and expectations for the future. Meaning apart, most scales are not sensitive enough as they simply ask respondents whether they have no or some difficulty with a task, or whether they are unable to perform it at all. The problem emerges of how limited does one have to be to answer in the affirmative? More sensitive scales with greater response choices based on degrees of severity require development.

Finally, caution is needed when deciding on which measures to use. Measures tend to be developed, administered and validated on one of two types of samples – people living in the community or in institutions. The measures are not necessarily interchangeable between samples. The measures must be appropriate for the population type. Many measures have been developed to be optimally suitable for a particular age group and may be inappropriate for use with other age groups.

THE OLDER AMERICANS' RESOURCES AND SERVICES SCHEDULE (OARS): MULTIDIMENSIONAL FUNCTIONAL ASSESSMENT QUESTIONNAIRE (OMFAQ)

The OARS OMFAQ was developed in order to measure the level of functioning and need for services of older people. It was developed at Duke University Center for the Study of Ageing and Human Development (Fillenbaum 1978, 1988 – updated 1996; Fillenbaum and Smyer 1981). The measure was developed for use with adults aged 55 and over and should be restricted to this age group. Gatz *et al.* (1987) tested OARS on a sample of over 1,000 people aged 26–86 and reported that the global test scores can be misleading when applied to different age groups. It can be used with community or institutional samples. When used with institutionalized samples some questions are omitted, and institution-relevant items are added.

OARS measures five dimensions of personal functioning, including mental impairment. Despite its popularity, little work has been done on the measurement properties of the mental health scale.

The numerous applications of the OARS during its construction are described in the OARS handbook (Fillenbaum 1978). One of the most well-known studies using the OARS questionnaire was the survey of social support in relation to mortality carried out in Durham, North Carolina (Blazer 1982). This was based on 331 people aged 65 and over, taken from a wider community sample survey of 997 people. This sub-sample was followed up 30 months after baseline interview which assessed functional status, social support, depressive symptoms, physical health status and cognitive functioning, stressful life events and cigarette smoking. Increased mortality risk was found for those with impaired social support and social interaction. The OARS questionnaire has been widely used throughout the USA and in other countries, including Australia. Two Spanish translations are available for use with Spanish-speaking people in America. A Brazilian version of the mental health subscale has been developed (Blay *et al.* 1988). The use of the OARS subscales of mental health and physical functioning (IADL) has been more common than the administration of the entire measure (Gatz *et al.* 1987; Pfeiffer *et al.* 1989; Doble *et al.* 1997). Administration time is on average 45 minutes but probably takes an hour generally to administer. The main limitation of OARS is its length (Perlman 1987).

A shorter version of OARS is available, known as the Functional Assessment Inventory (FAI), although this still takes approximately 35 minutes to administer. The shorter FAI contains the functional assessment items, but not the detailed service-use items (Pfeiffer *et al.* 1989). Interviewer training, which takes two days, is recommended. Its administration is also explained in a manual which can be purchased from the authors. As with most scales, OARS is copyrighted and permission for its use must be obtained from the authors; copies of the OARS manual, training materials, and questionnaires may be purchased from: http://centerforaging.duke.edu/services/141, accessed 12 October 2015.

Content

The questionnaire consists of two independent sections. Part A consists of the assessment of functioning in relation to five domains: social, economic, mental and physical health, and ADL. Interviewers also make ratings of ability. The responses to the items in each area are summarized on a six-point scale (e.g. level of functioning: 1 = excellent to 6 = totally impaired). These five ratings yield a profile showing concomitant functioning across the five areas. This scale contains 66 questions, plus 10 questions for completion by an informant. If sub-questions are included, the total number of items asked is 120, plus five interviewer summary ratings. Part B is a services assessment that directs enquiry into 24 generically defined services, determining for each the current use, the extent of use in the past six months, the type of service provider and perceived need. There is also a demographic section. Information is sought from the respondent, proxy interviews are permitted. Examples of the items are shown in Box 3.1.

Box 3.1 Examples from the OARS

Can you get to places out of walking distance?

2　Without help (can travel alone on buses, taxis, or drive your own car).
1　With some help (need someone to help you or go with you when travelling).
0　Or are you unable to travel unless emergency arrangements are made for a
　　specialized vehicle like an ambulance?
–　Not answered.

Can you go shopping for groceries or clothes (assuming subject has transportation)?

2　Without help (taking care of all shopping needs yourself, assuming you had
　　transportation).
1　With some help (need someone to go with you on all shopping trips).
0　Or are you completely unable to go shopping?
–　Not answered.

Can you prepare your own meals?

2　Without help (plan and cook full meals yourself).
1　With some help (can prepare some things but unable to cook full meals yourself).
0　Or are you completely unable to prepare any meals?
–　Not answered.

Can you do your own housework?

2   Without help (can scrub floors, etc.).
1   With some help (can do light housework but need help with heavy work).
0   Or are you completely unable to do any housework?
–   Not answered.

© Duke University Center for the Study of Aging and Human Development. Source: Fillenbaum, G.G. (1988) *Multidimensional functional assessment of older adults: the Duke Older Americans Resources and Services Procedures*. Hillsdale, NJ: Erlbaum, updated 1996 (available only from Center for the Study of Aging and Human Development, Duke University Medical Center, Durham, NC 27710). With permission of the developer. Permission is required for use. Copies of the OARS manual, training materials, and questionnaires may be purchased from: http://centerforaging.duke.edu/services/141, accessed 12 October 2015.

Scoring

There are various methods of aggregation. The 1–6 ratings on each of the five scales may be summed (5: excellent functioning in each area to 30: total overall impairment), although summing is problematic as was indicated earlier. Alternatively, the number of areas of functioning that are impaired can be counted. To do this, it is necessary first to establish which level of functioning indicates impairment. Ratings of 1 and 2 may be combined and compared with ratings of 3–6 (i.e. nonimpaired versus impaired) or the contrast may be between ratings of 1–3 and 4–6. Summed over areas, this yields a 6-class system (0 areas of functioning impaired to 5 areas impaired). A more complex classification based on a trichotomized scale (1 + 2/3 + 4/5 + 6) which takes account of both number of areas of impairment and severity of impairment has also been developed; full details are contained in the handbook. It is also possible to examine the responses to each individual question and treat the items as separate units. For clinical purposes it might be important to maintain the distinctions but not for population purposes.

However, a classification based on summed information assumes that areas are equivalent; at present the validity of this assumption has not been established. Consequently a classification system that maintains distinctions between areas may be preferred.

Validity

OARS and the shorter FAI were extensively tested for validity at the various stages of development (Fillenbaum 1978; Cairl et al. 1983). Both instruments appear to have face and content validity, although discriminant and predictive validity have not yet been adequately tested.

Criterion validity was tested on 33 patients from a family medical practice. Spearman correlation between separate criterion ratings and the economic items was 0.68, 0.67 for mental health, 0.82 for physical health and 0.89 for self-care ability. On another study of 82 community residents, the Spearman correlation between independent psychiatrists' ratings and the mental health items was 0.62, and between physician assistants' ratings and the physical health items was 0.70. Detailed results for reliability and validity of OARS can be found in Fillenbaum (1978) and Fillenbaum and Smyer (1981), and results for the FAI can be found in Cairl *et al.* (1983).

Fillenbaum (1978) analysed the factor structure of the OARS instrument and reported that it represented three factors within social resources, one in economic resources, four in mental health (life satisfaction, psychosomatic symptoms, alienation, cognitive deficit), and one in each of the physical functioning subscales confirming their division into ADL and IADL. The mental health items have been used separately, in an instrument known as the Short Psychiatric Evaluation Schedule, and factor analyses of this subscale have indicated that its 15 subscale items represent three distinct factors: alienation, somatic symptoms and depression (Gatz *et al.* 1987).

Reliability

OARS and the FAI have been extensively tested for reliability. Tests of agreement of the raters' assessments have been carried out involving 11 raters who assessed 30 patients. Intra-class correlations ranged from 0.66 for physical health to 0.87 for self-care. Raters were in complete agreement for 74 per cent of the ratings (Fillenbaum 1978). Reliability ratings of the Community Service Questionnaire gave inter-rater Kendall coefficients of concordance between 0.70 and 0.93. Test-retest reliability, conducted 12–18 months apart, gave correlations of between 0.47 and 1.00. Five-week test-retest correlations based on ratings of 30 elderly people gave results of 0.82 for the physical ADL questions, such as personal care, 0.71 for the IADL questions, such as housework, and 0.79 for the economic resources items. For social resources the correlation was 0.71 and for subjective questions it was 0.53. Coefficients for life satisfaction and mental health were lower: 0.42 and 0.32 respectively.

Although much of the data on reliability and validity refers to previous versions of the instrument, the OARS appears to be a superior measure to most others, and it was regarded as a valuable contribution by McDowell and Newell (1996) and McDowell (2006) in their detailed reviews of measures. Haywood *et al.* (2005) conducted systematic literature searches for their review of the evidence of the measurement properties of multidimensional measures of health status specific to older people. They reported that the most evidence was found for the OARS. It has been translated and used in many countries (translations include English, Afrikaans, Chinese, Dutch, German (Austria, Germany), Greek, Italian, Korean, Malay, Portuguese (Brazil), Spanish (Puerto Rico, Cuba, Castilian), Swedish; sections in French; instrumental ADL in Japanese and Vietnamese – see http://centerforaging.duke.edu/services/141, accessed 12 October 2015).

THE STANFORD ARTHRITIS CENTER HEALTH ASSESSMENT QUESTIONNAIRE (HAQ)

Fries *et al.* (1980) developed the HAQ on the basis that outcome should be measured in terms of the patient's value system. Functional ability (e.g. the ability to walk) is a component of this but sedimentation rate is not. The framework used for the development of the HAQ was based on the belief that a patient desires to be alive, free of pain, functioning normally, experiencing minimal treatment toxicity, and financially solvent. Patient outcome was thus represented by:

1 death,
2 discomfort,
3 disability,
4 therapeutic toxicity,
5 dollar cost.

The HAQ was one of the first broader, patient-based measures of functioning.

In the process of developing this measure, 62 potential questions were selected from questionnaires in use in the rheumatic diseases field and elsewhere, including the Uniform Database for Rheumatic Diseases (Fries *et al*. 1974; Convery *et al*. 1977); the Barthel Index (Mahoney and Barthel 1965); and the ADL (Katz *et al*. 1963). Testing the measure for reliability and validity with patients with rheumatoid arthritis reduced it to 21 questions, grouped into nine components, and graded in ordinal fashion from 0 to 3. Individual items with correlations of 0.85 or higher were eliminated in the interests of conciseness, on the assumption that this suggested redundancy between components. Correlations of remaining items range between 0.35 and 0.65 (Fries *et al*. 1980). The resulting instrument was subsequently administered in more than two dozen settings.

The HAQ is suitable for use in community settings and has been frequently administered to patients with rheumatoid arthritis and osteoarthritis, systemic lupus and ankylosing spondylitis. It is coherent and concise and can be administered face to face or self-administered, so it does not rely on skilled personnel to administer (it is therefore relatively cheap). Administration takes 5–10 minutes and manual scoring can be completed within a minute. The full HAQ is the most commonly used, although a short two-page HAQ is also available, which includes the functional ability scale (HAQ Disability Index), the visual analogue pain scale, and visual analogue patient global health scale (Bruce and Fries 2003a, 2003b).

Content

Functional ability is measured by 20 questions within eight components relating to movements of the upper extremity, locomotor activities of the lower extremity and activities that involve both extremities: dressing and grooming, rising, eating, walking, hygiene, reach, grip, outside activity. Sexual activity was included in an earlier version. Each of these components consists of two or three relevant questions. Pain, discomfort, drug toxicity and financial costs are also assessed. The functional ability scale is the most commonly used, rather than the full HAQ. Examples of questions are shown in Box 3.2.

Scoring

In relation to functional ability, the ordinal scoring of 0–3 is based on the following scale: without difficulty = 0 (no disability), with some difficulty = 1, with much difficulty = 2 and unable to do = 3 (completely disabled). The index is calculated by the addition of scores and then dividing the score by the total number of components answered. Higher scores reflect greater limitations. The authors reported reluctance among patients to report

---

Box 3.2 Examples from the HAQ

Are you able to:

Dress yourself, including tying shoelaces and doing buttons?
Stand up from an armless chair?
Get in and out of bed?
Walk outdoors on flat ground?
Do chores such as vacuuming, housework or light gardening?

The range of answers is 'without any difficulty (0); with some difficulty (1); with much difficulty (2); unable to do (3)'.

© Stanford University. With permission of developer. The HAQ is downloadable and free to use, although independently translated copies may carry a charge: http://aramis.stanford.edu; http://aramis.stanford.edu/HAQ.html, accessed 12 October 2015.

---

sexual activity (Fries *et al.* 1980), and some investigators omitted this item (Fitzpatrick *et al.* 1988); thus it has been removed from the current version of the HAQ.

The scales of pain and drug toxicity range from 0 to 3. The HAQ VAS pain scale asks about pain over the last week, and consists of a horizontal visual analogue scale (VAS) anchored at each end with 0 (no pain) to 3 (severe pain). A scale of 0 to 100 may be used instead. The global health status scale is a 15 cm VAS anchored with 0 (very well) to 100 (very poor). The drug toxicity index is composed of questions about the adverse effects from drugs and treatment ranging from none = 0 to severe = 3.

In the personal cost section (applicable to private health care systems), medical and surgical costs are calculated for the past year. The number and type of medications, X-rays, surgery, physician and paramedical visits, appliances, number of laboratory tests, and hospitalizations are detailed. The average cost in the area covered by the research team (Stanford, California) was determined and used for the computation of the dollar values. This section can be applied only in countries and areas where costs are known. Social costs are calculated by determining changes in employment, income, the need to employ domestic help, the cost of transport for medical care and all arthritis-related costs over the past 12 months (Fries *et al.* 1980). The cost questions have not yet been satisfactorily tested; initial tests for validity suffered from poor patient recall. Most investigators only use the scales of functioning.

Fitzpatrick *et al.* (1989), in their comparison of the HAQ and the Functional Limitation Profile (FLP) (derived from the Sickness Impact Profile), reported that nothing appeared to be achieved in relation to precision by the complex scoring system utilized by the FLP in comparison with the simpler ordinal assumptions of the HAQ. It takes less than 10 minutes to administer.

Validity

It has been extensively validated. Correlations of the HAQ against observed patient performance ranged from fair to high (0.47–0.88) (Fries *et al.* 1980, 1982; Fries 1983;

Kirwan and Reeback 1983), and it correlated highly with a range of clinical and laboratory measures (Fries *et al.* 1980, 1982; Ramey *et al.* 1992, 1996; Bruce and Fries 2003a).

Several studies have tested the validity of the HAQ, in particular by correlation of the results of the HAQ with the Arthritis Impact Measurement Scales (AIMS) (Fries *et al.* 1982; Brown *et al.* 1984). These two instruments were shown to measure the same dimensions of disability; the correlation coefficient reported by Fries *et al.* (1982) was 0.91. Inter-correlations within the three parts of each instrument relating to physical disability, psychological state and pain were high and those across these three dimensions were weak. Patient self-assessed global arthritis scores were also strongly associated with disability score and less strongly to pain. These correlations are consistent with current knowledge within the speciality of rheumatology, that disability is a large component of arthritic patients' concerns. HAQ scores correlated in the expected direction with the direct medical costs of treatment for rheumatoid arthritis (Michaud *et al.* 2003), and were able to predict outcome at six months in an exercise programme for people with osteoarthritis of the knee (Dias *et al.* 2003).

The HAQ has been reported by Liang *et al.* (1985) to correlate well with other well-tested scales of health status, such as the Sickness Impact Profile (Bergner *et al.* 1981). A study in the UK by Fitzpatrick *et al.* (1988) of 105 patients with rheumatoid arthritis reported high inter-measure correlations between the HAQ, the Functional Limitations Profile (FLP) (Charlton *et al.* 1983), and between observations of grip strength and the articular index (e.g. the correlations between grip strength and the HAQ on two occasions were −0.73 and −0.68). The HAQ appears to be a valid measure of function in rheumatoid arthritis. Liang *et al.* (1985) also reported good correlations between the HAQ and other scales of health status and functional ability, including the Sickness Impact Profile (Bergner *et al.* 1981) and the Functional Status Index (Denniston and Jette 1980; Jette 1980).

HAQ scores have been reported to be predictive of outcome among patients with rheumatoid arthritis, and other conditions. Sultan *et al.* (2004) reported that a baseline HAQ disability score of less than the median was predictive of at least a 20 per cent improvement in condition at one and two years (odds ratios 1.77 to 5.05) in four out of five outcome measures used in a drug treatment trial of patients with early diffuse scleroderma. The HAQ was reported in early studies to be sensitive to change in patients' conditions (Fries 1983). Fitzpatrick *et al.* (1989), in their UK study, reported that the HAQ performed better than the FLP in relation to specificity and sensitivity, although at best this can only be said to be moderate. The large standard deviations in the scores of both measures indicated the presence of many 'false positives' for both improvement and deterioration of patients over time.

The validity of the HAQ pain scale and global health status scale has been demonstrated in many studies (Ramey *et al.* 1996; Bruce and Fries 2003b). However, initial tests for the validity and reliability of the drug toxicity section revealed weak results, and this component requires further testing (Fries *et al.* 1980).

Principal components analysis has shown factor loadings along the first 'disability' component, which explains 65 per cent of the variance, and a second component with positive loadings for fine activities of the upper extremity and negative loadings for weight-bearing actions of the lower extremity, which explains an additional 10 per cent of the variance (Fries *et al.* 1980, 1982). From this, it was inferred that the resulting disability index (an equal weight sum) is well focused and appropriate for measuring overall arthritis severity.

Reliability

The earliest tests for reliability were reported by Fries *et al.* (1980). In addition to the reporting of mean values, these included correlations of HAQ scores with the results of direct observations by a nurse of patients' performance of 15 household and personal care tasks, mobility and grip; and of self-administered and interview-based HAQ completion. These early tests were based on just 20 patient volunteers attending a rheumatoid arthritis clinic. The correlations for individual items for self-administration versus interview-administered HAQ range from average (or 'respectable') at 0.56 to excellent at 0.85. The corresponding correlations for the disability score was 0.85, indicating good reliability for this component.

The inter-item correlations ranged from average at 0.47 to excellent at 0.88. The weaker items (e.g. reach) were subsequently reworded to minimize variability in responses – for example, this question originally read 'reach and get down heavy objects'. People's ideas of 'heavy' varied, so respondents are now asked about a standardized item: 'reach and get down a 5 lb bag of sugar which is above your head'. The authors also compared overall questionnaire and evaluator agreement; these agreed exactly on 59 per cent of the responses and were within one point in 93 per cent of cases (the weighted kappa statistic result, using rank disagreement rates, was 0.52, implying 'moderate' agreement).

Fries *et al.* (1982) reported mean values from a diverse English-speaking community population of 331 respondents suffering from rheumatoid arthritis. The authors also reported the test-retest correlation of 0.98, based on this population. The mean values showed stability on repeat testing. Responses are similar when the instrument is self-completed, administered by a nurse or doctor. Many studies have since replicated or improved upon these correlations indicating excellent levels of reliability (Ramey *et al.* 1996).

The HAQ is a good measure of function and has been extensively tested for reliability and validity. It is sensitive to change, can be self- or interviewer-administered and is suitable for use in the community. It is often the preferred tool for use because it is concise, short and easy to administer (Lubeck 2002). It has been used in population-based studies as well as evaluations of treatment outcome (Bruce and Fries 2003b). However, it does not capture disability associated with sensory dysfunction, patient satisfaction or social role functioning. An eight-item HAQ has also been developed (Lorig *et al.* 2001) (and see http://aramis.stanford.edu/HAQ.htm, accessed 12 October 2015).

Pincus *et al.* (1983) developed an abbreviated version of the HAQ with one question for each of the eight disability domains, plus new questions on satisfaction and transition items on changes in ability. Its test-retest reliability was high (0.91), although correlations with grip strength, walking time and functional classification were more moderate (0.44–0.60). Other modified versions have been developed for use in other disease-specific contexts, including AIDS (Lubeck and Fries 1992). The HAQ has been extensively used among clinicians in the USA and the UK (Ramey et al. 1992), is available in more than 60 languages and is supported by a bibliography of more than 500 references (Bruce and Fries 2003a, 2003b). Subsequent versions of the HAQ have been developed in order to reduce ceiling or facilitate scoring in clinical settings (e.g. Wolfe et al. 2004; Pincus et al. 2005).

While freely available and considered to be in the public domain, the HAQ is strictly copyrighted by Stanford University (http://aramis.stanford.edu) in order to prevent unauthorized modifications and to preserve its validity and the standardization of assessments across studies.

THE ARTHRITIS IMPACT MEASUREMENT SCALES (AIMS)

The AIMS instruments were developed in people with rheumatoid arthritis and osteoarthritis for the assessment of their outcomes of health care.

The original AIMS1, and the revised AIMS2, were developed by Meenan et al. (1980) and Meenan and Mason (1990). A shortened version of the AIMS1 was produced with good psychometric properties (Wallston et al. 1989). AIMS2 was developed in an attempt to produce a more comprehensive and sensitive version of AIMS1 (Meenan et al. 1992). Expanded and shortened versions of AIMS2 (AIMS2-SF), as well as a short form of AIMS2 (AIMS2-SF) have also been developed. These have good psychometric properties, similar to those in the full AIMS2 (Guillemin et al. 1997), as well as an expanded version.

Both AIMS1 and AIMS2 cover physical, social and emotional well-being, and were developed to assess patient outcome in arthritis and other chronic diseases. AIMS1 was partly adapted from Katz's Index of Activities of Daily Living, the RAND and BUSH scales (Patrick et al. 1973a; Brook et al. 1979a, 1979b; Ware et al. 1979; Bush 1984). AIMS1 and AIMS2 were well tested for reliability and validity, and sensitivity to change. Its applications have been predominantly in clinical settings (with arthritis and rheumatism patients) as an assessment of outcome after therapy. The instrument can be self-completed. The AIMS takes 15 minutes to complete. The self-completion time for AIMS2 is an average of 23 minutes (Meenan et al. 1992). AIMS2-SF takes 10 minutes. AIMS has been translated into many languages.

Content

The original AIMS1 had 45 multiple-choice items, with nine subscales. It assessed nine dimensions of health and functional ability: mobility, physical activity (walking, bending, lifting), ADL, dexterity, household activities (management of money, medication, housekeeping), pain, social activity, depression and anxiety. An additional 19 items covered general health, health perceptions and demographic details (e.g. questions, including a visual analogue item, that assess the effect of arthritis, other medical problems and their treatment). Items were based on the RAND Health Insurance Survey questionnaire, the Quality of Well-Being Scale, and Katz's Index of Daily Living, plus items on dexterity and pain.

AIMS2 is a longer, 78-item questionnaire than AIMS1 (which contained just 45 items). It has some new items and others have been revised or deleted. The three new sections evaluate arm function, work and social support. Sections were added to assess satisfaction with function, attribution of problems to arthritis, and self-designation of priority areas for improvement. The first 57 items form 12 scales: mobility level, walking and bending, hand and finger function, arm function, self-care tasks, household tasks, social activity, social support, pain from arthritis, work, level of tension and mood. The remaining items relate to satisfaction with health status in each of the areas of functioning measured, functional problems due to arthritis, prioritization of the three areas in which the respondent would most like to see improvement, general health perceptions, overall impact of arthritis in each of the areas of functioning measured, type and duration of arthritis, medication usage, co-morbidity and sociodemographic characteristics (Meenan and Mason 1990, 1994). Most questions refer to problems experienced within the last month. Box 3.3 shows examples of items.

Box 3.3 Examples from the AIMS2

How often were you in a bed or chair for most or all of the day?
Did you have trouble doing vigorous activities such as running, lifting heavy objects, or participating in strenuous sports?
Could you easily button a shirt or blouse?
How often did you get together with friends or relatives?
How often did you have severe pain from your arthritis?
How often were you unable to do any paid work, housework or schoolwork?

All days (1)/Most days (2)/Some days (3)/Few days (4)/No days (5)

How often have you felt tense or strung up?
How often have you been in low or very low spirits?

Always (1)/Very often (2)/Sometimes (3)/Almost never (4)/Never (5)

With permission of the developer. Availability and access: the AIMS, AIMS2 and user manuals are in the public domain and free to use in part or whole without permission. They are available from Professor Meenan: Robert F. Meenan, Boston University School of Public Health, 715 Albany Street, T-C-306, Boston, MA 02118. Contact: Professor Robert F. Meenan, MD, MPH, MBA, Special Assistant to the President, Boston University, 141 Bay State Road, Boston, MA 02215, USA; tel.: (617) 877-7536; email: rmeenan@bu.edu, and see also at: https://eprovide.mapi-trust.org/ - click on box 'See for free' and then simply register to view, accessed 21 July 2016. Also see http://www. rheumatology.org/I-Am-A/Rheumatologist/Research/Clinician-Researchers/Arthritis-Impact-Measurement-Scales-AIMS, accessed 12 October 2015.

Scoring

Items in AIMS1 and AIMS2 are listed in Guttman scale order, so that a respondent who indicates a disability on one item will also indicate disability on section items falling below it. AIMS1 had a combination of dichotomous 'yes/no' and scaled response categories. AIMS2 has mainly scaled response choices, for example: 'All days' (1) to 'No days' (5); 'Always' (1) to 'Never' (5); or 'Very satisfied' (1) to 'Very dissatisfied' (5).

Scale scores are summed, the range of scores depends on the number of items in the subscale. No item weights are used. A 'normalization procedure' converts scores into the range 0–10, with 0 representing good 'health status' and 10 representing poor 'health status' (in AIMS1 and AIMS2). The scale is ordinal in type. Users' guides for scoring are available.

Validity

Extensive studies of the validity and reliability of AIMS1 were conducted, demonstrating its good psychometric properties (Meenan et al. 1980, 1982, 1984; Meenan 1982, 1985; Brown et al. 1984; Meenan and Mason 1990, 1994; Weinberger et al. 1990). The scaling properties, validity and reliability of the AIMS2 have also been reported to be good.

Meenan et al. (1992) reported that patients' subjective assessments of problems and areas in need of improvement were significantly associated with a poorer AIMS2 score in that area. Haavardsholm et al. (2000), on the basis of a community survey of over 1,000 rheumatoid arthritis patients, reported that the components of the AIMS2 and AIMS2-SF had substantial to near perfect agreement.

Both AIMS2 and AIMS2-SF correlated well with other measures of health status (Medical Outcomes Study Short Form-36 and a modified Health Assessment Questionnaire) supporting their convergent validity, and with an indicator of patient assessed change in health status (Haavardsholm et al. 2000). De Joode et al. (2001) also reported that the physical health component of the Dutch version of the AIMS2 scale correlated significantly with clinical data in patients with haemophilia, and also with the Sickness Impact Profile (SIP) (Pearson's $r = 0.53$; $p < 0.05$). However, the psychological health and social interaction components of the Dutch AIMS2 did not correlate significantly with the psychosocial components of the SIP; possibly they were tapping different conceptual parts.

Meenan et al. (1992) reported that, in samples of patients with osteoarthritis and rheumatoid arthritis, all within-scale factor analyses produced single factors, except for mobility in patients with osteoarthritis. Sala et al. (2000), used the Italian version of AIMS2 in a study of patients with osteoarthritis of the knee, and reported a three-factor health status model explaining 63 per cent of the variance between patients. Three factors (physical function, psychological, pain) have also been replicated in other studies.

Reliability

Meenan et al. (1992) reported, on the basis of a study of 408 respondents with rheumatoid arthritis or osteoarthritis, that the internal consistency coefficients for the 12 AIMS2 scales were 0.72–0.91 in the rheumatoid arthritis group and 0.74–0.96 in the osteoarthritis group. Haavardsholm et al. (2000), on the basis of their large community survey, also reported that internal consistency was high in all components for AIMS2 and AIMS2-SF.

Test-retest reliability at two weeks (postal survey) was 0.78–0.94. Sala *et al.* (2000) reported high internal consistency for the Italian version of AIMS2, and that test-retest reliability at six months exceeded 0.80 for 8 of the 12 subscales. De Joode *et al.* (2001) reported that the Dutch version of the AIMS2 scale and subscales had moderate to high internal consistency in patients with haemophilia (Cronbach's alpha = 0.62–0.92).

In sum, the AIMS has good measurement properties, has been extensively tested for validity and reliability, and the identified dimensions explain the majority of illness impact estimated by patients. AIMS2 appears to be a superior instrument to AIMS1. The full length versions of AIMS are time consuming to complete, but the short-form version (AIMS2-SF) is quicker to complete, and more practical for self-administration.

The AIMS instruments have been validated for use in many countries (Sala *et al.* 2000; de Joode *et al.* 2001). Dutch and Italian translations are available, see more at: http://www.rheumatology.org/I-Am-A/Rheumatologist/Research/Clinician-Researchers/Arthritis-Impact-Measurement-Scales-AIMS#sthash.JweCZNa1.dpuf, accessed 12 October 2015.

THE INDEX OF ACTIVITIES OF DAILY LIVING (ADL)

One of the oldest, and best known, of the disability scales is the ADL index developed by Katz *et al.* (1963, 1966, 1968, 1970, 1973; Katz and Akpom 1976). This is also known as the Index of Independence in Activities of Daily Living. Katz designed the index in order to describe, for clinical purposes, the functional status of elderly and chronically ill patients.

Content

The index consists of a rating form that is completed by a therapist or other observer on the basis of observation and interview. In each of the activities assessed, the patient is rated by the observer on a three-point scale of independence for each activity. The index assesses independence in functioning in six areas: bathing, dressing, toileting, transferring from bed to chair, continence and feeding. On the basis of more than 2,000 evaluations of states of patients, the authors observed that these functions decreased in order. They claimed to have a measure of fundamental biological functions, a claim questioned by those using Guttman scales (Williams *et al.* 1976). The evaluation form is shown in Box 3.4.

Box 3.4 Katz Index of Activities of Daily Living

Bathing (sponge bath, tub bath, or shower)
Receives no assistance (gets in and out of tub by self if tub is usual means of bathing)
Receives assistance in bathing only one part of the body (such as back of a leg)
Receives assistance in bathing more than one part of the body (or not bathed)

Dressing

Gets clothes and gets completely dressed without assistance

Gets clothes and gets dressed without assistance except for assistance in tying shoes

Receives assistance in getting clothes or in getting dressed, or stays partly or completely undressed

Toileting

Goes to toilet room, uses toilet/cleans self, arranges clothes, and returns without any assistance (may use cane, walker or wheelchair and may manage night bedpan or commode)

Receives assistance in going to toilet room or in using toilet/cleaning self or arranging clothes

Doesn't go to toilet room

Transfer

Moves in and out of bed and chair without assistance (may use cane or walker)

Moves in and out of bed or chair with assistance

Doesn't get out of bed

Continence

Controls urination and bowel movement completely by self

Has occasional accidents

Supervision helps keep urine or bowel control; catheter is used, or is incontinent

Feeding

Feeds self without assistance

Feeds self except for getting assistance in cutting meat or buttering bread

Receives assistance in feeding or is fed partly or completely by using tubes or intravenous fluids

Reproduced from Katz, S. *et al.* (1970) Progress in Development of the Index of ADL, *The Gerontologist*, 10 (1 Part 1): 20–30. By permission of Oxford University Press on behalf of the Gerontological Society of America.

The authors later developed a survey instrument for obtaining health status data containing questions about the need for and use of health services and attitudes towards medical care. Five categories of 'need' were defined and ranked: no disability, restricted activity with no chronic conditions, restricted activity with chronic condition, mobility limitations and bed disability. These were chosen to permit comparisons with existing national surveys (Katz *et al.* 1973).

Scoring

Patients are graded on ordinal three-point scales by interviewers in relation to their ability in bathing, dressing, transferring, toileting, continence and feeding. Scores on individual scales are translated into 'dependent'/'independent' classifications, and then the overall level of functioning is summarized on an eight-point scale (A–G, plus 'Other' – see below).

An alternative scoring system simply counts the number of activities in which the person is dependent: 0 (independent in all six functions) to 6 (dependent in all six functions), removing the need for the 'Other' category. Some investigators have reversed the scoring so that a score of 6 indicates full functioning, 4 indicates moderate functioning, and 2 or less indicates severe functional impairment. Thus each method produces a single total score, and all items are treated as equal. The use of a single index results in a loss of information about variability, because different patterns of restriction, with different implications, can be reduced to the same score.

The eight-point scale is:

A   Independent in feeding, continence, transferring, going to toilet, dressing and bathing
B   Independent in all but one of these functions
C   Independent in all but bathing and one additional function
D   Independent in all but bathing, dressing and one additional function
E   Independent in all but bathing, dressing, going to toilet and one additional function
F   Independent in all but bathing, dressing, going to toilet, transferring and one additional function
G   Dependent in all six functions
Other   Dependent in at least two functions, but not classifiable as C, D, E or F.

Full definitions of activities are given by Katz et al. (1970).

Validity

Despite the scale's widespread popularity among clinicians worldwide, there is little evidence of the validity of the scale. Katz et al. (1970) administered the ADL and other instruments to 270 chronically ill patients. The ADL correlated weakly to moderately with a mobility scale (0.50) and with a scale of home confinement (0.39).

The index of ADL was shown to predict the long-term course and social adaptation of patients with a number of conditions, including strokes and hip fractures, and was used to evaluate outpatient treatment for rheumatoid arthritis (Katz et al. 1966, 1968). It has also been shown to predict mortality (Brorsson and Asberg 1984). There is other early evidence of its predictive validity, reported by Katz and Akpom (1976). There are more studies which support the ability of the scale to discriminate between groups in the hypothesized direction. For example, it was able to distinguish between people aged 77 <85, 85 <90 and 90 and over in a community survey, with the oldest members having the poorest ADL scores (von Strauss et al. 2003). However, such concise indices tend to be insensitive to small changes in disease severity and to focus on physical performance measures. It is also of limited value in community surveys of elderly people because, like other short scales, it does not take adaptation to environment into account. It apparently underestimates dysfunction in community populations (Spector et al. 1987). LaPlante (2010) applied Guttman and item response theory (IRT) scaling methods to the scale, based on a household survey of 25,470 people aged 18+ and reported the ADL measure to be substantially biased by age, compared to an expanded measure.

Reliability

Little testing for reliability has been carried out; this is again surprising given the popularity of this scale, particularly by clinicians. Katz *et al.* (1963) assessed inter-rater reliability; they reported that discrepancies between raters occurred in 1 in 20 observations.

A Swedish study of Guttman analyses on 100 patients yielded coefficients of scalability of 0.74–0.88, suggesting that the index is a successful cumulative scale (Brorsson and Asberg 1984).

The Katz is one of the earliest indices used in the evaluation of the care of elderly and chronically ill patients, and hence one of the best known. The items included in the scale have formed the basis for ADL scales used in major national surveys in Britain (Bridgwood 2000). It is still a popular and useful index with a restricted range of patients, particularly those living in nursing and care homes, or clinical populations. However, the range of disabilities included in the instrument is not comprehensive and thus the populations to which it can be administered are restricted. It focuses on basic activities for daily living. The single index also means that the information derived from the index is limited. Wade (1992) concluded that while this was once the most popular scale used by neurologists, it has since been overtaken by the Barthel Index.

TOWNSEND'S DISABILITY SCALE

Townsend's Disability Scale is frequently used in population surveys of older people in the UK. It comprises a list of ADL, derived from early research on disabled people of all ages in the UK and the USA (Haber 1968; Sainsbury 1973) and from Townsend's own early survey work on elderly people (Townsend 1962; Shanas *et al.* 1968). It was also used in Townsend's later poverty survey (Townsend 1979). It is still popular because it is concise and simple, and focuses on tasks which are relevant to people living at home. Sainsbury (1973) stated that the list of tasks of daily living initially selected was chosen on the basis of a 'subjective' decision 'of the more important daily and social activities'. Its advantages are its brevity and acceptability to elderly people. Although the scale is also useful in that needs for particular types of health and social services can easily be inferred from the items, it still requires more detailed testing.

Content

The index deliberately focuses on a narrow range of activities, in order that the concepts underlying them are generally applicable to a wide section of the population and for ease of application within a survey framework of the general population:

(a) activities which maintain personal existence, such as washing, cutting own toenails;
(b) activities which provide the means to fulfil these personal acts, such as shopping, preparing hot meals and doing heavy housework.

The scale asks respondents if they have difficulty doing a range of ADL (none = 0, some difficulty = 1, or unable to do alone = 2). It can be self- or interviewer-administered, is easily completed and concise. Examples are shown in Box 3.5.

Box 3.5 Examples from Townsend's Disability Scale

Do you or would you have any difficulty (or find it troublesome, exhausting or worrying):

(a)   Washing down (whether in bath or not)?
(b)   Removing a jug, say, from an overhead shelf?
(c)   Tying a good knot in string?
(d)   Cutting toenails?

The remaining questions are not asked of children under the age of 10 or the bedfast:

(e)   Running to catch a bus?
(f)   Going up/down stairs?
(g)   Going shopping and carrying a full basket of shopping in each hand?
(h)   Doing heavy housework?
(i)   Preparing a hot meal?

The instrument is in the public domain, no permissions are needed and there is no charge for its use: see http://www.incamresearch.ca/content/townsend-disability-scale, accessed 21 September 2015.

Scoring

Difficulty with each activity is given equal weighting; changes in individual capacity from day to day and season to season are ignored. 'No difficulty' is scored as 0, 'with some difficulty' is scored as 1, and the score is 2 if the reply was 'unable to do alone'. The overall score has a range of 0–18. Townsend, as a result of early validation work, regards people with a score of 0 as having no disability, 1–2 as slightly affected, 3–6 some disability, 7–10 as appreciable disability and 11–18 as severe/very severe. The basis for this does not appear to have been tested any further.

Validity and reliability

None of the original studies which used the scale provided adequate details of the initial testing of the measure (Haber 1968; Sainsbury 1973). Bowling and Gabriel (2004), used the original version of the scale with a national sample of people aged 65 and over living at home; they reported that it had high internal consistency and a Cronbach's alpha of 0.91. Bowling (2005b) also used it, along with additional items, in a national population survey of people aged 65+ living at home, and reported the Cronbach's alpha as 0.91; it also correlated with perceived health stats as expected, supporting its construct validity (r 0.49, p <0.001).

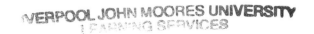

There are numerous examples in the UK of applications of the scale, or adaptations of it (both item and response-scale wording), and population norms are available (e.g. Vetter *et al.* 1982; Vetter and Ford 1989; Bowling *et al.* 1992, 2002; McGee *et al.* 1998). The scale is popular because it is simple and covers a range of activities which are relevant to living at home, although more extensive testing for its reliability, validity and factor structure is still required. It was used on the assumption that it represents one factor, although it covers three domains of functioning (mobility; personal care (ADL); and domestic activities (IADL)). McGee *et al.* (1998) confirmed the construct validity of the scale as an indicator of physical ability, but cautioned that the instrument may overestimate disability for a small number of people.

Adaptations

The limitations of this scale have led to adaptation by many researchers, in terms of adding other ADL (e.g. Bowling 2005b) or removing others. For example, some of the items are not appropriate for use with a frail population (e.g. 'running to catch a bus'). Adaptation of the scoring is also common. Bowling and Grundy (1997) increased the number of items and also the range of responses to: no difficulty with the task, slight, moderate or severe difficulty, unable to do alone, and unable to do at all (even with help). Each response was then scored from 0 (no difficulty) to 5 (unable to do at all) and the scores summed to produce a total score. The sub-sections representing mobility, ADL and IADL can also be scored separately. It was initially scored from 1 to 6, but the score of '0' was judged to be more useful as the number of people with no problems with any of the tasks is then evident in the raw total score, and is simpler to manipulate statistically. The scoring methods still require validation.

The extended scale items by Bowling and Grundy (1997) are shown below (as with the original, there are also no charges for its use and no permissions are needed):

Mobility
Getting in/out of bed
Transferring from a chair/wheelchair
Going up/down stairs
Getting on/off toilet
Getting in/out of bath
Getting about indoors
Getting about outdoors
Using public transport

Personal care
Washing self/shaving (men)
Bathing self
Dressing self
Brushing/combing hair
Washing hair
Cutting toenails

Domestic
Cooking/preparing meal
Housework
Laundry
Shopping
Doing odd jobs

Two other items were initially included, brushing or managing teeth and handling money, but these appeared ambiguous. They were excluded after factor analysis. On the basis of community surveys with 662 people aged 85 and over living in London, and almost 700 people aged 65+ living in Essex and London, inter-item correlations coefficients between tasks ranged from around 0.13 (this was for shopping and managing teeth or dentures which would not be expected necessarily to correlate highly) to around 0.74 (for difficulties with washing self and with dressing self which would be expected to correlate more highly); split half reliability: 0.78–0.91 between samples. The inter-item correlation (alpha) for the personal care task section was 0.70–0.75; for the domestic-task section was 0.80–0.85; and for the mobility section was 0.81–0.89. Testing of the scale was carried out across the three samples, and results were highly statistically significant, indicating that the scale has good reliability. The ADL scale items correlated moderately to well with comparable items on dressing self, trouble with steps/stairs, walking outdoors, and walking indoors from the Nottingham Health Profile (Hunt *et al.* 1986), which was used for a sub-sample (0.635, p <0.0001; 0.565, p <0.0001; 0.350, p <0.004; and 0.472, p <0.0001 respectively). The scale, and items from it (e.g. difficulties getting about outdoors), was also highly significantly associated with relevant physical health problems (e.g. aches, pains, stiffness in joints, muscles), health and social service use, life satisfaction and mental health, and predictive of worsening emotional well-being, supporting its convergent and predictive validity (Bowling *et al.* 1992, 1993, 1994a, 1994b). The convergent validity of the scale is further supported by its ability to independently predict quality of life rating in the expected direction, in a British survey of 999 people aged 65 and over living at home (Bowling *et al.* 2002).

A similar scale was developed by the Institute for Economic and Social Research at York University and used in a wide range of surveys (Morton-Williams 1979). Their scale encompasses a wider range of self-care activities than the original Townsend scale, with alternative rankings of: able to do easily, with a little difficulty, with a lot of difficulty, unable to do without someone helping, unable to do even with someone helping. Testing of this modified scale is also incomplete.

Another adaptation of the scale was undertaken by Bond and Carstairs (1982) in their survey of 5,000 elderly people in Scotland. These authors distinguished between functional criteria for dependency (mobility, self-care and home-care capacity) and clinical criteria for dependency (incontinence, mental state), and they attempted to measure these. They selected items from the original Sainsbury scale, on the basis of inter-item correlations, which were then subjected to a Guttman scaling analysis. The items selected were based on a hierarchical concept: having difficulty with an activity is associated with having difficulty with earlier scale items. This modification finally covered nine ADL (washing all over, cutting toenails, getting on a bus, going up and down stairs, doing heavy housework, going shopping and carrying heavy bags, preparing and cooking hot meals, reaching an overhead shelf and tying a good knot in a piece of string). Each activity carries a score of 0 (no difficulty), 1 (can do but with difficulty), or 2 (not able). The scores are summed to give a total, which is then subdivided into five groups: 0 (no incapacity), 1–2 (slight incapacity), 3–6 (some incapacity), 7–10 (appreciable incapacity) and 11 or more (severe incapacity). A person classified as physically disabled (score of 11+) would need help with at least two of the specified activities, and have some difficulty with some/all of the rest. This version, and its scoring, was also used by Melzer *et al.* (2000), along with a measure of dementia, in a prevalence study of disability in over 10,000 people aged 65+ living in Cambridgeshire, Newcastle, Nottingham and Oxford. In support of construct validity, they reported that the prevalence of disability overall and need for 'constant care' was lower in men and women in higher social classes I and II, compared with those in lower social class groups.

THE KARNOFSKY PERFORMANCE INDEX (KPI)

The KPI (sometimes called the Karnofsky Performance Scale) emphasizes physical performance and dependency. It has been frequently used to measure patients' prognosis. It was originally designed for use with lung cancer patients in relation to assessing palliative treatments (Karnofsky *et al.* 1948; Karnofsky and Burchenal 1949). It is a descriptive, ordinal scale ranging from 0 to 100 (normal to dead), developed for use in clinical settings. Patients are assigned to categories by a clinician or other health care professional. It is widely used in the USA and Europe. It has undergone some adjustments since its development in 1949 (Péus *et al.* 2013).

An early literature review, examining the frequency of measurement of QoL in clinical trials of outcome of care in six international cancer journals, showed that only 6 per cent attempted to measure it, and that the vast majority of this 6 per cent used the original performance criteria of Karnofsky (Bardelli and Saracci 1978), although it only taps a narrow, physical dependency dimension of QoL.

Content

The 11-point scale is heavily weighted towards the physical performance and dependency dimensions of life. Examples of some of the classifications, which are made by professionals, and scores, are shown in Box 3.6.

Box 3.6 Examples from the KPI

Normal; no complaint; no evidence of disease (index: 100).
Requires occasional assistance from others but able to care for most needs (index: 60).
Disabled; requires special care and assistance (index: 40).

Moribund; fatal processes progressing rapidly (index: 10).
Dead (index: 0).

No permissions are required for use, and no charges are applied: see this website which displays two versions of the scale, and scroll down to 'functional ability tools': http://www.acsu.buffalo.edu/~drstall/assessmenttools.html, accessed 21 September 2015.

Scoring

Each of the 11 components of the scale is given a notional percentage score (100 = normal/no evidence of disease/no symptoms; 0 = dead). A score of 70–100 has been interpreted as favourable (Christakou *et al.* 2013). Various categorizations exist.

Karnofsky ratings are often reported as a mean score, although there is no evidence that the intervals between the 10 categories represent the same degree of dysfunction (O'Brien 1988). Interpretations of the scale's classifications are likely to vary, as the points cover different conceptual elements.

Validity

The disadvantage of the KPI, apart from its limited content, is that it involves categorization of patients by another person. This is a fundamental flaw, given the evidence of discrepancies between patients' and physicians' ratings of functioning and QoL. In Evans *et al.*'s (1984) study, for example, there were wide discrepancies between patients' self-assessments, based on the Sickness Impact Profile, and physicians' assessments, based on the KPI, with the latter rating patients as being less impaired than the former.

However, it is still very popular among clinical researchers, especially in oncology (Hwang *et al.* 2003; Llobera *et al.* 2003; Tentes *et al.* 2003). Mor *et al.* (1984) used the scale in a national hospice evaluation study. They reported that the convergent validity of the scale was achieved: it was strongly related to two other independent measures of patient functioning (Katz's ADL scale and another QoL assessment). It was also able to predict longevity (0.30) in the population of terminally ill cancer patients, thus indicating that it has predictive validity. Firat *et al.* (2002) also reported, on the basis of a sample of patients with lung cancer, that the KPI was independently associated with overall survival, and was a better predictor (along with comorbidity) than clinical tumour stage. Thus, the KPI is a successful predictor of survival. Llobera *et al.* (2003) also reported that it was predictive of dependence and deterioration of cancer patients during their terminal stages.

Mor (1987), again in a study of cancer patients (total: 2,046), reported a moderate correlation between the Karnofsky and the Spitzer Quality of Life Index; the correlation was probably moderate because the latter is multidimensional. One of its most well-known early applications has been in the US National Heart Transplantation Study (Evans *et al.* 1984). Results from this study showed a marked shift in the distribution of Karnofsky scores before and after transplantation. In a study of 139 lung cancer patients, Schaafsma and Osoba (1994) reported weak associations between observer-rated

Karnofsky scores and self-rated QoL using the core European Organization for the Treatment of Cancer 30-item Questionnaire (Aaronson 1993). Early and more recent research has shown that the Karnofsky has prognostic value, especially for cancers (e.g. Sperduto *et al.* 2012; see Péus *et al.* 2013).

Reliability

The results of testing for inter-rater reliability have varied widely, with some studies reporting low reliability at 29–43 per cent, with Cohen's kappa, and others reporting higher (Pearson's) correlations of 0.66–0.69 (Hutchinson *et al.* 1979; Yates *et al.* 1980). Mor *et al.* (1984), on the basis of a national hospice evaluation, reported that the inter-rater reliability coefficient of the 47 interviewers employed at test-retests at four-month intervals was 0.97. Schag *et al.* (1984) asked doctors and mental health professionals to assess 293 cancer patients with the KPI. The reliability of the KPI between these two different groups of assessors was high at r = 0.89, with doctors generally giving higher scores than the mental health professionals. Slevin *et al.* (1988) reported a study involving 108 cancer patients in which two different groups of patients self-completed the Karnofsky index, and other measures, on a single day, and then daily for five consecutive days. Although the Karnofsky was more robust than the other measures tested (Spitzer's Quality of Life Index, the Hospital Anxiety and Depression scale and LASA visual analogue scales), the same score was achieved on only 54 per cent of occasions, despite the fact that only the top five points on the Karnofsky were covered.

Yates *et al.* (1980) carried out the first objective validation of the scale and concluded that the index is not appropriately scaled and that scale values may bear no relation to clinical significance. Research has since focused on the difficulties inherent in interpreting scores for people with reduced 'performance status' because scores of 10–40 per cent have been used to indicate the need for hospital admission. This reflects the different structures of care in the 1940s – now there are more alternatives to avoid hospitalization (Péus *et al.* 2013). An attempt to reformulate the Karnofsky criteria for values between 10–40 per cent was made in the Australian-modified Karnofsky Performance Status (AKPS) scale: 40 per cent (in bed more than 50 per cent of the time); 30 per cent (almost completely bedfast); 20 per cent (totally bedfast and requiring extensive nursing care by professionals and/or family); 10 per cent (comatose or barely arousable) (Abernethy *et al.* 2005). These authors then used the Karnofsky and their modified version, with 26 trained nurses assessing 306 palliative care patients at 1,600 time-points within a clinical trial. The KPS and AKPS scores correlated strongly, although the AKPS scores were more powerful predictors of patients' survival (Abernethy *et al.* 2005).

The Eastern Cooperative Oncology Group developed an alternative performance status measure (ECOG PS), derived from the Karnofsky (Oken *et al.* 1982), and both measures are generally used as selection criteria and stratification methods in studies of patient cohorts (Péus *et al.* 2013). Other versions of the scale have been developed, but these have shown no obvious improvements in effectiveness over the original version (Zubrod *et al.* 1960; World Health Organization 1979; Nou and Aberg 1980).

Although it is frequently described as an indicator of QoL (Sitjas *et al.* 2003), it is a measure of functioning, not QoL, and can only capture narrow aspects of this broad concept.

The scale has generally been uncritically applied in a large number of clinical settings. It has even been used in settings where its applicability can be questioned (bone marrow transplantation in children) (Hinterberger *et al.* 1987).

In sum, its limitation is that it requires assessments to be made by another person, rather than being a patient-based self-assessment measure, and it is a measure of performance (and not QoL, which users have frequently claimed). Although advanced measurement approaches have been developed, a literature review of the history of the use of the KPI from the 1940s to the 1990s by Timmermann (2012) reported on its popularity.

THE BARTHEL INDEX

The Barthel Index was developed by Mahoney and Barthel (1965). The Index is a popular measure in neurology, and is widely judged to be useful and able to predict outcomes, particularly in stroke patients. It is not a comprehensive measure of functioning. It omits tasks of daily living such as cooking and shopping and other everyday tasks essential for life in the community. It is based on observed functions, and thus assesses performance, not ability. The Index was developed to measure functioning before and after intervention treatment, and to indicate the amount of nursing care required. It was designed for use with long-term hospital patients with neuromuscular or musculo-skeletal disorders, and has been used more generally to evaluate treatment outcomes since.

Content

The Barthel Index is based on a rating scale of 10 domains completed by a therapist or other observer. It measures capacity to perform 10 basic ADL: self-care (feeding, grooming, bathing, dressing, bowel care, bladder care and toilet use) and mobility (ambulation, transferring – from bed to wheelchair – and climbing stairs). The dimensions covered are shown in Box 3.7.

Box 3.7 Examples from the Barthel Index

Dimensions:

Feeding
Moving from wheelchair to bed and return
Personal toilet (wash face, comb hair, shave, clean teeth)
Getting on and off the toilet
Bathing self
Walking on level surface (or if unable to walk, propel wheelchair)
Ascend and descend stairs
Dressing
Controlling bowels and controlling bladder

Source: Mahoney, F.I. and Barthel, D. (1965) Functional evaluation: the Barthel Index. *Maryland State Medical Journal*, 14: 56–61. Reprinted with permission of MAPI Research Trust. Barthel Index © MedChi 1965. All Rights Reserved. The Maryland State Medical Society. Permission is required to modify the Barthel Index or to use it for commercial purposes. It may be used freely for non-commercial purposes with the following citation: Mahoney, F.I., Barthel, D. Functional evaluation: the Barthel Index. *Maryland State Medical Journal* 1965; 14: 56–61. Contact information and permission to use: MAPI Research Trust, Lyon, France; PROinformation@mapi-trust.org; https://eprovide.mapi-trust.org/ accessed 21 July 2016.

The scale takes approximately five minutes to complete.

Scoring

Different values are assigned to different activities. Individuals are scored on 10 activities which are summed to give a score of 0 (totally dependent) to 100 (fully independent). Index scores are >90 minimal or no disability; 55–90 moderate disability, <55 severe disability.

The authors of the scale provide detailed instructions for assessing and scoring patients; for example:

> Doing personal toilet: 5 = patient can wash hands and face, comb hair, clean teeth, and shave. He may use any kind of razor but must put in blade or plug in razor without help as well as get it from drawer or cabinet. Female patients must put on own make-up, if used, but need not braid or style hair.

A modified scoring method was also developed that gives a maximum score of 20 to patients who are continent, able to wash, feed and dress themselves and are independently mobile (Collin *et al.* 1988).

The scores are intended to reflect the amount of time and assistance a patient requires. However, the scoring method is inconsistent in that changes by a given number of points do not reflect equivalent changes in disability across different activities. Moreover, as its authors point out, the scale is restricted in that changes can occur beyond the end points of the scale.

Validity

The original Barthel Index was tested for validity by Wade *et al.* (1985, 1992) and Collen *et al.* (1990), in their evaluations of therapies for stroke patients. The results have been more fully described by Wade (1992). Mattison *et al.* (1991) used the Barthel Index with 364 patients attending day centres for the physically disabled. They compared it with the PULSES Scale and the Edinburgh Rehabilitation Status Scale (ERSS) (Affleck *et al.* 1988) and reported that the correlation between the Barthel and these two scales was 0.65 and r = −0.69 respectively. Good results were reported by Wade and Collin (1988). Most studies of its validity compare it with the PULSES profile, which give correlations of −0.74 to −0.90 (Granger *et al.* 1979; Mattison *et al.* 1991). Wilkinson *et al.*'s (1997) study of the long-term outcome of stroke patients reported that the Barthel Index correlated highly with the physical functioning dimension of the SF-36 (r = 0.810), the physical mobility dimension of the Nottingham Health Profile (r = −0.840), the London Handicap Scale (r = 0.727) and the Frenchay Activities Index (r = 0.826). They concluded that the use of the Barthel Index is still justified in long-term follow-up studies of stroke patients. A review of the evidence by Quinn *et al.* (2011) concluded that the Barthel Index is a valid measure of activities of daily living.

The Barthel Index has been reported to have predictive validity as it correlates well with various prognostic scores of stroke patients (Kalra and Crome 1993), length of hospital stay and mortality (Wylie and White 1964). It has been reported to be sensitive to their recovery (Wade and Langton-Hewer 1987). However, it was insensitive to clinical change among elderly patients attending a day hospital (Rodgers *et al.* 1993; Parker *et al.* 1994). It may not be sensitive to improvements of deteriorations beyond the end points of the scale ('floor' and 'ceiling' effects) (McDowell and Newell 1996; Quinn *et al.* 2011). Yohannes *et al.* (1998) assessed the sensitivity and specificity of the Barthel Index in a study of people with and without chronic airflow limitation (CAL) (outpatients and people in the community). They reported that the Index underestimated disability in CAL and that the Nottingham extended ADL index discriminated between groups better than the Barthel Index. It has been reported that the Barthel Index has less powerful end points than the earlier developed Rankin Scale when used in clinical trials of stroke patients (Rankin 1957), with the implication that it weakens trial power for a given trial size, or requires a larger sample size to obtain statistical power, than the Rankin Scale (Young *et al.* 2003).

De Haan *et al.* (1993) reported that the Barthel Index factor analysis showed that the items described one common trait, which explained 81 per cent of the variance in their study of stroke patients. This supports earlier factor analyses which showed that it measures a single domain, although two factors have also been reported – mobility and personal care (Wade and Langton-Hewer 1987).

Reliability

Sherwood *et al.* (1977) reported alpha reliability coefficients of 0.95 to 0.97 for three samples of hospital patients, suggesting that the scale is internally consistent. Collin *et al.* (1988) tested it for reliability on 25 stroke patients, and analysed observer agreement, using groups of two, three and four observers. They reported that difficulties in agreement were lower for the middle category, and consequently they refined the instructions for observers. De Haan *et al.* (1993), in a study of neurology outpatients with stroke, also reported that the Barthel Index had high internal consistency (Cronbach's alpha = 0.96) and concordance of total scores by three observers (mean kappa = 0.88, range 0.82–0.90), and single-item scores (mean values for kappa = 0.82–1.00). Granger *et al.* (1979) reported a test-retest reliability of 0.89 with severely disabled adults, and an inter-rater agreement exceeding 0.95. Other studies of doctors' and nurses' ratings of elderly nursing-home patients have reported poor agreement, particularly for patients with some degree of cognitive impairment (Ranhoff and Laake 1993).

Despite its acknowledged limitations, there is a large body of literature supporting its use with specific groups of disabled patients, such as those with neurological disability

(Collin *et al.* 1988; Wade and Collin 1988). As the Barthel Index is a measure of what the patient actually does, rather than ability, scoring may also be location dependent (McMurdo and Rennie 1993).

Quinn *et al.*'s (2011) review concluded that the Barthel Index is one of the most widely used measures in stroke trials, and its reliability is acceptable – but they also reported that sensitivity to change is limited at extremes of disability (see above). They queried whether the Barthel Index was appropriate for contemporary multicentre stroke trials.

Modifications

Several modified versions of the Barthel Index have been developed (Granger *et al.* 1979; Fortinsky *et al.* 1981; Granger 1982; Granger and McNamara 1984; Shah *et al.* 1989; Gompertz *et al.* 1993a, 1993b). Although the Barthel Index is narrow in scope, modifications have not always been shown to have greater validity or responsiveness to change in condition (Guyatt *et al.* 1993). Granger and his colleagues now regard their early modifications of the scale (which was extended to cover 15 topics) to be obsolete and have replaced it with the Functional Independence Measure (18 items) and Functional Assessment Measure (12 items) (FIM+FAM) (Stineman *et al.* 1994). A five-item short form of the Barthel Index has been developed, and assessed, along with the Barthel Index, and the Functional Independence Measure by Hsueh *et al.* (2002) in a prospective study of stroke patients. The psychometric properties were similar, except for a more notable floor effect for the short form Barthel Index in patients with severe disabilities.

THE FUNCTIONAL INDEPENDENCE MEASURE (FIM) AND FUNCTIONAL ASSESSMENT MEASURE (FAM)

The FIM

The FIM measures the level of assistance needed for people to complete basic ADL. There are two domains: motor (developed from the Barthel Index) and cognitive. Clinicians score patients on a seven-point scale. The FIM was developed after a review of functional assessment scales. It was intended to be sensitive to individuals' changes over the course of rehabilitation.

Content

The FIM is an 18-item, ordinal level rating scale of disability, covering motor (13 items) and cognitive (5 items) dysfunction: self-care (eating, grooming, bathing, dressing, toileting); sphincter control (bladder and bowel management); mobility (transferring – bed, chair, wheelchair; toilet; tub or shower); locomotion (walking or using wheelchair; stairs); communication (comprehension; expression); social cognition (social interaction; problem solving; memory). Patients are asked to complete each activity in order to produce a score. Patient burden has been estimated at 30–45 minutes. See summary example in Box 3.8.

Box 3.8 Example from the FIM® instrument motor items

Summary of transfers (version 5.2)

Transfers: bed, chair, wheelchair. Includes all aspects of transferring from a bed to a chair and back, or from a bed to a wheelchair and back, or coming to a standing position if walking is typical mode of locomotion.

Transfers: toilet. Includes all aspects of transferring on and off a toilet. This includes safely approaching, sitting down on, and getting up from the toilet.

Transfers: tub/shower: includes getting into/out of tub or shower stall.

Source: Uniform Data System for Medical Rehabilitation 2009. The FIM System® Clinical Guide, Version 5.2. Buffalo: UDSMR. Reprinted with permission. Contact for licensing information, guidelines and updates: Uniform Data System for Medical Rehabilitation, 270 Northpointe Parkway, Suite 300, Amherst, NY, 14228, USA; info@udsmr.org; website: http://www.udsmr.org, accessed 21 September 2015.

Scoring

Scores for each variable range from 1 (total assistance) to 7 (complete independence), and are summed, yielding a total score range of between 18 (complete dependence) and 126 (complete independence). It is one of the most widely used measures of basic functional activities in intensive care units, although some components cannot be assessed in such settings (e.g. stairs) (Christakou *et al.* 2013).

Reliability and validity

Intra-class correlations for pairs of clinical raters, rating 263 patients (for the seven-point rating scale) ranged from 0.93 to 0.96; mean kappa for level of agreement was 0.71 (Hamilton *et al.* 1991). Cronbach's alphas of between 0.93 and 0.95 were reported, on admission and discharge in a study of 11,102 patients, except for the locomotor subscale (alpha 0.68) (Dodds *et al.* 1993). Content validity was tested by clinical assessments of its scope at the development stage (Keith *et al.* 1987). Dodds *et al.*'s (1993) study confirmed that scores improved between admission and discharge. The FIM has been reported to correlate with other functional measures, including the Barthel Index (0.84), and the Katz Index of ADL (0.68) (Rockwood *et al.* 1993). FIM scores have correlated with age, comorbidity, place of discharge and other measures of functioning (see White *et al.* (2011)).

FIM+FAM

The FAM contains 12 items, with the same seven-point rating scale as the FIM. It was intended as an adjunct to the FIM, to address major areas of functioning not included in the FIM. The FAM includes cognitive, behavioural, communication and community functioning (Hall 1997). The total 18-item scale is known as the FIM+FAM, and takes approximately 35 minutes to administer.

Reliability and validity

FIM+FAM has been generally reported to have good reliability, including inter-rater reliability, and validity (Ottenbacher *et al.* 1994; Kidd *et al.* 1995; Turner-Stokes *et al.* 1999, and see brief review by Christakou *et al.* 2013). Hall (1992) reported rater agreement to be 89 per cent, and the kappa score was 0.85. However, Riazi *et al.* (2003a) reported that the FAM mobility subscale had lower internal consistency reliability (Cronbach's alpha 0.78) than the SF-36 physical subscale in a clinical trial of patients with multiple sclerosis. Ceiling effects have been reported, limiting its usefulness in assessing change post-discharge/rehabilitation (Hall *et al.* 1996). It can have floor effects, due to its combination of all transfer types (bed, mobility to standing transfers) into one task, possibly limiting its use in chronically critically ill populations (Christakou *et al.* 2013). Hobart *et al.* (2001) compared the Barthel Index with the FIM, and FIM+FAM in rehabilitation patients. Each instrument demonstrated similar levels of reliability and validity in measuring physical disability and similar levels of responsiveness to change.

A UK version has been developed, and ensuing modifications to enhance the objectivity of the scoring have resulted in improved team and individual accuracy in scoring (Turner-Stokes *et al.* 1999). The FIM+FAM is increasingly used, although the original Barthel Index is still very popular, particularly in studies of stroke (Wilkinson *et al.* 1997; Fjartoft *et al.* 2003). A UK users group was set up which aimed to improve the objectivity of the scoring and developed a UK version of the FAM. For more information about the FAM, contact Jerry Wright at tbiscibi-sci.org or Lynne Turner at lynne.turner-stokes@dial.pipex.com.

LONDON HANDICAP SCALE (LHS)

The LHS is a handicap classification questionnaire covering six domains: mobility, physical independence, occupation, social integration, orientation and economic self-sufficiency (Harwood *et al.* 1994; Harwood and Ebrahim 1995). It includes a table of severity weights to enable an overall interval-level handicap score to be calculated. Handicap was defined by the scale developers as the disadvantage for a person that results from ill health. The scale was based on the WHO (1980) *International Classification of Impairments, Disabilities and Handicaps*. The weights for scoring were obtained from two samples of lay people (n = 34 and 79), 97 medical doctors and 14 health professionals who were asked to rate the severity of hypothetical descriptions.

Content, administration and scoring

Each of the six domains contains a single item question, with standardized six-point response choices, and detailed descriptions of the meaning of the subscale response items. The appropriate score from a matrix is applied to each response, and entered into the score formula to obtain the overall handicap score. The score is an estimate of the relative desirability (utility) of the state of health described. A score of 100 indicates no handicap, while a score of 0 represents maximum handicap. The scale is self-completed; a proxy version for completion by a third party is available for people who are unable to complete the questionnaire themselves. A handbook is available which describes the scale and includes the scoring instructions. Examples from the LHS are shown in Box 3.9.

Box 3.9 Examples from the LHS

Physical independence
Looking after yourself. Think about things like housework, shopping, looking after money, cooking, laundry, getting dressed, washing, shaving and using the toilet.

Does your health stop you looking after yourself?

Not at all: You do everything to look after yourself.
Very slightly: You need a little help now and again.
Quite a lot: You need help with some tasks (such as heavy housework or shopping), but no more than once a day.
Very much: You do some things for yourself, but you need help more than once a day. You can be left alone safely for a few hours.
Almost completely: You need help with everything. You need constant attention, day and night.

© Rowan H. Harwood / Shah Ebrahim. Source: Harwood, R.H. and Ebrahim, S. (1995) *Manual of the London Handicap Scale*. Nottingham: University of Nottingham, Department of Health Care of the Elderly. Reprinted with permission of the developer. Contact: MAPI Research Trust at: https://eprovide.mapi-trust.org/ accessed 21 July 2016. PROInformation@mapi-trust.org. Developer contact information: Prof. Rowan H. Harwood, Consultant Geriatrician & Professor in Geriatric Medicine, Nottingham University Hospitals NHS Trust, QMC, Nottingham NG7 2UH; tel.: (0115) 924 9924, ext. 61412 (secretary ext. 64186); email: rowan.harwood@nuh.nhs.uk.

Validity and reliability

The LHS, together with several other scales, was administered to 89 survivors of stroke at 12 months and between 24 and 36 months after the index stroke. The Scale was moderately strongly associated with the other scales used (r = 0.4 to 0.7), which included the Barthel Index (Mahoney and Barthel 1965), the Nottingham Extended ADL Scale (Nouri and Lincoln 1987), the Nottingham Health Profile (Hunt *et al.* 1986) and the Geriatric Depression Scale (Yesavage *et al.* 1983). In a further study of 58 patients, the scale was administered six months after hospital admission for stroke. The scale correlated highly (r = 0.78) with the modified Rankin Scale (Rankin 1957), supporting its concurrent validity (Harwood and Ebrahim 1995). The scale was associated with pre-stroke disability, initial stroke severity and mood at one, and two to three years follow-up of 316 acute stroke patients (Harwood *et al.* 1994, 1997). In a study of long-term outcome of stroke by Wilkinson *et al.* (1997), the LHS was reported to correlate highly with the Barthel Index (r = 0.726). Dubec *et al.* (2004), in a study of 75 people aged 60+ living at home, reported, however, that the LHS had large ceiling effects.

It has been shown to be sensitive to improvement after hip replacement in a study of 81 patients. Principal components analyses showed one or two factor solutions (with the first representing handicap, but there was no particular pattern to the loadings on the second factor) (Harwood and Ebrahim 1995).

In a study of 37 stroke patients who recompleted the scale at two weeks post-baseline assessment, the reliability coefficient was 0.91. A three-month follow-up study of 79 rheumatology patients yielded a reliability coefficient of 0.72. The reliability coefficient from mixed groups of patients (13 hip replacement, four knee replacement and six angioplasty patients) was 0.77 (Harwood and Ebrahim 1995).

The weighted and unweighted (simple summation of scores without weights) scale scores were tested in a study of stroke patients by Jenkinson *et al.* (2000). Cronbach's alpha for the LHS was 0.83 indicating good internal consistency. The weighted and unweighted versions of the LHS correlated highly with each other (r = 0.98). Both versions correlated similarly with the Dartmouth Coop Charts, the Frenchay Activities Index, the Barthel Index and the Hospital Anxiety and Depression scale, and the correlations supported their convergent validity and discriminative ability. Thus the simple summation of scores of the LHS did not lead to any change in the measurement properties of the instrument, compared with standard weighted scoring. Hence the authors recommended that unweighted scores should be used as these are easier to calculate and interpret.

The scale has been used in several descriptive studies of handicap (Harwood *et al.* 1996, 1998a, 1998b; Prince *et al.* 1997, 1998). In sum, it is a relatively recently developed scale showing good psychometric abilities to date.

THE QUALITY OF WELL-BEING SCALE (QWBS)

The QWBS was developed in order to operationalize 'wellness' for a general health-policy model. This was an attempt to develop an alternative to economic cost-benefit analysis for resource allocation – for example, by comparing the health status of groups of individuals for the evaluation of health care programmes (Kaplan *et al.* 1976; Bush 1984). Hence it provides an estimate of the value of health status which is necessary for cost-utility analyses (Hays *et al.* 1996).

It can be used with general populations and applied to any type of disease. The items in the interview schedule were drawn mainly from the US Health Interview Survey and from the Social Security Administration Survey, but the schedule has been extensively tested on large groups of nurses and graduate students and revised. The QWBS combines mortality with estimates of QoL. It quantifies the health output of a treatment in terms of years of life, adjusted for their diminished quality, that it is responsible for. First, the assessment of health begins with an assessment of functional status, based on the individual's performance. Second, a value reflecting the relative desirability (utility) is assigned to each functional level (Fanshel and Bush 1970).

Responses to a branching questionnaire are used to assign subjects to one of a number of discrete function states. It is based on a model of health which encompasses symptom/problem, mobility, physical activity and social activity. The QWBS has been used in many evaluative studies of pulmonary disease and in drug trials (Toevs *et al.* 1984; Bombardier *et al.* 1986; Kaplan 1994). Several areas of application have been reported by Bush (1984), most of which are unpublished. The scale includes death. This avoids the problem inherent in other indices where, as death is frequently ignored, the death of a disabled person appears to improve the population estimate of health status (Kaplan *et al.* 1994).

Third, information is also collected about future changes (prognosis). This permits a distinction between two people with equal functional disability, one of whom is terminally ill.

Interview and self-administered formats are available as well as two- and four-page versions.

Content

The QWBS consists of three ordinal scales on dimensions of daily activity. Combinations of each of the three scales of mobility, physical and social activity were initially taken to define 29 function levels. Subsequent modification has increased the number of function levels to 43. Each function level can be linked with a separate classification of symptoms and problems. Questions are based on performance, not capacity. Four aspects of function are covered – mobility/confinement, physical activity, social activity (e.g. work, housekeeping) and self-care. The categories on each scale range from full independence to death. The physical ability scale has four categories and the others have five.

Respondents are given a list of 22 'symptom/problem' complexes and asked to identify all that applied to them during the preceding six days. They are then asked to indicate which of these has 'bothered them most'. Next, they are asked about mobility, physical and social activity. Actual ability rather than capacity to perform is asked about. Examples of the scale items are shown in Box 3.10.

Box 3.10 Examples from the QWBS V1.04

Time frame: Over the last 3 days:

No days/Yesterday/2 days ago/ 3 days ago

Part II – Self-care

5a. Did you spend any part of the day or night as a patient in a hospital, nursing home, or rehabilitation centre?

Part III – Mobility

6a. Which days did you drive a motor vehicle?

Part IV – Physical activity

7a. Have trouble climbing stairs or inclines or walking off the curb?

Source: Kaplan, R. *et al.* (1993) The Quality of Well-Being Scale: rationale for a single quality of life index, in S.R. Walker and R.M. Rosser (eds) *Quality of Life Assessment: Key Issues in the 1990s.* Dordrecht, The Netherlands: Kluwer Academic Publishers, pp. 65–94. With permission. Copyright © 1996 by Robert M. Kaplan, Theodore G. Ganiats, and William J. Sieber. All rights reserved. Health Policy Project, University of California at San Diego. qwb@ucsd.edu; https://eprovide.mapi-trust.org/ accessed 21 July 2016.

Scoring

Respondents' functional status is classified for each day on the scales of mobility, physical and social activity. The QWBS score is calculated by combining this information with the symptom/problem responses, using a set of preference weights. The latter were developed on the basis of interviews with 800 respondents in a household survey in which respondents were asked to rate different health states on a 10-point scale ranging from death to perfect health. The ratings were used in a multiple-regression analysis to obtain weights for different responses. Scores are calculated separately for each of the six days, and the QWBS score is expressed as the average of these. The final score ranges from 0 (equated with death) to 1 (perfect health) (Patrick *et al.* 1973a, 1973b). For each of the 43 function levels a 'preference weight' has been established empirically, ranging from 1.0 (complete well-being/full function) to 0.0 (death). The appropriate preference weight is assigned to the respondent's functional ability level, and the resulting score is known as the quality of well-being score. The authors noted that it is possible to provide a score below zero to represent a state 'worse than death' (Kaplan and Bush 1982). The weights assigned represent preferences of the relative importance that members of society assigned to each functional level. The third stage of rating involves adjusting for prognosis (Kaplan *et al.* 1976, 1979). QWBS scores can be translated into quality-adjusted life years (QALYs) for policy analysis purposes.

Validity

The content validity of the QWBS has been stated by Kaplan *et al.* (1976). Its content validity as an index of disability is enhanced by incorporating death. Kaplan *et al.* (1976) reported correlations of −0.75 between the QWBS and number of reported symptoms, and of 0.96 between the QWBS and the number of chronic health problems. The correlation between the QWBS and the number of physician contacts in the preceding eight days was 0.55. It correlated well (0.76) with self-rated quality of life. A review of the literature showed that it correlated with functional ability and broader health status scales from 0.17 to 0.71, with most correlations at 0.50 or more (Revicki and Kaplan 1993). Thus it was said by its authors to have convergent validity. More recent studies have confirmed the good convergent validity of the QWBS when tested against other measures of health status (Groessl *et al.* 2003). It is able to successfully predict outcome among people with HIV infection (Kaplan *et al.* 1995), and has been widely reported as having good convergent validity when tested against other HIV health status measures (Hughes *et al.* 1997). Its predictive value has been reported to be between 0.95 and 0.98 and sensitivity at 0.90, on the basis of data from 1,324 subjects with a range of diseases and injuries. It is able to discriminate between changes in life quality over time (Kaplan *et al.* 1976).

The QWBS was used by Leighton Read *et al.* (1987) in a study of 400 outpatients in Boston, Massachusetts, USA. The authors tested this scale, the SIP and the RAND Corporation's General Health Rating Index (GHRI) for convergent validity, content and discriminant validity. The findings for convergent validity were similar to those achieved by the developers of the scales – the correlations between scales were moderately high (0.46–0.55). They reported the GHRI to be the easiest to use, as they found both the SIP and the QWBS required a major commitment to interviewer training. All were equally acceptable to respondents. The QWBS contained more items than the others on specific symptoms; in contrast the SIP contained more detail on dysfunction. The authors concluded that each scale was a valid measure of health status. Anderson *et al.* (1998) compared the results of the QWBS with those of the SF-36 in characterizing the health of patients (mainly cancer and AIDS) over two and a half years. They reported that while the QWBS indicated a decrease in the functioning of patients over time, the SF-36 did not. Apparently, this was because the QWBS counted patient deaths as an outcome, whereas the SF-36 counted them as missing data. Hence the authors recommended the QWBS as better able to capture the outcomes of serious illness over time than the SF-36. Validation of the scaling technique was reported by Kaplan and Ernst (1983).

Kuspinar and Mayo (2014) reviewed and compared the psychometric properties of the EQ-5D, HUI2/HUI3, the QWBS and the SF-6D in multiple sclerosis patients. They reported that the QWBS was not able to discriminate between moderately and severely disabled patients with multiple sclerosis, and had only small to moderate correlations with instruments measuring impairments, and slightly stronger correlations against measures of activity limitations/participation restrictions and health-related QoL. Frosch *et al.* (2004) tested the self-administered version of the QWBS with 334 rheumatology and 562 family medicine clinic patients, and confirmed its construct validity (it was significantly associated with the AIMS and HAQ), and discriminative ability between patient groups.

Reliability

The reliability coefficient obtained when judges reassessed scale values for 29 function levels was 0.90 (Kaplan and Bush 1982). Test-retest reliability is between 0.93 and 0.98 (Kaplan *et al.* 1978; Bush 1984). The internal consistency reliability estimates for the QWBS overall score have been reported for four populations and reliability estimates have exceeded 0.90. The means and variances of preferences for attributes of QoL did not change over time (Kaplan *et al.* 1978). Details of the early reliability studies are reported in Kaplan *et al.* (1988).

The QWBS is advantageous in that it incorporates mortality. Kaplan (1994) and Kaplan *et al.* (1994) recommended that the QWBS is useful for policy analysis and clinical research because of its unidimensionality, but its unidimensional approach makes it less informative for clinical studies, where a multidimensional scoring approach is preferable. The complexity of the original interviewer-administered scale has inhibited its use in research on health outcomes. At the other extreme it has also been used with patients where its appropriateness is questionable, such as with paediatric cancer patients (Bradlyn *et al.* 1993). The short form (QWBS-SA) also has good psychometric properties and may be preferred as a less expensive and complex instrument to use than the interviewer-administered version when estimating the effectiveness and cost-effectiveness of treatments (Pyne *et al.* 2003). Fryback *et al.* (2007) published population norms for the USA, based on almost 4,000 people participating in the National Health Measurement study.

THE CLIFTON ASSESSMENT PROCEDURES FOR THE ELDERLY (CAPE)

The CAPE is the most extensively tested measure of dependency in widespread use in the UK, particularly in relation to psychological assessments of the elderly. The scales were developed for use with elderly people living in institutions, and tested for validity by Pattie and Gilleard (1975, 1979). A manual is available which provides details of use and also normative data for a range of patient populations (Pattie and Gilleard 1979). The CAPE consists of two schedules, designed to measure behaviour and cognitive performance, known as the Behaviour Rating Scale and the Cognitive Assessment Scale. The Cognitive Assessment Scale was originally known as the Clifton Assessment Scale, and can be completed by an elderly person in 5 to 15 minutes. The Behaviour Rating Scale is a short version of the Stockton Geriatric Rating Scale, designed for use with elderly people in hospital. The whole test can take between 5 and 30 minutes, depending on the mental and functional ability of the respondent. It is designed to be completed by a third party who knows the respondent well. Interviewer training is necessary. A shortened version of the two subscales was also developed (Pattie 1981).

Content

The Cognitive Performance Scale consists of a battery of tests which include items such as the person tracing a circular route with a pencil, avoiding obstacles; the information/orientation items include the usual memory tests of own place of residence, name of the prime minister, date, etc., and, more unusually, knowledge of the colours of the British flag.

The Behavioural Rating Scale contains 18 items. Four items relate to mobility, continence and ADL. The remaining items relate to confused behaviour. The scale asks about current-level functioning. It focuses heavily on the behavioural problems of those elderly people who are mentally infirm. The rater is instructed to rate people according to their level of current functioning, and to take into account behaviour over the past two weeks. The CAPE relates to four subscales: physical disability, apathy, communication difficulties and social disturbance. Examples of the behaviour rating scale are shown in Box 3.11.

Box 3.11 Examples from the CAPE

When bathing or dressing, he/she requires:

0   No assistance
1   Some assistance
2   Maximum assistance

With regard to walking, he/she

0   Shows no signs of weakness
1   Walks slowly without aid, or uses a stick
2   Is unable to walk, or if able to walk, needs frame, crutches or someone by his/her side

He/she is confused (unable to find way around, loses possessions, etc.)

0   Almost never confused
1   Sometimes confused
2   Almost always confused

His/her sleep pattern at night is

0   Almost never awake
1   Sometimes awake
2   Often awake

Source: Pattie, A.H. and Gilleard, C.J. (1979) *Manual of the Clifton Assessment Procedures for the Elderly*. Sevenoaks: Hodder & Stoughton. With permission of the developer. There is a charge for the forms and manual: http://www.nzcer.org.nz/pts/clifton-assessment-procedures-elderly-cape, accessed 21 September 2015.

Scoring

The 18 items are added to form a total score, or selected items are added to produce subscale scores. Each item has a range of scores from 0 (no/few problems) to 2 (frequent/constant problems). Four subscales can be created from the items relating to physical disability, apathy, communication difficulties and social disturbance. The total scale range of scores is from 0 to 36. A score of 0–3 indicates independence; 4–7 indicates low dependency; 8–12 indicates medium dependency; 13–17 indicates high dependency and 18–36 is maximum dependency. No item weights are used.

Validity

Early versions were shown to correlate with clinicians' assessments about appropriate levels of care for females but not males. The sample size was small, 38. The authors also report correlations with other scales such as the Wechsler Memory Scale, but sample sizes were too small to be conclusive. Pattie and Gilleard (1975) reported that the CAPE correlated highly with psychiatric diagnoses and was able to discriminate between patients who were discharged home and those who were not. In relation to behaviour, Pattie and Gilleard (1979) reported that the CAPE can discriminate between elderly people requiring differing degrees of help, with different levels of social adjustment following admission to a residential home, and between mentally infirm people who survive and those who die.

   Smith *et al.* (1981) reported early on that evidence of concurrent and convergent validity was limited. The evidence base on convergent and predictive validity has improved slightly. Black *et al.* (1990) compared the diagnostic ability of the CAPE, in relation to dementia, with the diagnosis made by the computer program AGECAT and a clinical diagnosis made by a psychiatrist. The sample was an elderly sample of patients from a general practice (112 were selected from 378 who had been tested three years previously when aged 70+ using a 13-item mental-function test). The authors reported that the sensitivity of the CAPE was low, probably because it identified only the more severe cases. The CAPE only detected about half the number of known cases. McPherson *et al.* (1985) reported that the shortened survey version was able to distinguish between patients with severe, moderate, mild and no dementia, and patients with physical disability. Aspray *et al.* (2006) used the CAPE, among other measures, in a cross-sectional study to assess predictors of fracture risk and treatment for osteoporosis in over 300 elderly care home residents in Newcastle upon Tyne, UK. They reported that of the measures used to assess function, only the CAPE predicted low bone mineral density in the homes for the elderly mentally infirm.

In relation to behaviour, Pattie and Gilleard (1979) reported that the CAPE discriminated between elderly people requiring differing degrees of help, with different levels of social adjustment following admission to a residential home, and between mentally infirm people who survived and those who died. In a study by Moran *et al.* (1990), 261 patients admitted consecutively to a geriatric psychiatric assessment ward, most with a diagnosis of dementia, were assessed using the CAPE. They reported that the CAPE predicted survival at 36 months.

Results of factor analyses showed that two factor structures emerged for three groups of elderly people tested, and no clear factor structure emerged for non-psychiatrically ill elderly people (Pattie and Gilleard 1979). The four subscales suggested by the authors for analysing the Behaviour Rating Scale data were not supported. Factor analyses carried out on the CAPE by Twining and Allen (1981), on the basis of 903 people in residential homes for the elderly, also failed to support the four suggested subscales.

Reliability

Pattie and Gilleard (1979) reported inter-item correlations, and all are fairly high. This suggests that items are consistent and are measuring the same dimensions of dependency. Inter-rater reliability for the four subscales was tested on psychiatric and psychogeriatric patients, and people in residential homes for the elderly; the correlations were all 0.70 or higher with the exception of the correlation for 'communication difficulties' which was low. Tests for inter-rater reliability for the total scale showed wide variations. Smith *et al.* (1981), in their study of 38 elderly mentally handicapped patients, reported an inter-rater reliability coefficient of 0.58 between two nursing sisters.

Test-retest reliability coefficients ranged from 0.56 to 0.90 at retests over two to three days with 38 hospital patients aged 65 and over, and at retests over two to three months. The six-month test-retest reliabilities, based on 39 new admissions to homes for the elderly, ranged from 0.69 to 0.84 (Pattie and Gilleard 1979).

Evidence to support the psychometric properties of the CAPE is still limited. Wilkin and Thompson (1989) drew attention to ambiguities in the wording – for example, the terms 'sometimes' and 'frequently' are not defined, and therefore likely to be interpreted differently by different raters. Mulgrave's early review (1985) reported that the CAPE's main advantages are that the scales are short and easily administered.

EXAMPLE

An example of the use of measures of functional ability is shown in Box 3.12.

Box 3.12 Example of before-after study using functional ability measures

Mikołajewska (2013) carried out a study which aimed to evaluate a rehabilitation programme for patients after they suffered an ischemic stroke. The study group consisted of 60 patients after ischemic stroke who participated in the programme of rehabilitation. No control group was included.

The study outcome was patients' ability to perform selected ADL. Selected items from the Barthel Index were used to measure this.

Patients' outcomes were assessed on admission (before the therapy) and after the last session of the therapy.

The results showed that statistically significant and positive changes in functioning post-intervention, using the selected Barthel items, supported the effectiveness of the rehabilitation programme. However, as no control group was used this finding needs further investigation.

CHAPTER 4

MEASURING BROADER HEALTH STATUS

MEASUREMENT

Broader measures of health status generally focus on individuals' subjective perceptions of their health. Subjective or perceived health may be defined as an individual's experience of mental, physical and social events as they impinge upon feelings of well-being (Hunt 1988). Many studies in medical sociology have indicated the importance of the perceptual component of illness in determining whether people feel ill or whether they seek help.

Scales of broader health status are more stable, and have better reliability and validity than single-item questions and are the preferred instruments to use. On the other hand, some single items, despite some instability, are popularly used in general, multi-topic population surveys. A popular single-item measure consists of simply asking respondents to rate their health as 'Excellent, Good, Fair or Poor'. In order to increase the question's ability to discriminate between groups, researchers often insert a 'Very good' category in between 'Excellent' and 'Good', as most respondents are influenced by social desirability bias and rate their health at the 'good' end of the scale spectrum (Ware 1984; Ware et al. 1993). Also, the tradition in social gerontology is to ask respondents to rate their health in relation to their age (see national surveys by Cartwright and Anderson 1981; Bowling and Cartwright 1982; Bowling et al. 2002). This prevents older respondents from assessing their health with reference to younger age groups as well as their own.

This single-item measure of self-perceived health status has long been reported to be significantly and independently associated with use of health services, changes in functional status, mortality and rates of recovery from episodes of ill health (National Heart and Lung Institute 1976; Singer et al. 1976; Kaplan and Camacho 1983; Goldstein et al. 1984; Idler and Kasl 1995; Greiner et al. 1999; Siegel et al. 2003). DeSalvo et al. (2006) conducted a systematic review of the association between a single item assessing general self-rated health and mortality. Their meta-analysis found a statistically significant relationship between worse general self-rated health and an increased risk of death, even after adjustment for functional status, depression and co-morbidity. This relationship persisted in studies with a long duration of follow-up, for both males and females, and irrespective of country of origin.

This measure may be contextual and vary over time with people's varying expectations. Thus, self-ratings of health are often criticized as subjective, although their subjectivity is their strength because they reflect personal evaluations of health. People experiencing psychological distress may be more likely to perceive their health status to be poor, although the association is bi-directional as poor perceived health also leads to increased psychological distress (Farmer and Ferraro 1997).

Crossley and Kennedy (2000) analysed the stability of the commonly used question on self-assessed health in a large national survey. Respondents to one of the Australian National Health Surveys were asked to rate their health in general as 'Excellent, Very good, Good, Fair or Poor'; and a sub-sample of these respondents was asked the question twice – before and after other questions about their health. They found that 29 per cent of respondents changed their self-assessed health rating at the repeat question. This also partly reflects the biasing effects of question order. But while self-assessed health status was associated, in the expected directions, with age and income, response instability was also associated with age, income and occupation. In a similar exercise, Bowling and Windsor (2008) analysed wave 1 of the English Longitudinal Survey of Ageing, comprising 11,000 respondents aged 50+ living at home. They reported that the self-assessed health status question asked after, rather than before, a module of questions about health, resulted in more optimal health assessments, although the effect size was small.

Given that subjectivity is a major criticism levelled at this type of indicator, it merits some discussion. Health indicators have largely been developed within the era of science, based on the logical positivist paradigm. This can lead to suspicion when data are presented which are based on subjective experience. This is despite the research questioning the reliability of 'objective' data. The concordance rate of clinical and pathological diagnoses has been shown in classic studies to be as low as 45.3 per cent (Heasman and Lipworth 1966); several early studies reported on the arbitrary nature of normal values in biochemistry (Grasbeck and Saris 1969; Bradwell et al. 1974), and of the problem of establishing a dividing line between sick and healthy in relation to diabetes, hypertension and glaucoma (Cochrane and Holland 1971).

There are also classic studies reporting wide discrepancies between patients and clinicians in relation to preferences for treatments (McNeil et al. 1978, 1981; Liddle et al. 1993; Schneiderman et al. 1993), and between their ratings of the patients' outcomes after specific therapies. One Swedish outpatient study also found that there was only 50 per cent agreement between doctors and patients on whether treatment had been successful (Orth-Gomer et al. 1979). Similar results have been obtained in relation to low back pain and outcome of surgery, blood pressure treatment, results of surgery for peptic ulcer, the effect of cancer treatment and other treatments (Hall et al. 1976; Orth-Gomer et al. 1979; Thomas and Lyttle 1980; Jachuck et al. 1982; Slevin et al. 1988). Research has indicated that doctors and patients use different criteria in their assessments, which may explain discrepancies between assessments (Demyttenaere et al. 2009). Discrepancies can also be found between cancer patients' assessments of their own quality of life (QoL) and assessments of them by their families, as well as clinical staff (Moinpour et al. 2000; Addington-Hall and Kalra 2001). While people's own self-ratings may be subject to optimism, social desirability and other biases (Brissette et al. 2003), so proxy ratings can carry their own biases. As Addington-Hall and Kalra (2001) stated, proxies' scores may be influenced by their own feelings about, and experiences of, caring for the patient, as well as whether patients normally talk about their feelings to their proxies.

Other measurement formats, which are commonly used in studies of health status, are symptom checklists. These also have their limitations, but are generally considered to be useful tools if used in conjunction with scaled measurement techniques. There are numerous examples of checklists of symptoms presented to respondents in surveys. Respondents are typically asked to indicate which, if any, they currently suffer from. General symptom checklists can be found in George and Bearon (1980), in Cartwright's classic national surveys (Dunnell and Cartwright 1972; Cartwright and Anderson 1981; Bowling and Cartwright 1982) and in the RAND Health Insurance Study Questionnaires (Stewart et al. 1978). Disease-specific QoL questionnaires usually contain a list of symptoms relevant to the condition under study (see Bowling 2001). However, questions that ask about symptoms tend to produce a high proportion of affirmative responses, given the presence of a large amount of minor morbidity in a population. Items focusing on trivial problems are unlikely to have much discriminatory power in terms of monitoring change between groups over time. They may include not only response errors, but diagnostic errors (many people do not present their symptoms to doctors for investigation, and patients are not always fully investigated by their doctors) (Bond *et al.* 2003). Reporting of morbidity, and consultation patterns, depend on symptom tolerance levels, pain thresholds, attitude towards illness and self-care, the expectations and demands of others (family, employer, friends), knowledge and understanding of symptoms experienced and other social and cultural factors.

Given that a subjective measure of health status is required, and single-item measures can be limited, the issue becomes that of which measure to choose. The researcher also has to decide whether a general and/or specific measure is required, depending on the nature of the study. There is little point in including a health measure if it is unlikely to detect the effects of the treatment or symptoms specific to the condition. Some specific disease-related scales do exist, although the Nottingham Health Profile and the Short Form-36 have also been used as more general measures of health status and are apparently successful at distinguishing between patient types.

The case for using general, rather than specific, indicators of health status in population surveys was clearly argued by Kaplan (1988). For example, detailed information about specific disease categories may appear overwhelming to many respondents not suffering from them. Also, the use of disease-specific measures precludes the possibility of comparing the outcomes of services that are directed at different groups suffering from different diseases. Policy analysis requires a general measure of health status. Broader measures of physical, social and psychological functioning exist, but their use in the UK has been limited. If necessary, as in the case of a study of a specific disease group, global measures can be supplemented with disease-effect questions.

The following sections describe the most well-known and best-tested measures of broader health status that are currently available.

THE SICKNESS IMPACT PROFILE (SIP)

One of the best instruments developed in the USA has been the SIP (Deyo *et al.* 1982, 1983; Bergner 1988, 1993). The SIP was developed as a measure of perceived health status, for use as an outcome measure for health care evaluation across a wide range of health problems and diseases, across demographic and cultural groups. Sickness is measured in relation to its impact on behaviour. The profile emphasizes sickness-related dysfunction rather than disease. It was designed to be sensitive to differences in health status in terms of minor morbidity (Bergner *et al.* 1976a, 1976b, 1981; Gilson *et al.* 1979).

The SIP concentrates on assessing the impact of sickness on daily activities and behaviour, rather than feelings and clinical reports. The justification was that feelings are difficult to measure and subjective and thus difficult to validate, and clinical reports can be provided only where someone has sought medical care. The authors felt that behavioural reports were less subject to bias than feelings, although reported behaviour can be influenced by perceptual bias and behaviour can be influenced by feelings. The authors acknowledged that the SIP does not measure positive functioning. The SIP was developed on the basis of a literature review and after extracting statements from health professionals, healthy and ill lay people, which described 'sickness related behaviour dysfunction' (Bergner et al. 1981).

The populations and patient groups involved in its development varied widely and included inpatients, outpatients, and home-care patients with chronic diseases, patients in intensive care units, patients undergoing hip replacements and arthritis patients. It may be self- or interviewer-administered. It takes 20–30 minutes to complete. Deyo et al. (1983) recognized the problem of its length and suggested that attempts to shorten it might augment patient acceptability. A sub-sample of the participants in their study were asked about their opinions of the SIP and, while most said it was acceptable, the few complaints elicited concerned its length and the fact that it was not disease specific. The authors suggest that the subscales could be used independently if desired (e.g. the physical function subscale consists of only 45 of the 136 items). A study asking interviewers to make ratings of the ease of application of the SIP by Read et al. (1987) found that the length of the SIP was reported to be tedious, largely because of the repetition it contained. They also reported that the SIP involved a major commitment to interviewer training time (at least a week). More optimistic findings were reported by Hall et al. (1987). The SIP was used in a general study of patient outcome, based in a general practice setting in Sydney, Australia, by Hall et al. (1987). The SIP was used along with the General Health Questionnaire and the RAND Health Insurance Battery; 160 questionnaires were completed by patients, and only 3 per cent did not complete all the questions across the three scales.

There have been many applications of the SIP to a wide range of patient groups, mainly in the USA, but also in the UK and other parts of the world. One application in the UK was by Fletcher et al. (1988) in a randomized controlled trial (RCT) of outcome of drug treatment of angina patients. The SIP has been widely used in the US heart-transplantation evaluations. Many applications of the SIP have been described by Wenger et al. (1984). The advantage that this wide application provides is that scores for many population groups are available for comparison.

The SIP incorporates 136 questions, not only on functioning, but also on feelings of emotional well-being and social functioning. The items refer to illness-related dysfunction in 12 areas: work, recreation, emotion, affect, home life, sleep, rest, eating, ambulation, mobility, communication and social interaction. A typical set of questions from the SIP requests respondents to tick statements, which apply to them on a given day and are related to their state of health – see examples of items in Box 4.1.

Box 4.1 Examples from the SIP

I spend much of the day lying down in order to rest.
I sit during much of the day.
I am sleeping or dozing most of the time – day and night.
I stand up only with someone's help.
I kneel, stoop, or bend down only by holding on to something.

I am in a restricted position all the time.
I do work around the house only for short periods of time or rest often.
I am doing less of the regular daily work around the house that I would usually do.
I am not doing any of the house cleaning that I would usually do.
I am going out less to visit people.
I am not going out to visit people at all.
I am doing fewer social activities with groups of people.

Content

Only those questions to which the respondents answer 'yes' are recorded; thus there is no way of knowing in the analysis whether the columns left blank represent 'no' replies or whether the respondent/interviewer omitted them deliberately or in error.

Scoring

The responses to the 136 items can be scored by component, by physical or psychosocial dimension or as a single score with a range of 0–100. The lower the score the better the respondent's health status. The overall score for the SIP is calculated by adding the scale values for each item checked across all categories and dividing by the maximum possible dysfunction score for the SIP. This figure is then multiplied by 100 to obtain the SIP overall score. The two sub-scores (physical and psychosocial) are calculated using a similar formula, but limiting the calculations to the relevant items.

Item weights indicate the relative severity of limitation implied by each statement. The weights were derived from equal-appearing interval-scaling procedures involving more than 100 judges. The judges rated each item on an equal-interval 11-point scale from 'minimally dysfunctional' to 'severely dysfunctional'. The scaling technique has been justified and described by Carter et al. (1976). However, Jenkinson et al. (1991) argued that Thurstone's scaling method was unsuccessful as the distributions of the SIP were similar whether the scale items were weighted or simply added.

The study based in Sydney by Hall et al. (1987) reported that results were skewed towards the healthy end of the SIP scale. Eighteen per cent of patients scored 0 on all components. There were no scores above 25 (range of possible scores 0–100). This pattern was repeated within components. Although the many studies using the SIP have provided population norms for comparison, it is unclear what each score represents. Many other scales also suffer this problem. It is known that a normal population may score only 2 or 3 on the SIP, increasing to the mid-30s for terminally-ill cancer and stroke patients, but the precise definition of scale points has not so far been tackled.

Validity

The early validation studies of the SIP tested it against self-assessments of health status, clinicians' assessments of health status and functional assessment instruments; 278 people were assessed. SIP scores discriminated between four subgroups divided according to severity of sickness, and correlations between measures were better for patients' self-assessments than physicians' assessments (0.69 with a self-assessment of limitation; 0.63 with a self-assessment of sickness; 0.50 with a clinician's assessment of limitation; and 0.40 with a clinician's assessment of sickness). The combined SIP score was tested against the Katz ADL scale with a correlation of 0.64; and the correlation between the SIP and the National Health Interview Survey Instrument was 0.55 (Bergner *et al.* 1981).

Convergent and discriminant validity was evaluated using the multi-trait-multi-method technique. Clinical validity was assessed by comparing clinical judgements with SIP scores; all achieved good results. These have been described in some detail by Bergner *et al.* (1981). More recent evidence pointing to its strong validity properties has been provided by Read *et al.* (1987). However, the correlations between the SIP score and clinical status have tended to range between 0.40 and 0.60, probably due to the broad nature of the SIP; this may not be a high enough correlation for the successful use of the scale in studies of clinical outcome of health care interventions (Anderson *et al.* 1993).

The Australian study by Hall *et al.* (1987) reported that, with the use of a correlation threshold of −0.30, the SIP correlated with instruments from RAND. The RAND mental-health index correlated with the SIP items relating to social interaction, emotional behaviour and alertness; and ambulation from the SIP correlated with the RAND physical abilities scale. Home management and social interaction items from the SIP correlated with the role-functioning items on the RAND battery. However, the correlations ranged from 0.32 to 0.54. Other research has reported moderate correlations (0.40–0.60) between the SIP and scales of anxiety and depression, reflecting the behavioural focus of the SIP (Linzer *et al.* 1991).

However, the SIP has reportedly been used successfully in clinical trials (Bergner *et al.* 1976a, 1976b, 1981) and is valuable for assessing the impact of illness on the chronically ill. It has been used in an RCT of early exercise and counselling for patients with myocardial infarction. This study reported that the SIP showed that the group undergoing exercise plus counselling reported better functioning (Ott *et al.* 1983). It has also been used to evaluate treatment for patients with end-stage renal disease, with the result that transplantation patients had better SIP scores (Hart and Evans 1987). In a cross-sectional longitudinal study of 99 women with rheumatoid arthritis, the SIP was reported to be sensitive to one-year pre- and post-treatment changes, showing both improvement and deterioration (Sullivan *et al.* 1990). Grady *et al.* (2003) reported that it was able to discriminate between different groups of heart patients at three months after surgery.

More negative results relating to sensitivity were reported by Hall *et al.* (1987) who tested the SIP against the RAND Health Insurance Study batteries. The RAND and the SIP were reported to be measuring different aspects of health. The range of scores for the RAND measures was less skewed than for the SIP. The problem with an instrument, which registers high scores, is that it may be unable to measure improvements in health. Thus the RAND measures have better discriminative abilities than the SIP. A follow-up study of 185 stroke patients by Schuling *et al.* (1993) reported that the SIP was 'time consuming and tiring' with these patients, and it was insensitive to improvement in condition at eight weeks, in contrast to the cruder Barthel Index which did detect improvement. Katz *et al.* (1992) also found that the SIP was less sensitive to clinical change among patients undergoing hip replacement than shorter measures, including the SF-36 and a short version of the Arthritis Impact Measurement Scales. A review of studies using the SIP by de Bruin *et al.* (1992) reported research demonstrating that the SIP was insensitive to small changes and improvements. A European study by Stummer *et al.* (2015) of 532 consecutive stroke patients from four rehabilitation centres, with follow-up at six months, reported that all three dimensions of the SIP at six months were predicted by the Barthel Index score on admission.

In relation to factor structure of the full SIP, de Bruin *et al.*'s (1992) review also questions the SIP's construct validity as the results of factor analyses have been inconsistent.

Reliability

Work began on the SIP in 1972, and tests for reliability and validity continued to be conducted by its authors for over a decade. Patients studied included those with hypothyroidism, rheumatoid arthritis and hip replacements. The details of the reliability tests conducted on the SIP are reported by Bergner *et al.* (1981). Earlier reliability tests on SIPs of differing lengths before the development of the 136 version are reported by Pollard *et al.* (1976, 1978).

Test-retest reliability was high (0.88–0.92). Internal consistency was also high (0.81–0.97). The interviewer-administered versions scored better in each case than mailed or self-completed versions. Deyo *et al.* (1983) applied the SIP to 79 patients with arthritis and found that test-retest reliability for 23 patients tested was 0.91. It was found to have better reliability than the traditional functional scales of the American Rheumatism Association and patients' self-ratings of function. Test-retest reliability was better for the overall score than for each of the dimensions. Results of studies of the reliability of the SIP throughout Europe and the USA indicate similarly high levels of internal consistency (0.91–0.95), test-retest correlations (0.75–0.85) and also inter-rater reliability (0.87–0.92) (de Bruin *et al.* 1992). Nanda *et al.*'s (2003) study of people with disability found retest correlations were greater than 0.75 for all dimensions except physical disability (0.61).

68-item version of the SIP

Given that the length of the SIP (136 items) has been one barrier to its use, there have been attempts to shorten it. De Bruin *et al.* (1993) have constructed a 68-item version using multivariate techniques, reporting that its psychometric properties were similar to the longer 136-item version. In Post *et al.*'s research (1996, 2001) with rehabilitation patients, the SIP-68 had evidence of good internal consistency (Cronbach's alpha 0.88 to 0.92); it correlated well with the Barthel Index (0.74) and moderately with a life satisfaction measure (0.52). Nanda *et al.* (2003) assessed the psychometric properties of the short, 68-item version of the SIP in comparison with the full version (136 items), among a sample of people with disabilities. They reported that the correlation between the SIP and SIP-68 was 0.94; and they were moderate between the SIP-68 and comparable subscales of the SF-36. A factor analysis of the SIP-68 reproduced a factor structure that included 65 of the items. It still needs more evidence of reliability and responsiveness.

Adaptations

Although patient acceptance of the SIP was judged by the US authors to be good, it has been rejected for use in evaluations of some treatment programme evaluations in the UK on the grounds of its length, and the more concise Nottingham Health Profile selected in preference (Buxton 1983; O'Brien 1988).

A modified version of the SIP was developed at St Thomas's Hospital, London, for a community disability survey. The modified version is called the Functional Limitations Profile (FLP) (Patrick 1982; Charlton *et al.* 1983). Linguistic changes were made and scale weights were recalculated, although these agreed closely with the original weights of the US version. The translation has been criticized by Hunt *et al.* (1986) on the grounds that language changes alone do not satisfy the requirements for cross-cultural adaptations. The changes made are fairly minimal and the FLP is still 136 items long, is designed to be interviewer-administered and contains the same range of scores from 0 (low) to 100 (high), although the weighting is different. The authors later reported that FLP and SIP items grouped satisfactorily into five global measures: physical, psychosocial, eating, communication and work. They found the items related to age and number of medical conditions but were poor predictors of service use (Charlton *et al.* 1983). Another UK application of the FLP was a study of 92 patients with chronic obstructive pulmonary disease by Williams and Bury (1989) who reported poor to good correlations between the FLP physical sub-section and clinical data of 0.38–0.90. Fitzpatrick *et al.* (1988) also used the FLP in their study of 105 patients with rheumatoid arthritis assessed over a 15-month period. They used both the FLP and the HAQ, but reported only modest levels of sensitivity and specificity in relation to data on clinical change for each. Although the authors acknowledged that the FLP provided more information and was more precise than the short HAQ, they cautioned that this has to be weighed against the simpler measurement assumptions and shorter time required to administer the HAQ. Fitzpatrick *et al.* (1988) concluded that the SIP/FLP is less sensitive to improvement than to deterioration. McColl *et al.* (1995) reported that the FLP had a high level of item of non-response and also had ceiling effects. The conclusion relating to the FLP is that it requires far more testing for reliability and validity before it can be considered the UK alternative to the SIP.

Some investigators have adapted the SIP to specific clinical conditions, and used a selection of the items. Ada *et al.* (2003) used 30 items from the SIP in their study of outcome of rehabilitation programmes for stroke, but reported that they did not detect documented improvements in patients' walking speed and capacity. Vetter *et al.* (1989) used their own adaptation of the SIP along with the Barthel Index to assess rehabilitation outcomes among a pilot sample of 59 elderly people receiving either home or day hospital care in Wales. The authors substantially changed the style of the SIP. They reported that respondents found the 'I' format (e.g. 'I dress myself, but do so very slowly') confusing. They became confused about who the 'I' was referring to. The statements were, therefore, changed to actual questions (e.g. 'Do you dress yourself, but do so very slowly?'). A further problem they found with the SIP was that some questions were not applicable to all patients. Thus the question 'Are you unable to walk up and down hills?' in the original profile could be answered only 'yes' or 'no'. The researchers thus added a 'not applicable' category to avoid confusion, for example, for those who were bed-/chair-fast. The physical dimension scale of the SIP was found to have acceptable validity and was judged as a suitable measure of outcome (other dimensions are yet to be tested), although the correlations were unreported. The SIP was also found to be a stable measure when repeated eight weeks later on the patients (they were not expected to change in relation to physical state).

The advantages of the SIP and its adaptations are that it can be self-administered or interview based, it can be used with chronically or acutely ill patients, it has been adapted for use in the UK as the FLP, and it is well tested for reliability and validity. McDowell and Newell (1996), in their review of health status measures, noted the thoroughness and care with which the SIP was developed, and its frequent use as a gold standard against which scales are evaluated. Its limitations are its length and the fact that it can be used only with people who are regarded or who regard themselves as ill; also, its factor structure and responsiveness to change have not been adequately demonstrated. International versions of the SIP have been reviewed by Anderson *et al.* (1993).

THE NOTTINGHAM HEALTH PROFILE (NHP)

The conceptual basis of the NHP was that it should reflect lay rather than professional definitions of health. It was developed after interviews with a large number of lay people about the effects of illness on behaviour. Hunt *et al.* (1986) commented that their pilot interviewing to develop the NHP demonstrated that lay people had a limited range of language for describing good health and well-being, which would have made the creation of a comprehensive health index difficult. The NHP is not an index of disease, illness or disability but relates rather to how people feel when they are experiencing various states of ill health. As a survey tool it is useful in assessing whether people have a (severe) health problem, although diagnostic data would be required to point to the kind of health problem. The measure was not intended by its developers to measure health-related QoL, nor to detect health conditions or states of mild symptom severity (Hunt 1984). It is too short to assess the impact of a condition on QoL. For this, combinations of measures are required: a functional-disability scale, symptom and pain indices, a measure of psychological disturbance, quantitative and more qualitative methods of the impact on social functioning (e.g. work, interpersonal relationships and social support, domestic life, etc.). The NHP can provide only a shallow profile of effects on these aspects.

Pilot work with the NHP in the UK led to the identification of relevant concepts. Statements were drawn which exemplified those concepts and, after further piloting, statements were finally categorized into six areas: physical mobility, pain, sleep, energy, emotional reactions and social isolation. The NHP is designed for self-completion, is concise and easily administered and was the first measure of perceived health which was extensively tested and developed for use in Europe. Hunt *et al.* (1986) reported that, when the NHP is based on a postal survey, people are unlikely to return it if they have a high number of zero scores (no problems). People felt they had nothing to contribute to the study. Pilot work has been undertaken with positive items as dummies: 'I sleep soundly at night'; 'I am usually free of any pain'.

The NHP is short and simple, and it can be used with groups of patients or a general population. Although it is suitable for people who are not necessarily unhealthy or ill, like many others, it focuses on negative rather than positive experiences. Population norms exist for the instrument, as do scores on individual patient groups (Hunt *et al.* 1984b).

Content

The NHP measures perceived or subjective health status by asking for yes/no responses to 38 simple statements of six dimensions (as noted above: mobility, pain, energy, sleep, emotional reactions and social isolation). Each dimension has a range of possible scores of 0–100.

The original NHP included a Part I (which is the current NHP) and a Part II asking about any effects of health on seven areas of daily life: work, looking after the home, social life, home life, sex life, interests, hobbies and holidays, with scored yes (1)/no (0) responses. The authors carried out later developmental work on Part II and recommended that it should not be used.

Examples of the remaining NHP items, which ask about the applicability of statements to the respondent at the present time, include the items in Box 4.2.

Box 4.2. Examples from the NHP

I'm tired all the time.
I have pain at night.
Things are getting me down.
I have unbearable pain.
I take tablets to help me sleep.

© NHP is owned and licensed by Galen Research. Contact information: http://www.galen-research.com/measures-database, accessed 24 August 2015.

The authors of the NHP published a book describing the development of the scale, and early studies of its reliability and validity, NHP items and a user guide (Hunt *et al.* 1986).

Scoring

The NHP is scored with scores ranging from 0 (no problems) to 100 (where all problems in a section are affirmed). The weighted scores are summed for each NHP domain, but an overall score is not obtainable. It has been extensively tested for reliability and validity, and results were reported by the authors to be good. The weights for the NHP were derived using Thurstone's method of paired comparisons. Judgements were obtained from several hundred people and converted into weights using the appropriate formula (McKenna *et al.* 1981). However, Jenkinson *et al.* (1991) provided evidence that the use of Thurstone's scaling method was unsuccessful as the distributions of the NHP were similar whether the scale items were weighted or simply added. They also detected inconsistencies in the scoring system with the score for a person with walking difficulties erroneously exceeding the scores for those who were totally unable to walk.

The NHP scores are not 'true' numbers but are obtained from a scaling technique; thus the appropriate statistical tests for testing hypotheses are non-parametric. Its highly skewed distribution of scores (see column 2 below) means that careful consideration needs to be given to the application of statistical tests as many assume that the results are normally distributed, although statistical transformations can be applied to skewed data, thus permitting the application of parametric statistics.

The NHP requires respondents to indicate 'yes' or 'no' according to whether the statement applies to them 'in general at the present time'. Relative weights are applied to these. All statements relate to limitations on activity or aspects of distress. Dimension scores of 100 indicate the presence of all limitations listed, and a zero score the absence of limitations, but these two extremes do not reflect the extremes of death or perfect health.

There can be problems with the sensitivity of the NHP as a survey instrument because of the zero modal response, which means that the NHP does not discriminate for a substantial proportion of the adult population. The problem with using the NHP within a population survey is that the sample would include a large number of relatively fit members who would gain low NHP scores. As it is a severe measure, minor illnesses are not detected by the instrument, and therefore minor improvements over time are unlikely to be detected. This problem was acknowledged by its authors: 'The NHP is clearly tapping only the extreme end of perceived health problems. Such a distribution was built into the NHP during its development. At an early stage it was decided that it would be undesirable to include health problems which would be affirmed by a large proportion of the population' (Hunt *et al.* 1986).

Hunt (1988) reported on the proportion of zero scorers from combined data from several community studies using the NHP:

Section	*Proportion of zero scores*
Pain	83
Social isolation	82
Physical mobility	78
Energy	75
Emotional reactions	61
Sleep	56

As she admits, this instrument only taps the more extreme end of a distribution.

Kind and Carr-Hill (1987) used the NHP with 1,598 people in a follow-up study of the Rowntree Poverty Survey in York. The sample was weighted towards older and retired adults. Negative responses to all categories of the NHP exceeded 60 per cent, and for social isolation the figure rose to 89 per cent, in evidence of its negative skew. Three items in particular only received 2 per cent endorsement: 'I find it hard to dress myself', 'I'm unable to walk at all', and 'I feel that life is not worth living'. Also, three of the most often cited items were drawn from the sleep category and three of the least frequently cited items were from the physical mobility category. The authors argued that the skewness of the distribution of responses does not appear to be based on any logic. For example, nearly half of those who made just one positive response selected 'I'm waking up early in the morning', 17.5 per cent also chose 'I lose my temper easily' but no other item was chosen by more than 5 per cent of this group. In contrast, among those who scored heavily (11 or more positive responses), six items were more popular than 'I lose my temper easily'. They reported no simple relationship between the overall score and the probability of responding to any one item and that there appeared to be considerable redundancy among items. The scale and its scoring system have frequently been criticized for inconsistencies and anomalies (Anderson *et al.* 1993).

Validity

The NHP was well tested for face, content and criterion validity by its developers, and has generally been reported to be a satisfactory measure of subjective health status in physical, social and emotional spheres. The face and content validity of the subjective items were established by the developers on the basis of the method for devising the scale: the items were drawn from lay experiences and respondents were able to relate to them and understand the relevance of the items (Hunt *et al.* 1986).

Testing for discriminative ability took place with four groups of people aged 65+; 40 people participating in a research exercise programme; 19 patients from a general practitioner's (GP's) list who had no known disability or illness and who had not contacted a doctor within the prior two months; 49 people with a variety of health and social problems attending a local authority-run luncheon club; 54 chronically ill patients on GPs' lists; and 352 randomly selected patients from GPs' lists. Results showed that the NHP was able to discriminate between groups of 'well' and 'ill' people, and in terms of physiological fitness; high and low GP consulters; social classes, age groups and sexes and that the content of the questions was understood by, and acceptable to, elderly people. Perceived health status was also associated with objective health status (Hunt *et al.* 1980, 1986). Jenkinson *et al.* (1988) assessed the sensitivity of the NHP with 39 rheumatoid arthritis sufferers and 43 migraine sufferers. The NHP was able to distinguish between the two patient groups: the arthritis patients scored worse in relation to effects on energy levels and mobility. Discriminant analysis showed that the NHP was able to discriminate between 79 per cent of arthritis and 93 per cent of migraine patients. Other investigators have also reported good results with the NHP with coronary patients (Permanyer-Miralda *et al.* 1991), and have supported the ability of the NHP to discriminate between a normal population and those with a range of serious medical conditions (van Agt *et al.* 1993).

The NHP was shown to be sensitive to change. One unpublished study cited by Hunt *et al.* (1986) was based on a sample of 80 pregnant women. The NHP was administered to the women at three stages during their pregnancy – 18, 27 and 37 weeks. The NHP was sensitive to changes during pregnancy. It was also administered to 141 patients attending a fracture clinic and an equal number of control subjects. Scores were obtained soon after the fracture occurred and eight weeks later. Scores were sensitive to changes in perceived health, concomitant with the healing of the fracture (McKenna *et al.* 1984). O'Brien *et al.* (1988) used the instrument to measure QoL before and after combined lung and heart transplantation in the UK. It was again sensitive to changes and correlated well with clinical measures such as exercise capacity (correlation coefficient for the latter not given). The results indicated significant reductions in NHP scores for patients at 3 months after surgery; no further differences were recorded at 6 and 12 months post-operatively. In a study of 196 heart transplant patients, the NHP was reported to be sensitive to deterioration in patients' condition prior to transplant and to post-transplant improvement. It was able to predict outcome in relation to length of hospital stay, return to work and leisure activity at three months after transplantation (Buxton *et al.* 1985; Caine *et al.* 1990). Caine *et al.* (1991) also used the NHP to study the QoL of 100 males aged under 60 before and after coronary artery bypass grafting. The NHP was sensitive to improvements in health following the procedure (at three months and one year later). The instrument was reported to be sensitive to improvements in patients' condition following transplantation and coronary artery bypass surgery (Buxton *et al.* 1985; Wallwork and Caine 1985). However, its performance in relation to respiratory disease, and clinical measures of respiratory function, has been variable (Alonso *et al.* 1992). While the scale appears sensitive to changes following dramatic treatment interventions, its performance with less dramatic, and more minor, treatments is less certain (Hunt *et al.* 1984a; Brazier *et al.* 1992). Jenkinson *et al.* (1988) used both the NHP and Goldberg's General Health Questionnaire (GHQ) on a population of 39 rheumatoid arthritis and 43 migraine patients and reported a moderate correlation of 0.49 between the GHQ and the emotional-reactions scale of the NHP for both samples. The implication is that the NHP was providing no more than a moderately accurate measure in this domain.

Tabali *et al.* (2012) used the NHP in a prospective multicentre observational study in 11 nursing homes in Germany, in which 286 newly admitted residents were included. Questionnaires were completed during interviews with residents. The convergent validity of the NHP was supported by significant associations with cognitive function in the expected direction. They concluded that the NHP could be administered in nursing home settings to residents with normal cognitive function and moderate cognitive impairment.

There has been some criticism that each section of the NHP does not represent just one dimension (Kind and Carr-Hill 1987; Kind undated). In particular, fairly high correlations between the pain and physical mobility categories were reported. While covariation might be expected for items within categories, covariation between items in different categories raises difficulties in interpretation of a cross-category profile.

Reliability

Modest inter-correlations (0.32–0.50) between the NHP dimensions of pain, energy and sleep were reported by over 1,000 patients with zoster (reactivation of the varicella zoster virus), as reported by Mauskopf *et al.* (1994) (the other dimensions of the NHP were weaker). The developers reported on two studies which tested the reliability of the NHP, using the test-retest technique. These were based on 58 patients with osteoarthritis and 93 with peripheral vascular disease. The questionnaires were repeated with these two groups at four and eight weeks after the first administration respectively. Both demonstrated a fairly high level of reliability with correlations of between 0.71 and 0.88, with the exception of the items on home life (0.64), social life (0.59), interests and hobbies (0.44) for patients with osteoarthritis; and social life (0.61), looking after the home (0.64) and work (0.55) for patients with vascular disease (Hunt *et al.* 1981, 1986). Kutlay *et al.* (2003) tested the reliability of the NHP with haemodialysis patients. They reported that test-retest Pearson's correlation coefficients (at two weeks apart) were 0.61 or greater. Cronbach's alpha coefficients for the dimensions of the NHP ranged between 0.61 and 0.79 (the energy, sleep and social isolation dimensions were well below 0.70). The NHP has been reported to be less stable in relation to rheumatology patients (Fitzpatrick *et al.* 1992). In the Tabali *et al.* (2012) study using the NHP with residents in nursing homes, Cronbach's alpha met the 0.70 threshold in four domains, but not in two domains (although higher than 0.60 in both). The intra-class correlation in all domains was >0.70. They reported an administration rate ranging from 76 per cent for normal residents to 6 per cent for residents with a severe cognitive impairment. Frequently missing items were for the pain domain. A study of 145 patients with dementia and their families and formal caregivers in France (as proxy respondents) reported that 94 per cent of the NHP items were correctly filled in, although an interviewer had to be present due to problems with comprehension or attention. The test-retest reliability (with 32–39 respondents) was good (intra-class correlation coefficients: energy 0.83; pain 0.78; sleep 0.77; physical mobility >0.73) except for emotional reactions (0.62) and social isolation (0.45) (Bureau-Chalot *et al.* 2002). The internal consistency coefficients (Cronbach's alpha) met the threshold for acceptability (0.70) for all domains (alphas between 0.74 and 0.85) except social isolation (0.54) and energy (0.63).

Part II of the NHP did not obtain as good results as Part I, which explains its earlier withdrawal. For example, Hunt *et al.* (1981) reported that the test-retest reliability coefficients on the osteoarthritis patients ranged between 0.77 and 0.85 for Part I in comparison with a wider range for Part II at 0.44 to 0.86. The authors note that any changes in perceived health between the two administrations will consequently reduce the correlations (Hunt *et al.* 1981). The NHP does not meet the requirements for carrying out split-half reliability as it is too short and the items are not homogeneous. The authors also argue that it is not possible to test it against an acceptable gold standard as no suitable measure exists.

A study of its adaptation into French by Bucquet *et al.* (1990) confirmed the immediate intelligibility of the French version, although it was not without problems. The authors used the same methods of calculating item weights as McKenna *et al.* (1981) for the original version, based on Thurstone's paired comparisons; their study was based on a quota sample of 625 people (judges). However, Bucquet *et al.* (1990) did report that the respondents had difficulties making these ratings, especially in relation to the pain, mobility, energy and sleep sections. They did not all grasp the concept of a 'general view' easily when comparing the health statements. International versions of the scale have been reviewed by Anderson *et al.* (1993).

In sum, the advantages of the NHP are that it is short, simple and inexpensive to administer, it can be self-administered or interview-based, and it has been well tested for validity. However, it provides only a limited measure of function, and some disabilities are not assessed at all (e.g. sensory defects, incontinence, eating problems). It also lacks an adequate index of mental distress and requires supplementation if used as a broader measure of health-related QoL. The measure was not intended by its developers to measure health-related QoL, nor to detect health conditions or states of mild symptom severity (Hunt 1984). It is too short to test for split-half reliability, and it is a severe measure with a highly skewed distribution – it may not measure minor improvements in health. The result of the focus on severe conditions is that some people who are in distress may not show scores on the profile. Similarly, normally healthy persons or those with few ailments may affirm only a small number of statements on some sections. This makes it difficult to compare their scores over time. People who score zero cannot be shown to improve over time. It is a negative measure of health.

It is still often used in clinical studies (e.g. Aydemir *et al.* 2006), although its use has declined as the use of the SF-36 has become more widespread. It was used successfully as an outcome measure with patients undergoing heart surgery (O'Brien 1988; O'Brien *et al.* 1988), correlates well with clinical judgements of morbidity and prognosis and is simple to administer and analyse. The NHP has been a popular measure of health status and outcome in Europe, and has been adapted for use in other languages (e.g. Bucquet *et al.* 1990; Lovas *et al.* 2003; Uutela *et al.* 2003).

The measure is strictly copyrighted with charges for its use (with some exceptions, e.g. student use). See http://www.galen-research.com/measures-database, accessed 24 August 2015.

THE McMASTER HEALTH INDEX QUESTIONNAIRE (MHIQ)

The MHIQ was developed in Ontario, Canada, as a measure of physical, social and emotional functioning, underpinned by the WHO (1947, 1958) definition of health. The measure was intended to provide independent measurements of these separate areas, given the authors' recognition that two individuals with the same level of physical disability may differ widely in their social and emotional functioning (Chambers *et al.* 1976; Chambers 1998). The aim was to produce a health status questionnaire suitable for administration to general populations that could be used to predict a health professional's clinical assessment of a person's health. It was developed on the basis of a literature review of health status measurement, brainstorming sessions and consultation of experts.

The Social Function Index section was developed after consideration of existing scales, including the Spitzer Mental Status Schedule, the Cornell Medical Index and the Katz Adjustment Scale (Brodman *et al.* 1949; Herron *et al.* 1964; Spitzer *et al.* 1964), and a range of survey instruments. Review of sociological studies of leisure and social participation produced an additional list of social function questions. The selection criteria for item inclusion were positive as well as negative discriminative ability (i.e. good as well as poor functioning was intended to be identified); general applicability and acceptability; low cost and quick administration; and quantifiable responses.

The Health Index section of the questionnaire included additional items on physical function and items relating to symptoms (respiratory symptoms) and behaviour (cigarette use). Clinical assessments of social function from 'very poor' to 'very good' were included. The original version contained 172 items. The best 59 items were identified after assessing responsiveness to change, prediction of physicians' assessments and multivariate analyses, using physicians' assessments as the criterion variable. These items were tested initially on 70 patients in an acute medical ward and repeated after their discharge. The draft questionnaire was reported to be quick and simple to administer, acceptable to respondents and sensitive to changes in health status (values unreported). Clinical assessments were repeated by an independent physician on 54 patients. Consistency ratings resulted in a Goodman-Kruskal Index of Agreement value of 0.90.

Further testing with over 200 patients registered with a family physician reported high consistency between social functioning items (dichotomizing responses into good and poor). The sensitivity of the instrument was assessed to be good. Self-completion of the final version of the MHIQ takes 20 minutes. The MHIQ has been used on a number of different patient populations, including psychiatry outpatients, diabetic patients, respiratory disease patients, patients with myocardial infarction and patients with rheumatoid arthritis (see review by Chambers 1984).

Content

While the early version of the scale contained 150 items, it was later abbreviated to 59 items. It contains 24 physical function items (physical activity, mobility, self-care, communication (sight, hearing), global physical function); 25 social function items (general well-being, work/social role performance/material welfare, family support/participation, friends' support/participation and global social function); and 25 (overlapping with social function items) emotional function items (self-esteem, feelings toward personal relationships, thoughts about the future, critical life events and global emotional function). The overlapping items are thus counted twice in the scoring, and carry twice the weight of other items. Validation of this method is required.

All the physical function items are designed to evaluate the patient's functional level on the day the MHIQ is administered. The social function items are explicitly concerned with a specific time period (usually the present). The agree–disagree emotional function items are phrased in the present tense. Other emotional function items refer to the recent past as specifically defined within the question (e.g. within the last year). The emphasis is on ability, rather than performance ('Can you . . .?' rather than 'Do you . . .?'). The aim was to elicit information on activities that could be observed at the time the MHIQ was completed. Examples of questions are shown in Box 4.3.

Box 4.3 Examples from the MHIQ

Physical

Today, are you physically able to take part in any sports (hockey, swimming, bowling, golf, and so forth) or exercise regularly?
1   No
2   Yes

Do you have any physical difficulty at all driving a car by yourself?
1   No
2   Yes

Is this because of a physical difficulty?
1   No
2   Yes

Emotional health

(strongly agree 1———strongly disagree 5)

I sometimes feel that my life is not very useful.

People feel affectionate towards me.

Social health

(good 1———poor 5)

How would you say your social functioning is today? (By this we mean your ability to work, to have friends, and to get along with your family.)

How much time, in a one-week period do you usually spend watching television? (none———more than two hours a day).

Reproduced from original provided by the author.

Scoring

A score of 1 is given to 'good function' responses for each item, and 0 is assigned to 'poor functioning' responses. The scores are summed, although alternative weighting schemes have been developed (Chambers *et al.* 1982).

Validity

The authors reported, without publishing the values, that the MHIQ correlated well with other scales: the physical function item correlated well with rheumatologists' and occupational therapists' assessments based on the Lee Index of Functional Capacity; the MHIQ index of emotional, physical and social function correlated well with Bradburn's measures of psychological well-being. The physical function index also correlated well with analogue pain scales and with clinical and biological results (Chambers *et al.* 1982).

Assessments with a group of 96 physiotherapy patients showed a change in MHIQ scores between first visit and discharge, indicating sensitivity to change (Chambers *et al.* 1982) (numbers and values unreported). A subset of the items has been successfully used to predict patient outcome in an RCT trial of patients treated by nurse practitioners and doctors (Sackett *et al.* 1974). Self-completion of the MHIQ has been reported to be superior in terms of sensitivity to change than the other methods (Chambers *et al.* 1987). Ninety-six patients in a physiotherapy clinic were administered the MHIQ at four points in time. Patients were randomly assigned to different modes of administration: interviewer administered, self-completion or telephone interview. Self-completion was superior in terms of sensitivity to change than the other methods (Chambers 1984). However, the measure has been reported to be less sensitive to changes in rheumatoid arthritis patients' conditions than the disease-specific McMaster-Toronto Arthritis and Rheumatism (MACTAR) questionnaire (Tugwell *et al.* 1987).

Reliability

Chambers (1984) reported that reliability was assessed by asking 30 physiotherapy outpatients to complete the MHIQ on two occasions within a one-week period. Patients were not expected to change in their functional status. The correlation between the physical and emotional function values was 0.80. Intraclass correlation coefficients ranged from 0.48 to 0.95 for the physical, emotional and social scores. Internal consistency coefficients between the physical, emotional and social functional indices were 0.76, 0.67 and 0.51 respectively. Reliability was not affected by self- or interviewer-administered scales. Inter-rater agreement between four raters for the physical dimension of the early version of the scale was 0.71 (Kendall's coefficient of concordance) (Chambers 1993).

In sum, while more studies of its reliability and validity are needed, and the use of the scale is declining, the advantages of the scale are: its flexibility – it can be used in different settings; it is amenable to mathematical scoring construction; it focuses on present ability; it is positive in orientation; it is simple and inexpensive to administer, and acceptable to patients. It also has an acceptable level of reliability. However, it is of questionable applicability to frailer older people (e.g. the question on sports participation in the physical index).

THE RAND HEALTH INSURANCE/MEDICAL OUTCOMES STUDY BATTERIES

The RAND Corporation's health batteries were designed for the RAND Health Insurance Study (HIS), which was an experiment of health outcome following the random allocation of adults to various insurance plans in the USA. The HIS was based on a sample of about 8,000 people in 2,750 families in six sites across the USA. The Medical

Outcomes Study (MOS) involved the more detailed assessment of health outcome and led to further development of the batteries (Stewart and Ware 1992). The batteries were developed for use in population surveys, and more specifically as outcome measures to detect changes in health status that might be expected to occur as a result of health service use within a relatively short period of time. The batteries cover physical health, physiological health, mental health, social health and perceptions of health. The measures were intended to be sensitive to differences in health in general populations (Ware and Karmos 1976; Stewart *et al.* 1978, 1981, 1989; Ware *et al.* 1979, 1980; Stewart and Ware 1992). The HIS batteries were developed after extensive research into existing measures, testing of adaptations of existing measures, or of new measures developed on the basis of extensive reviews of the literature. Each section can be used independently. Many investigators across the world also used the RAND batteries (e.g. Hall *et al.* 1987). Each battery can be used independently. The authors have a wide range of publicly available reports of findings to date, and some published papers which show the interrelationships between the HIS batteries (Stewart *et al.* 1989; Wells *et al.* 1989a, 1989b). A short 20-item version of the batteries was developed (Stewart *et al.* 1988), although this was soon overtaken by a 36-item version (the Short Form-36), which is now used worldwide, with good results for tests of reliability and validity (Anderson *et al.* 1990; Stewart and Ware 1992). The International Quality of Life Assessment (IQOLA) Project translated and adapted the widely used SF-36 Health Survey Questionnaire in several countries, and provided norms for the new translations, in order to facilitate their use in international studies of health outcomes (Aaronson *et al.* 1992).

The batteries are described below to provide the context for the RAND 36-Item Short Form Survey (see later), which is probably the most widely used measure of broader health status (often referred to as a measure of health-related QoL) survey instrument in the world (Hayes and Morales 2001). All the surveys and tools from RAND Health are public documents, available without charge (terms and conditions, the downloadable questionnaire, scoring and references are available at http://www.RAND.org/health/surveys_tools/mos/mos_core_36item.html, accessed 24 August 2015).

RAND PHYSICAL HEALTH BATTERY: FUNCTIONAL LIMITATIONS BATTERY AND PHYSICAL ABILITIES BATTERY

Physical health in the HIS was operationalized in terms of functional status. A review of the literature revealed six categories of functional activity for which performance has been assumed to reflect physical health: self-care (e.g. feeding, bathing), mobility, physical activities, role activities (e.g. employment), household activities and leisure activities. These six areas were thus incorporated into the RAND battery, called the Functional Limitations Battery. These items in the Functional Limitations Battery were based on items from the US National Health Interview Survey and Patrick *et al.*'s (1973a, 1973b) work on developing functional ability scales. Performance was measured by three separate batteries of items: functional limitations, physical abilities and disability days.

An advantage of the RAND Functional Limitations Battery over a number of other scales is that it relates the scale to the cause of the physical incapacity. The RAND

Physical Health Battery includes the Physical Abilities Battery in addition to the Functional Limitations Battery. These are similar to each other and were intended to be administered to respondents at different stages of the longitudinal HIS.

Content

Fourteen HIS items assess activities in self-care, mobility, physical, household and leisure activities, and role activities. Response choices are either 'yes' or 'no' or 'yes, can do', 'yes, can do but only slowly' or 'no, unable to do'. Positive responses to problems lead to further items on length of restriction.

Examples from the (revised) Functional Limitations Battery and Physical Abilities Battery are shown in Box 4.4.

Box 4.4 Examples from the RAND Functional Limitations Battery and Physical Abilities Battery

Does your health limit the kind of vigorous activities you can do, such as running, lifting heavy objects, or participating in strenuous sports?   Yes   1/No   2

Do you have any trouble either walking several blocks or climbing a few flights of stairs, because of your health? Yes   1/No   2

Do you need help with eating, dressing, bathing, or using the toilet because of your health? Yes   1/No   2

Can you do hard activities at home, heavy work like scrubbing floors, or lifting or moving heavy furniture? Yes   1/Yes, but only slowly   2/No, I can't do this   3

If you wanted to, could you participate in active sports such as swimming, tennis, basketball, volleyball, or rowing a boat? Yes   1 /Yes, but only slowly   2/No, I can't do this   3

© The RAND Corporation. The RAND Functional Limitations Battery and Physical Abilities Battery is reproduced here (in part) with permission from the RAND Corporation. RAND's permission to reproduce the survey is not an endorsement of the products, services, or other uses in which the survey appears or is applied. All of the surveys and tools from RAND Health are public documents, available without charge, http://www.rand.org/health/surveys_tools/mos/mos_core.html, accessed 21 September 2015. Contact information: RAND_Health@rand.org. RAND Health, RAND Corporation, 1776 Main St, Santa Monica, CA 90407-2138; tel.: (310)393-0411; http://www.rand.org/health/

Many of these items are inapplicable to very elderly people (e.g. strenuous sports activity) or are too general (e.g. asking about several limitations in the same question) to be useful in surveys where discriminative ability is important.

Scoring

Item score ranges vary: 0–3 (none to more severe limitations) for mobility; 0–4 for physical limitations; 0–2 for role limitations. Items can be scored in groups: mobility limitations, role limitations, self-care limitations (the latter included only one item). An overall score – the Functional Status Index – utilizes all items and is an index of the number of categories in which a person has one or more limitations (0–4). This has not been fully tested for validity.

Results from the RAND study showed that the physical health measures yielded skewed distributions: most sample members had no functional limitations or physical disabilities. This is a limitation regarding its suitability for use in population surveys.

Validity

The authors judged the measure to have acceptable content validity as the content of items included in the physical health measures reflected the range of content reported in the literature. Construct validity was assumed by the authors as associations between the Functional Limitations Battery and the Physical Abilities Battery were moderate to strong (0.49–0.99), indicating an underlying general construct, presumably physical health.

Reliability

Reliability was estimated for the physical abilities measures using internal consistency coefficients. The internal consistency and reproducibility coefficients for HIS measures of physical health were high (0.90 or above); test-retest coefficients (at four months apart) were also high (0.92–0.99).

RAND MENTAL HEALTH BATTERY

As a result of an extensive literature review, ranging from assessments of depression scales to general well-being schedules, the measurement of symptoms of affective (mood) disorders (e.g. depression, anxiety) was considered important, as well as well-being and self-control of behaviour, moods, thought and feelings. The HIS Mental Health Battery contains items hypothesized to measure these constructs. It has been revised since its development in order to extend the range of measurement (particularly with anxiety and depression).

Content

The Revised Mental Health Battery is constructed from the General Well-Being Questionnaire. A new subscale has been added defining loss of behavioural/emotional control. The revised version was based on factor analyses. The General Well-Being Questionnaire comprises 46 questions with four to six response choices for each item, ranging from extremely positive to extremely negative evaluations. The Mental Health Battery utilizes 38 of these questions; the remaining eight items are used to estimate socially desirable responses. Examples of items are shown in Box 4.5.

Box 4.5 Examples from the RAND Mental Health Battery

How much have you been bothered by nervousness or your 'nerves' during the past month?

Extremely so – to the point where I could not work or take care of things	1
Very much bothered	2
Bothered quite a bit by nerves	3
Bothered some – enough to bother me	4
Bothered just a little by nerves	5
Not bothered at all by this	6

During the past month, have you had any reason to wonder if you were losing your mind, or losing control over the way you act, talk, think, feel, or of your memory?

No, not at all	1
Maybe a little	2
Yes, but not enough to be concerned or worried about it	3
Yes, and I have been a little concerned	4
Yes, and I am quite concerned	5
Yes, and I am very much concerned about it	6

In general, would you say your morals have been above reproach?

Yes, definitely	1
Yes, probably	2
I don't know	3
Probably not	4
Definitely not	5

How often have you felt like crying, during the past month?

Always	1
Very often	2
Fairly often	3
Sometimes	4
Almost never	5
Never	6

Scoring

Eight items measure social desirability and should be scored separately from the 38 Mental Health Index items.

Some items are recoded for scoring purposes. Subscales can be created relating to a life satisfaction item; a psychological distress scale; a psychological well-being scale and the mental health index. This involves the simple addition of item scores and the recoded scores. High scores are interpreted differently for different subscales, according to the scale name; for example, a high score for a negative scale corresponds with an unfavourable score and a high score for a positive scale corresponds with a favourable score. Full details of the scoring method are available from the authors at RAND Corporation, Santa Monica.

Validity

The content validity of the HIS Mental Health Battery was assumed by the authors as it contained items represented in the literature. Construct validity is more questionable as correlations between these scales and those constructed for validity studies ranged from 0–0.01 to 0.94. This reflects doubt about the measurement of a common construct within the scale. The authors use these findings to support their decision to score and interpret separately the four construct-specific mental health scales. An Australian community survey by Hall *et al.* (1987) reported a correlation of −0.76 between the RAND Mental Health Battery and the General Health Questionnaire which largely assesses depression and anxiety.

Reliability

The reliability of the HIS mental health measures was estimated using internal consistency and test-retest coefficients. Internal consistency estimates were fairly high (0.72–0.94). Test-retest estimates ranged from 0.70 to 0.80, the time period between administrations being generally less than one week. A more recent development is a brief eight-item depression scale, with initially promising results for reliability and validity (Burnam *et al.* 1988; Wells *et al.* 1989a, 1989b).

RAND DEPRESSION SCREENER

This eight-item, short self-report measure was developed to screen for depression (major depression and dysthymia) in the RAND MOS in the USA. It was developed for use in a screening instrument of three chronic diseases, and it was intended that the whole battery should not take more than 10 minutes to complete (Burnam *et al.* 1988).

The scale was developed on over 5,000 people from a general population sample, mental health service and primary care users. The study measures included the 20-item Center for Epidemiologic Studies Depression Scale (CES-D) (Radloff 1977), which enquired about symptoms and frequency, and two items from the Diagnostic

Interview Schedule (DIS) on duration of symptoms (Robins *et al.* 1981). The full DIS was also used to assess psychiatric disorders (as a gold standard). To select the best items for the screener, logistic regression analyses were employed. The final set of items selected for the screener included six CES-D items and the two DIS items. The latter two items were important predictors of depression and had the largest coefficients in the final regression model. A six-item screener, with the latter two items removed was also tested – the six-item depression screener. This performed very similarly to the eight-item screener, but the eight-item screener performed slightly better overall.

Content

All the questions relate specifically to depressive symptoms. The response format ranges from yes/no choices for the first three depression questions, to a four-point response choice ranging from 0 = rarely, or none of the time, to 3 = most or all of the time (the scores are reversed for one positive item in the scale: 'I enjoyed life'). Examples are shown in Box 4.6.

Box 4.6 Examples from the RAND Depression Screener

11   In the past year, have you had two weeks or more during which you felt sad, blue or depressed; or when you lost all interest or pleasure in things that you usually cared about or enjoyed?
Yes/no

12A   Have you felt depressed or sad much of the time in the past year?
Yes/no

13   For each statement below, mark one circle that best describes how much of the time you felt or behaved this way during the past week.

During the past week:

(b) I had crying spells
(d) I enjoyed life

Rarely or none of the time (<1 day)/some or a little of the time (1–2 days)/ occasionally or a moderate amount of the time (3–4 days)/most or all of the time (5–7 days).

© The RAND Corporation. The RAND Depression Screener is reproduced here (in part) with permission from the RAND Corporation. RAND's permission to reproduce the survey is not an endorsement of the products, services, or other uses in which the survey appears or is applied. All of the surveys and tools from RAND Health are public documents, available without charge, http:// www.RAND.org/health/surveys_tools/mos/mos_core.html, accessed 21 September 2015. Contact information: RAND_Health@RAND.org. RAND Health, RAND Corporation, 1776 Main St, Santa Monica, CA 90407-2138; tel.: (310)393-0411; http://www.RAND.org/health/

Scoring

The individual items carry different weights, and two of the items relate to diagnostically relevant periods. These features distinguish it from other depression scales. There is, however, a complicated scoring equation because of the differential weights applied to the items (see Burnam *et al.* 1988 for details).

Validity

The test results showed that the screener had high sensitivity and good positive predictive value for detecting recent depressive disorders and those that met full DSM-III criteria (American Psychiatric Association 2013; Burnam *et al.* 1988). It was better at predicting depressive disorder in the past month than within the past 6 or 12 months. Varying the cut-off point for the screener improved the sensitivity for longer prevalence periods (6 months, 12 months and lifetime). Detailed results for the specificity and sensitivity of the instrument by cut-off points have been published (Burnam *et al.* 1988).

Reliability

The test-retest reliability of the two DIS items from the screener was tested on 230 adults living in the community (baseline interview with the DIS and telephone follow-up of the depression subsection of the DIS) and showed that the overall agreement between the two DIS items asked on a lifetime basis was 86 per cent for two weeks of feeling depressed, and 91 per cent for two years of feeling depressed. The authors stated that the screener is suitable for population surveys and surveys of health service users. It is a promising development; some minor alteration of wording (e.g. 'blue') will be required, and testing needed, before adoption elsewhere (Burnam *et al.* 1988).

Modifications of the Screener and similar depression screeners from the RAND batteries

Three key items in the screener have been adapted for inclusion in one of the US versions of the SF-36 (the SF-36D). The items relate to (1) depression in the past year for two weeks or more, (2) depression for most days over a two-year period, and (3) depression for much of the time in the past year. The complex scoring of the screener has not been attempted, but instead the patterns of yes/no responses are used to identify patients at risk for major depression or dysthymia. A 'yes' reply to question 1 indicates a risk for major depression, and a 'yes' answer to questions 2 and 3 indicates a risk for dysthymia. Similar questions tested in large community studies identified 89 per cent of adults with a psychiatric diagnosis of major depression or dysthymia (Health Outcomes Institute (previously Interstudy) 1990).

There have been other attempts to develop a short screening questionnaire based on the RAND Health Insurance Experiment Mental Health Inventory. Berwick *et al.* (1991) developed a five-item screening test which is able to detect the most significant DIS disorders, and it performed as well as the original longer (18-item) version, and as well as Goldberg's (1978) General Health Questionnaire (30-item version).

RAND SOCIAL HEALTH BATTERY

The Social Health Battery was developed alongside the other RAND health measures assessing physical and psychological status.

On the basis of the literature again, social health was operationally defined in terms of interpersonal interactions. The Social Health Battery measures social well-being and support, operationalized by measuring social interaction and resources. The two main dimensions of the 11-item battery are the number of social resources a person has, and the frequency with which he or she has contact with relatives and friends.

Content

The 11-item scale covers home, family, friendships, social and community life. It does not cover satisfaction with relationships. The scale has been described by Donald and Ware (1982). Examples of questions are shown in Box 4.7.

Box 4.7 Examples from the RAND Social Health Battery

About how many close friends do you have – people you feel at ease with and can talk with about what is on your mind? (You may include relatives.)

During the past month, about how often have you had friends over to your home? (Do not count relatives.)

Every day.
Several days a week.
About once a week.
Two or three times in the past month.
Once in the past month.
Not at all in the past month.

And how often were you on the telephone with close friends or relatives during the past month?

Every day.
Several times a week.
About once a week.
Two or three times.
Once.
Not at all.

© The RAND Corporation. The RAND Social Health Battery is reproduced here (in part) with permission from the RAND Corporation. RAND's permission to reproduce the survey is not an

An additional item asks about frequency of letter writing but the authors advise dropping this item as so few people answer in the affirmative at all.

Scoring

An overall social support score utilizes all the items (except letter writing and a general question asking about how the person gets on with others). This scoring has not been fully tested for validity.

Validity

Data about validity was drawn from 4,603 interviews from the HIS. The Social Health Battery is judged by its authors to have content validity in so far as it reflects the two major components of social health identified in the literature: interpersonal interaction and social participation. The authors do not attempt to include any of the other areas of social health; thus content validity is only partial.

Criterion validity was tested by using the items in the scale and a nine-item self-rating of health, a measure of emotional ties and a nine-item psychological well-being scale. The correlations were low. Further evidence of the validity of the battery is required.

Reliability

The inter-item correlations are low. Test-retest coefficients are moderate and range from 0.55 to 0.68. Further testing for reliability is required.

The results for reliability and validity are not so far convincing. Further testing is required. The large-scale and longitudinal nature of the RAND HIS study offers exciting possibilities for further testing and development of the measure.

RAND SOCIAL SUPPORT SCALE

The RAND social support questionnaire was developed during the MOS (Sherbourne and Hays 1990). It reflects more recent conceptual thought on the subjective components of social support. An early 17-item version was used on almost 2,000 patients with chronic diseases in the RAND MOS study. For this study, social support was operationalized by four multi-item measures of the availability, if needed, of four distinct types of functional support: tangible support, involving the provision of material aid or behavioural assistance; affectionate support, involving expressions of love and affection; positive social interaction, involving the availability of other persons to do pleasurable things with; and emotional/informational support, involving the expression of positive affect, empathetic understanding, and the offering of advice, guidance or feedback (Sherbourne and Hays 1990). The latter was judged to be important to include because the authors felt that this type of support would be beneficial to the health outcomes of people with chronic illnesses.

Although the authors initially used a 17-item scale to represent these dimensions, they subsequently developed a 19-item version, which involved dividing the emotional/informational support domain into two dimensions, and thus the scale then contained five, rather than four, dimensions of social support (Sherbourne and Stewart 1991; Sherbourne et al. 1992). The emotional and informational domains were later combined back into the emotional/informational support subscale following evaluation by multi-trait correlation matrix, which showed considerable overlap between the items (Sherbourne and Stewart 1991).

In the 19-item version, two single items on the structure of social support are included in order to compensate for the lack of focus on the structure of the network (the number of close friends and relatives, and marital status). The development of the 19-item support scale was based on the same conceptual framework, question type and response format as the 17-item scale, and was described by Sherbourne and Stewart (1991). The 19-item scale is the current version.

The items selected for inclusion were derived from a larger pool of 50 items constructed on the basis of a literature review (Sherbourne and Stewart 1991). The items deliberately reflect subjective impressions of social support, rather than objective network structures (the latter was omitted in order to reduce respondent fatigue).

Content

For each item (in both the 17- and 19-item versions), respondents are asked how often each kind of support was available to them if they needed it. The five-point choice response scale for each item ranges from 'none of the time', 'a little of the time', 'some of the time', 'most of the time' to 'all of the time'. Five points were chosen by the authors on the basis of their review of the research evidence that five to seven response categories are necessary for optimal assessment. Examples from the scale are shown in Box 4.8.

Box 4.8 Examples from the RAND Social Support Scale

Next are some questions about the support that is available to you.

1   About how many close friends and close relatives do you have (people you feel at ease with and can talk to about what is on your mind)? Write in number of close friends and relatives:

Circle one number on each line

None of the time	A little of the time	Some of the time	Most of the time	All of the time
(1)	(2)	(3)	(4)	(5)

2   Someone to help you if you were confined to bed
3   Someone you can count on to listen to you when you need to talk
4   Someone to give you good advice about a crisis
5   Someone to take you to the doctor if you needed it
10   Someone who hugs you
15   Someone to help with daily chores if you were sick
20   Someone to love and make you feel wanted

© The RAND Corporation. The RAND Social Support Scale is reproduced here (in part) with permission from the RAND Corporation. RAND's permission to reproduce the survey is not an endorsement of the products, services, or other uses in which the survey appears or is applied. All of the surveys and tools from RAND Health are public documents, available without charge, http://www.RAND.org/health/surveys_tools/mos/mos_core.html, accessed 21 September 2015. Contact information: RAND_Health@RAND.org. RAND Health, RAND Corporation, 1776 Main St, Santa Monica, CA 90407-2138; tel.: (310)393-0411; http://www.RAND.org/health/

Scoring

Each response ('none of the time' to 'all of the time') is scored 1 to 5, and summed to provide an overall score of social support (the higher the score, the greater the level of social support).

Validity

Sherbourne et al. (1992) used the 19-item scale in a study of the effects of social support and stressful life events, on long-term physical functioning and emotional well-being of 1,402 chronically ill people (with hypertension, diabetes, coronary heart disease or depression) participating in the RAND MOS. The authors reported that patients with high levels of social support had better levels of physical functioning and emotional well-being than those with low levels of support, supporting its discriminative ability. In relation to the same sample, the 19 items were reported by Sherbourne and Stewart (1991) to be correlated weakly to moderately with measures of loneliness, health perceptions, mental health and measures of family and social functioning. Bowling et al. (2002) used the instrument in a survey of the quality of life among people aged 65+ in Britain, and reported that the overall social support score was a significant, independent predictor of self-rated QoL, further supporting the construct validity of the measure. In further support of validity, associations have been reported between the measure and anxiety in pregnancy (Campos et al. 2008), depression, marital status and employment (Gjesfjeld et al. 2010), and homelessness (Lin et al. 2009).

Sherbourne et al.'s (1992) study reported that standardized factor loadings ranged from 0.76 to 0.93 for the tangible support factor, 0.86–0.92 for the affection factor,

0.82–0.92 for the emotional/informational factor, and 0.91–0.93 for the positive interaction factor. Results of principal components factor analysis of the 19 items also supported the construction of the overall index (the first unrotated factor showed high loadings for each of the items, ranging from 0.67 to 0.88). These results support the scale as containing four dimensions and as providing a common measure of overall support.

Reliability

Sherbourne and Stewart (1991) reported that the correlations (Pearson's) between the items and the subscales were strong. Item-scale correlations ranged from 0.72 to 0.87 for the tangible support scale, 0.80–0.86 for the affection scale, 0.82–0.90 for the emotional/informational scale, and 0.87–0.88 for the positive interaction scale. The additional item on number of close friends and relatives correlated low to moderately with each of the functional support items (0.18–0.23), indicating its distinct status; marital status was not associated with numbers of close friends or relatives (0.01), but was more highly correlated with the functional support items (0.69–0.82).

Gjesfjeld et al. (2010) reported Cronbach's alpha reliability coefficients of 0.96 for the total score; and 0.83 to 0.97 for the subscales. Lin et al. (2009) reported Cronbach's alpha correlation coefficients of 0.83 to 0.94 for the subscales, and Campos et al. (2008) reported Cronbach's alphas of 0.83 to 0.97 for the subscales and total scale (see review by López and Cooper 2011 for details and for reliability coefficients for the Spanish version).

Because of its concentration on subjective perceptions, this scale needs to be supplemented with an objective measure of the structure of the network (e.g. size, composition, frequency of contact, geographical proximity, contacts by telephone/mail). Although it requires supplementation, and far more extensive testing, it is a promising scale and merits wider use in order to more fully assess its psychometric properties and cross-cultural applicability. One advantage of this scale is that it contains more health-specific items than many of the more generic social support scales that have been developed. Most social support scales were developed in the USA and contain culture-specific items which would be unusual in other societies (e.g. about having someone who would loan the respondent a car). The measure has very good psychometric properties and has been tested in several languages, and it is one of the social support measures recommended by López and Cooper (2011), on the basis of their extensive review of the literature.

RAND GENERAL HEALTH PERCEPTIONS BATTERY

This asks respondents for an assessment or self-rating of their health in general (Stewart et al. 1978; Davies and Ware 1981). These were defined in the HIS with respect to time (perceptions of prior, current and future health) and with respect to three other constructs indicative of general health perceptions, including resistance or susceptibility to illness, health worry and concern, and sickness orientation (the extent to which people perceive illness to be a part of their lives).

A major strength of the General Health Perceptions Battery is ease of administration. Self-administration of this section takes approximately seven minutes. It is of potential use in studies attempting to predict the use of medical services.

Content

The battery contains 29 items, 26 of which were taken from the Health Perceptions Questionnaire developed by Ware and Karmos (1976) for the National Center for Health Services Research.

The items include statements of opinion about personal health (e.g. 'I expect to have a very healthy life'), accompanied by five standardized response categories defining a true–false continuum: definitely true, mostly true, don't know, mostly false, definitely false. These items are used to score six subscales assessing different dimensions of health perceptions: past health, present health, future health, health-related worries and concerns, resistance or susceptibility to illness and the tendency to view illness as part of life. Examples of items are shown in Box 4.9.

Box 4.9 Examples from the RAND General Health Perceptions Battery

I try to avoid letting illness interfere with my life.
I will probably be sick a lot in the future.
I don't like going to the doctor.
I'm not as healthy as I used to be.
When I'm sick, I try to just keep going as usual.
I expect to have a very healthy life.
When I think I am getting sick, I fight it.

© The RAND Corporation. The RAND General Health Perceptions Battery is reproduced here (in part) with permission from the RAND Corporation. RAND's permission to reproduce the survey is not an endorsement of the products, services, or other uses in which the survey appears or is applied. All of the surveys and tools from RAND Health are public documents, available without charge, http://www.RAND.org/health/surveys_tools/mos/mos_core.html, accessed 21 September 2015. Contact information: RAND_Health@RAND.org, RAND Health, RAND Corporation, 1776 Main St, Santa Monica, CA 90407-2138; tel.: (310)393-0411; http://www.RAND.org/health/

It is apparent from these questions that analyses need to control for age, especially in relation to expectations about the future and current health status.

Scoring

All items are scored to produce a global figure, although the scoring has not been fully tested for validity. Distributions appear to be fairly normal. Hall *et al.* (1987) reported the RAND measures to be less skewed than the SIP or GHQ.

Validity

The measure of health perceptions was reported by the authors to be correlated with the physical, mental and social health batteries (coefficients unreported). In the Australian study by Hall *et al.* (1987) the RAND batteries relating to general health perceptions were tested on 160 patients along with the SIP and the GHQ. A correlation of −0.30 was considered to be the threshold for assessment of relationships between the three instruments. The RAND mental health index was reported to correlate weakly to moderately well with three of the SIP components (emotional behaviour): −0.32 to −0.54. To some extent the same constructs are being measured, although these correlations are not high. If 0.50 is taken as the minimum correlation coefficient for validity acceptance for group studies, then the instruments tested do not achieve this (Ware *et al.* 1980). On the other hand, it was reported previously that the GHQ correlated highly with the RAND Mental Health Battery (−0.76) (Hall *et al.* 1987). The developers indicated that it can successfully discriminate between those with and without a chronic disease, is sensitive to individual differences in disease severity, and is sensitive to changes over time in both physical and mental functioning. Hall *et al.* (1987) reported that of the three instruments used in the Australian study (the RAND instrument, the SIP and the GHQ), the RAND measures had the best discriminative ability and were reported by the authors to be preferred as a general health status measure in a general population.

Reliability

The reliability of the Health Perceptions scale was estimated using internal consistency and test-retest coefficients. These were tested by its authors using a non-HIS population. Test-retest reliability estimates were based on data collected approximately six weeks apart from the same respondents. Results indicate that the scale was more reliable than single-item measures, although internal consistency coefficients (unreported) were lower than for test-retest. Internal consistency for the scale generally exceeded 0.50 (sometimes 0.90). The stability of the Health Perceptions Battery has been estimated for intervals of one, two and three years between administrations. The median stability coefficients for one, two and three years for adults are 0.66, 0.59 and 0.56 respectively.

36-ITEM VERSIONS: RAND 36-ITEM SHORT FORM SURVEY (RAND SF-36) AND SHORT FORM-36 HEALTH SURVEY (SF-36)

A 36-item health status questionnaire was developed at the RAND Corporation in the USA for use in the HIS Experiment/Medical Outcomes Study (HIS/MOS) (Stewart and Ware 1992; Ware *et al.* 1993). It is a concise 36-item health status questionnaire, and its use across the world has escalated since 1990. The authors aimed to develop a short, generic measure of subjective health status that was psychometrically sound, and that could be applied in a wide range of settings. It was constructed with the aim of satisfying the minimum psychometric standards necessary for making comparisons between groups. The eight dimensions it includes were selected from the 40 dimensions included in the MOS, and were selected to represent the most frequently measured concepts in health surveys and those most affected by disease and treatment. Most SF-36 items are based on instruments that had been used since the 1970s and 1980s, including Dupuy's (1984) Psychological General Well-Being Index.

Initially, the SF-20 (Short Form 20-item version) was designed. For this, 17 items were taken from the questionnaires used in the HIS and three new items were added (Ware *et al.* 1992). This was used in the MOS. The authors decided to extend the scale to make it more comprehensive and with better psychometric properties. This led to the longer SF-36 item version. The RAND SF-36 is made up of the items which loaded best on factor analyses from 149 items from the longer batteries, based on the results from over 22,000 patients in the RAND HIS/MOS studies. The RAND SF-36 takes 5–10 minutes to complete and is self-administered. Examples are shown in Box 4.10.

Box 4.10 Examples from the RAND 36-Item Short Form Survey, original, Version 1

4. During the past 4 weeks, have you had any of the following problems with your work or other regular daily activities as a result of your physical health?
Yes No
1   2

Cut down the amount of time you spent on work or other activities

Accomplished less than you would like

Were limited in the kind of work or other activities

Had difficulty performing the work or other activities (for example, it took extra effort)

© The RAND Corporation. The RAND General Health Perceptions Battery is reproduced here (in part) with permission from the RAND Corporation. RAND's permission to reproduce the survey is not an endorsement of the products, services, or other uses in which the survey appears or is applied. The RAND 36-Item Short Form Survey is available at no cost – see link for instrument, scoring and literature, http://www.RAND.org/health/surveys_tools/mos/mos_core_36item.html, accessed 21 September 2015. Contact information: RAND_Health@RAND.org, RAND Health, RAND Corporation, 1776 Main St, Santa Monica, CA 90407-2138; tel.: (310)393-0411; http://www.RAND.org/health/

The RAND SF-36 is the most frequently used measure of generic health status across the world (Hays and Morales 2001). It is also commonly used in research with older people (Michalos *et al.* 2001). The RAND SF-36 (Version 1) is distributed with no charge by RAND Health, RAND Corporation, Santa Monica, where it was developed. RAND owns the copyright; all the surveys and tools from RAND Health are public documents, available without charge (terms and conditions, the downloadable questionnaire, scoring and references are available at http://www.RAND.org/health/surveys_tools/mos/mos_core_36item.html).

A similar format of the instrument, called the Short Form-36 Health Survey (SF-36 Health Survey), was later distributed by the Medical Outcomes (Study) Trust (MOT) of the Health Institute at the New England Medical Center, Boston, where one of its developers, John Ware, was later based (Medical Outcomes Trust 1993; Ware *et al.* 1993). This version is strictly copyrighted (to QualityMetric), and users are requested to complete and submit an online licence application to QualityMetric Incorporated (now part of www.optum.com, accessed 24 August 2015). The QualityMetric SF-36 is Version two (V2). A variable fee is payable for the use of this instrument for funded, approved research. A manual and scoring algorithm are also available. This QualityMetric copyrighted instrument is used worldwide, although many researchers also continue to use the original RAND version, which is still freely distributed from RAND (see earlier). Differences between the versions, and the various scoring formats, have been described by Hays and Morales (2001).

Population norms for the SF-36 in many countries have been published (Aaronson *et al.* 1992; Ware *et al.* 1993, 1997; Bullinger 1995; Sullivan *et al.* 1995; Gandek and Ware 1998), including those for the UK (Brazier *et al.* 1992, 1993b; Garratt *et al.* 1993; Jenkinson *et al.* 1993, 1996, 1999). The only changes made to the original scale for the UK version include Anglicization of some of the language and a slight alteration of the positioning and coding of one of the social functioning items in order to improve reliability in the UK and ease of administration. A second version, compatible with the US version 2.0, developed by Ware *et al.* (1997) has been developed (Jenkinson *et al.* 1999). The second version improved the wording and layout of the original scale, and added more sensitive response categories to the role functioning subscale, which has increased its reliability, raised the ceiling and lowered the floor ends of the scale, and improved precision (Jenkinson *et al.* 1996, 1999). Several investigators have reported notable floor effects for the SF-36 (Riazi *et al.* 2003b). A manual for the UK version can be purchased (Jenkinson *et al.* 1996).

Content

Both versions of the SF-36 contains 36 items which measure eight dimensions: physical functioning (10 items), social functioning (two), role limitations due to physical problems (four), role limitations due to emotional problems (three), mental health (five), energy/vitality (four), pain (two) and general health perception (five). There is also a single item about perceptions of health changes over the past 12 months (in effect, providing a ninth domain). It claims to measure positive as well as negative health.

Two versions are available with varying time recall referents in the responses to current health status questions – respondents are asked about their health over the past four weeks (the most commonly used) or (in the case of acute conditions) over the past one week. The latter should be more responsive to recent changes. Examples of the SF-36 Health Survey (QualityMetric Inc.) are shown in Box 4.11.

Box 4.11 Examples from the Short Form-36 Health Survey (SF-36 Health Survey) (QualityMetric Inc.)

1 In general, would you say your health is:

Excellent/Very good/Good/Fair/Poor

Health and daily activities.

The following questions are about activities you might do during a typical day. Does your health limit you in these activities? If so, how much?

Yes, limited a lot/Yes, limited a little/No, not limited at all

Vigorous activities, such as running, lifting heavy objects, participating in strenuous sports
Moderate activities, such as moving a table, pushing a vacuum, bowling or playing golf
Lifting or carrying groceries
Climbing several flights of stairs
Climbing one flight of stairs
Bending, kneeling or stooping
Walking more than a mile
Walking half a mile
Walking 100 yards
Bathing and dressing yourself

The measures (SF-36, SF-12, SG-8) are licensed by QualityMetric Incorporated (software company: 24 Albion Rd, Lincoln, RI 02865, US; tel.: +1 401-334-8800), registration and payment is required for their use. Details can be found on their website, www.qualitymetric.com/download/InstallationGuide_ScoringSoftwareV4.pdf. Details can also be found on the OPTUM website (which QualityMetric is now part of): https://campaign.optum.com/optum-outcomes/what-we-do/health-surveys.html

---

Scoring

The previous mix of scaled and dichotomous response formats confused respondents and led to item non-response. Thus the second version has changed the dichotomous response formats at the 'role-physical' and 'role-mental' dimensions to five-level response choices, as well as changing the six-level response format on the mental health dimension to five levels.

The coding format requires recoding before each subscale can be summed. The subscales are not summed together to produce an overall score, instead the scores for each of the eight dimensions are reported. The scoring algorithms adopted for the SF-36 were published after careful study of a number of alternatives. The scoring method selected was chosen for its simplicity and to optimize the ability to make comparisons of results across studies (Ware *et al.* 1993). In the original scoring method, the item scores for each of the eight dimensions are summed and transformed, using a scoring algorithm, into a scale from 0 (poor health) to 100 per cent (good health).

The original 0–100 scoring algorithms of the SF-36 (based on summated ratings) have been improved on by norm-based scoring (the standardization of mean scores and standard deviations for the SF-36 scales), which has facilitated the speed and ease of interpretation of SF-36 scores. Ware *et al.* (1994) described how linear transformations were performed to transform the scale scores to a mean of 50 and a standard deviation of 10 (in the general US population). With this method, then, each scale is scored to have the same average (50) and the same standard deviation (10). Without the need to refer to norms, scale values below 50 are interpreted as below average, and each point is one-tenth of a standard deviation.

The results have conventionally been reported as mean scores for each subscale, rather than frequency distribution, despite the well-known tendency of means to distort results by reflecting small numbers of outlying values. While generally accepted, the validity of this method, and the common usage of parametric statistics to analyse the SF-36, has, however, been seriously questioned by Julious *et al.* (1995), given the non-normal distributions of the data.

Two summary scales can also be obtained – the Physical Component Summary Score (PCS-36) and the Mental Component Summary Score (MCS-36), with the advantage of enabling a reduction in the number of statistical comparisons conducted. These two summary scales capture about 85 per cent of the reliable variance in the eight scale SF-36 and yield average scores which closely mirror those in the 36-item scale (Ware *et al.* 1994, 1995, 1996b; Jenkinson *et al.* 1997).

Validity

The results of the studies which tested the longer RAND batteries were published by Stewart and Ware (1992), together with the history of the development of the SF-36 from these instruments. There is a vast number of publications of the psychometric properties of the SF-36. Garratt *et al.* (2002) judged it to be the most widely evaluated generic health status instrument. For consistency, and in order to avoid confusion, this review will focus on the results for the SF-36 Health Survey. Equally good psychometric properties have been reported for the original RAND SF-36 item Health Survey (e.g. King and Roberts 2002; Lowrie *et al.* 2003; Oga *et al.* 2003).

The manuals and bibliographies of the SF-36 Health Survey reference the main studies which report the instrument's psychometric properties (Ware *et al.* 1993, 1997; Shiely *et al.* 1996). The International Quality of Life Assessment Project published the psychometric properties of the translated and tested versions of the SF-36 in international use (Gandek and Ware 1998). The results of British studies of the reliability and validity of the SF-36 have been summarized by Jenkinson *et al.* (1996, 1999). Bowling *et al.* (1999) compared the various British norms for the SF-36 and critically discussed their variations by mode of administration, survey context and question order. Their conclusions were consistent with those of McHorney *et al.* (1994) and Lyons *et al.* (1999) who reported under-reporting of health problems using the SF-36 in personal interviews in comparison with postal approaches, especially in relation to emotional and mental health.

Brazier *et al.* (1992), on the basis of the results of a postal survey in the UK, reported that the SF-36 was found to be more sensitive to gradations in poor health than the

EuroQol (EuroQol Group 1990) and the Nottingham Health Profile (Hunt *et al.* 1986). The authors cautioned that there was a higher rate of item non-response among older people, a finding confirmed by Sullivan *et al.* (1995) on the basis of a Swedish postal survey sample (in contrast to interview surveys). However, reports are contradictory. A later postal survey by Walters *et al.* (2001) of almost 1,000 people aged 65 and over registered with 12 general practices found that the response rate was 82 per cent and dimension completion rates ranged between 86.4 per cent and 97.7 per cent. Research in the USA has found good responses among elderly people (Health Outcomes Institute 1990). Lyons *et al.* (1994, 1997) reported that item response was good among elderly people in the UK when the instrument was interviewer- rather than self-administered, and it distinguished between those with and without markers of poor health, supporting the instrument's construct validity.

The 10 items in the physical functioning sub-scale of the SF-36 have established reliability and validity, and scale properties have been supported using item response theory (Haley *et al.* 1994; McHorney *et al.* 1997; Raczek *et al.* 1998). Although popularly used with older populations, Dubec *et al.* (2004), in a study of 75 people aged 60+ living at home, reported that it had moderate ceiling effects. The SF-36 was criticized previously for inadequately assessing physical functioning in elderly people in the community (Brazier *et al.* 1992). Hill and Harries (1994) and Hill *et al.* (1995) also reported flaws in the SF-36 instrument when used to measure the outcomes of health care for people aged 65 and over in community settings. The respondents (who tended to have high levels of co-morbidity and poor physical functioning) often reported during interviews that the SF-36 did not reflect their values. In one district, the median physical functioning score for the group was zero (worst functioning), meaning that the group as a whole were pushed to the margins of the scale. While dramatic improvements in physical functioning in this group, and therefore improvements in scores, were unlikely, the measure was reported to miss some changes that were important to people. Parker *et al.* (2006) administered the SF-36 to 245 people aged 65+ from a range of inpatient, outpatient and community settings to ensure a range of disability levels. They reported that global, rather than specific mental or physical dysfunction, was associated with inability to complete the SF-36, apparently due to difficulties performing a 'complex task'. They concluded that non-completion may lead to overestimates of health status in populations using this questionnaire. These findings support the argument of Hunt and McKenna (1993) who argued that the development and testing of the SF-36 has relied too heavily on psychometric techniques at the expense of serious consultation of lay people for their views about the instrument.

Mangione *et al.* (1993), in a study of 745 major elective (non-cardiac) patients in Boston, reported that the SF-36 health perception scale had the greatest correlation with the energy and fatigue scale ($r = 0.45$), correlated moderately with mental health ($r = 0.35$), social function ($r = 0.32$), and physical function ($r = 0.33$), but correlated less well with pain ($r = 0.23$). These results support the distinctive components of the health perceptions subscale although, on the other hand, these moderate to weak correlations among variables which would be expected to be more highly correlated (health perceptions and the various domains of health status) also suggest that the health perceptions battery might have weak convergent validity.

Mangione *et al.* (1993) also reported that the SF-36 was able to discriminate between surgical groups (major elective, non-cardiac surgery), and between younger patients and patients who were aged 70 years and over in relation to role function, energy, fatigue and physical function (the older patients had poorer scores on these domains). Ware *et al.* (1993), in the manual of the SF-36, reported studies showing that in tests for validity, the SF-36 was able to discriminate between groups with physical morbidities (the physical functioning subscale performed best and the mental health subscale discriminated between patients with mental health morbidities the best). Investigators in Grampian reported that different common medical conditions (low back pain, menorrhagia, suspected peptic ulcer and varicose veins) achieved a distinct score profile, indicating that the SF-36 can discriminate between conditions (Garratt *et al.* 1993). Further papers by these authors reported the scale means for these patient groups and good responsiveness to change in clinical condition (Garratt *et al.* 1994; Ruta *et al.* 1994a). The mental health subscale has a particularly impressive validity. For example, it was reported to be correlated by between 0.92 and 0.95 with the full Mental Health Inventory from different samples from the HIS (Davies *et al.* 1988; Stewart and Ware 1992). Correlations between the SF-36 and the General Psychological Well-Being measure (Dupuy 1984) ranged from $r = 0.19$ to $r = 0.60$, with a median of $r = 0.36$. Ware *et al.* (1993) presented the data from several studies that show that the correlations for the subscales range from weak to strong, but strong correlations were reported between the physical functioning subscale and the equivalent subscales of the SIP, the AIMS and the NHP (0.52 to 0.85). Strong correlations were reported between the mental health subscale and other psychological subscales (the range was $r = 0.51$ to $r = 0.82$). Longitudinal population data in the UK showed that the SF-36 was sensitive to respondents' short-term changes in health status (Hemingway *et al.* 1997).

Not all results have been good (see review by Anderson *et al.* 1993). For example, the bodily pain scale has been reported to have poor convergent validity when tested against severity of illness and independent pain scores in the case of knee conditions (McHorney *et al.* 1993). Other studies have reported 'floor' effects in the role functioning scales in severely ill patients, where 25–50 per cent of patients obtained the lowest score possible, with the implication that deterioration in condition will not be detected by the scale (Kurtin *et al.* 1992). The comparable percentage in an HIV population is 63 per cent (Watchel *et al.* 1992). Anderson *et al.* (1993) suggested that the item codes can be subject to 'ceiling' effects as they appear too crude to detect improvements. The modifications to the item scores in the second version of the SF-36 should alleviate this problem.

Other investigators reported that it has little discriminatory power among women receiving different treatments for Stage II breast cancer (Levine *et al.* 1988; Guyatt *et al.* 1989). The physical functioning scale also focuses more on mobility at the expense of other pertinent areas of functioning (e.g. domestic), necessitating its supplementation with other scales in studies of people with chronic conditions which affect their functioning (e.g. rheumatoid arthritis). Its sensitivity may vary with disease type. The SF-36 and both summary scales have been reported to have good validity in other clinical areas: they were able to detect improvement in patients' conditions after heart surgery (Sedrakyan *et al.* 2003); the SF-36 was associated with severity of hearing loss in the expected direction (Dalton *et al.* 2003) and with the Crohn's Disease Activity Index (Kiran *et al.* 2003). The mental health scale and the MCS summary scale have been reported to be of value in screening for psychiatric disorders, particularly depression (Ware *et al.* 1994).

Reliability

In the UK, Brazier *et al.* (1992) reported internal coefficiency correlations for the eight scales as ranging from 0.60 to 0.81, with a median of 0.76. High inter-item correlations were reported for the subscales (e.g. mental health). Jenkinson *et al.* (1993) reported that it has high internal consistency between dimensions, with high Cronbach's alphas being obtained of between 0.76 and 0.90. Garratt *et al.* (1993) reported that the internal consistency between the items exceeded 0.80 with Cronbach's alpha, and inter-item correlations ranged from 0.55 to 0.78. All satisfied statistical criteria of acceptable levels. Walters *et al.*'s (2001) survey of people aged 65 and over reported that Cronbach's alpha exceeded 0.80 for all dimensions except social functioning. Ware *et al.* (1993) reviewed 14 studies in the USA which analysed the reliability of the SF-36. The reliability coefficients for internal consistency range from 0.62 to 0.94 for the subscales, for test-retest reliability the coefficents range from 0.43 to 0.90, and for alternate form reliability the coefficient was 0.92. In relation to internal consistency, all but 11 coefficients reported in studies in the USA and the UK exceeded the 0.70 standard suggested by Nunnally (1978). Reliability estimates for the two summary scores generally exceed 0.90 (Ware *et al.* 1994). Meyer-Rosenberg *et al.* (2001) reported that the SF-36 had higher internal consistency reliability coefficients than the Nottingham Health Profile, which was previously used widely in Britain and Europe, and correlations between the two instruments were moderate, giving some support to their convergent validity. However, the Nottingham Health Profile had additional items on pain and sleep which were more relevant to their population of pain patients. Seymour *et al.* (2001) tested the reliability of the SF-36 in a sample of over 300 elderly rehabilitation patients and found the results to be less good than those reported in earlier studies. The Cronbach alphas for the eight dimensions of the SF-36 ranged from 0.54 (social functioning) to 0.933 (bodily pain) for the cognitively normal patients; they were slightly lower for the cognitively impaired patients (range 0.413–0.861). The values were significantly higher among the normal group for the bodily pain, mental health and role-emotional dimensions. Test-retest reliability coefficients were also higher for the normal group (at least 0.7 was attained for five out of eight dimensions) than the impaired group (0.7 was attained for four out of eight dimensions).

Ware *et al.* (1993) also reported the results of a factor analysis of the SF-36, which provided strong evidence for the conceptualization of health underlying the SF-36, and indicated that some scales principally measure physical health, some measure mental health, and others measure both. Garratt *et al.* (1993) also reported the results of a factor analysis which confirmed the distinct scale dimensions.

The SF-36 is probably the most widely used health status scale across the world, largely due to its brevity and coverage of broader health status, as well as active dissemination by the developers. It has been translated in more than 50 countries as part of the international QoL project. This increasing standardization of measurement facilitates comparisons between populations and evaluations of patient outcomes. Due to its coverage of social, physical and emotional health, many investigators use it as a proxy measure of health-related quality of life. Many disease-specific scales also recommend its use as a generic core. Each translated scale has conformed to strict protocols of the process (information about translations, as well as an online scoring service, and missing data estimator, is available at http://www.SF-36.com or at www.qualitymetric.com).

The SF-36 can be self-, interviewer-, telephone- or computer-administered, and takes about five minutes to complete. Ryan *et al.* (2002) reported that 71 per cent of their respondents (healthy individuals and chronic pain patients) who completed both electronic and paper versions preferred the electronic version.

SHORT 12-ITEM VERSIONS

There is a 12-item version of the SF-36 (the SF-12, licensed by Quality-Metric) (Ware *et al.* 1995, 1996a, 1996b) and a 12-item version of the original RAND SF-36 (HSQ-12; redeveloped as RAND-12), along with summary scores for the physical and mental health components (Radosevich and Pruitt 1995). These are one-page versions of the SF-36, which take about a minute to complete. The RAND summary scores of the 12-item scale (RAND-12) performed better than the similar SF-12 summary scores (licensed by Quality-Metric) in distinguishing between patients with different severities of diabetes (Johnson and Maddigan 2004). The items which were included in the initial RAND HSQ-12 were derived by using regression analysis on the data from over 4,000 respondents to a 39-item version of the questionnaire. Stepwise linear regression was used to select preliminary sets of questions that accounted for approximately 90 per cent of the variability in overall scale scores (Radosevich and Husnik 1995). The developers decided to emphasize items from the physical functioning and mental health subscales as these have been shown to be the most sensitive in distinguishing medical and psychiatric conditions (McHorney *et al.* 1993). The instrument was then initially tested against their longer 39-item version of the (SF-36) battery among a group of cardiology patients and in a healthy working population (Radosevich and Pruitt 1995). Over 800 respondents took part in the reliability testing. Replicate reliability coefficients for the short (12 items) and long forms (39 items) were above 0.52 for all scales. Both the SF-12 and the HSQ-12 have been tested in Britain (Bowling and Windsor 1997; Jenkinson and Layte 1997; Jenkinson *et al.* 1997; Pettit *et al.* 2001). In a community psychiatric survey of almost 1,000 people in London, Pettit *et al.* (2001), reported that the HSQ-12, but not the SF-12, could distinguish between people with and without dementia. However, the HSQ-12 is no longer supported by its developers and the SF-12 in use now is licensed by Quality-Metric (part of Optum).

The 12 items for both versions included self-assessment of health; physical functioning; physical role limitation; mental role limitation; social functioning; mental health items and pain. Standard four-week and one-week (acute) recall versions are available. These 12 items yield the eight scale profiles of the SF-36, but with fewer levels and with less precise scores, as would be expected with fewer items (e.g. some subscales now have just one or two items). The SF-12 covers the same eight domains as the SF-36 Version 2.

Ware *et al.* (1996a, 1996b) reported that the 12 items that were selected for inclusion in the SF-12 (with an improved scoring algorithm), on the grounds of their psychometric properties, were able to reproduce at least 90 per cent of the variance in the physical and mental subscales of the SF-36, and reproduced the profile of the eight dimensions of the SF-36. They argued that, consequently, the population norms for the SF-36 summary measures (PCS-36 and MCS-36) can also be used as norms for the SF-12 summary measures. Because the SF-12 is a subset of the SF-36, the many translations available for the SF-36 can be used for the SF-12.

Results for its validity and reliability are good. Lim and Fisher (1999) used it with over 2,000 heart and stroke patients in Australia. The SF-12 was able to discriminate between age groups, emergency versus planned admission patients, males and females and patients with varying lengths of stay. However, they did report that it had a high non-completion rate, cautioning against its use with these patients. A study by Salyers *et al.* (2000) in the USA of a sample of people with severe mental illness found that the SF-12 distinguished this group from the normal population, and that it was stable over a one-week interval. In the UK, as well as the USA, the SF-12 reflects the revised version of the SF-36 (Version 2). Jenkinson and Layte (1997) reported that the SF-12 summary scores produced very similar results to the longer SF-36 summary scores.

A scoring algorithm, involving weighted item responses, is available with the manual; it is available in different modes of administration and in standard four-week or acute one-week time recall periods. As population norms are used in the scoring of each, this enables comparisons to be made. As the SF-12 is shorter, it is less precise than the SF-36, and is suitable for use with larger samples in which broader health outcomes are being monitored (Ware *et al.* 1996b). It takes two to three minutes to complete. It is available in several language translations.

The Optum website describes the 'Optum™ SF-12v2®' as ' . . . a shorter version of the SF-36v2® Health Survey that uses just 12 questions to measure functional health and well-being from the patient's point of view' (https://www.optum.com/optum-outcomes/what-we-do/health-surveys/sf-12v2-health-survey.html).

The measures (SF-36, SF-12, SF-8) are licensed by QualityMetric Incorporated (software company: 24 Albion Rd, Lincoln, RI 02865, US; tel.: +1 401-334-8800), and registration and payment is required for their use. Details can be found on the website (www.qualitymetric.com/.../InstallationGuide_ScoringSoftwareV4.pdf). Details can also be found on the OPTUM website (which QualityMetric is now part of): https://www.optum.com/optum-outcomes/what-we-do/health-surveys.html

THE SHORT FORM-8 HEALTH SURVEY QUESTIONNAIRE (SF-8)

The SF-8 is an eight-item version of the SF-36, and is licensed by QualityMetric (https://www.optum.com/optum-outcomes/what-we-do/health-surveys/sf-8-health-survey.html, accessed 24 August 2015). The SF-8 yields a comparable eight-dimension health profile and comparable physical and mental summary score estimates

(Ware *et al.* 2001). The SF-8 relies on a single item to measure each of the eight dimensions of health status contained in the SF-36.

It was constructed on the basis of empirical studies linking each questionnaire item to a comprehensive pool of commonly used questions, including the SF-36, which measured the same health concept. Each item was calibrated on the same metric as the corresponding SF-36 scale. As with the 36- and 12-item versions, four-week and one-week recall time reference versions are available, as well as a 24-hour recall version. It can be self- or interviewer-administered, and has been translated and validated for use in over 30 countries. The SF-8 takes one to two minutes to administer. It was translated, back-translated and reassessed for use in a survey by Roberts *et al.* (2008) in northern Uganda (1,206 adults in camps for internally displaced people). They reported acceptable item response, strong validity and good test-retest reliability (0.61 for physical and 0.68 for the mental components). In support of the measure's validity, Lefante *et al.* (2005) administered the SF-8 by telephone or internet to almost 2,000 people in chronically ill, low-income groups in Central Louisiana. They reported that the SF-8 physical and mental component subscales were associated, in the expected directions, with age and number of diagnoses, and with improvement in scores six months post-intervention.

It is regarded as a practical and efficient instrument for use in population studies (Turner-Bowker *et al.* 2003). This conciseness is inevitably at the expense of precision, compared to the longer versions. A user manual is available on scoring and interpretation. The measures (SF-36, SF-12, SF-8) are licensed by QualityMetric Incorporated (software company: 24 Albion Rd, Lincoln, RI 02865, US; tel.: +1 401-334-8800), registration and payment is required for their use. Details can be found on the website (www. qualitymetric.com/.../InstallationGuide_ScoringSoftwareV4.pdf). Details can also be found on the OPTUM website (which QualityMetric is now part of): https://www.optum.com/optum-outcomes/what-we-do/health-surveys.html

SHORT-FORM 6D (SF-6D)

The SF-6D is a generic preference-based health utility index. It aims to derive a single index from the SF-36 for use in economic evaluation studies, by producing a 'bridging' transformation between SF-36 responses and utilities (O'Brien *et al.* 2003).

The SF-6D was developed from 11 items from the SF-36 to minimize loss of descriptive information. It incorporates seven of the eight domains of the SF-36 (it excludes general health), and the 11 items form a six-domain classification of health states:

Physical functioning,
Role participation (combined role-physical and role-emotional),
Social functioning,
Bodily pain,
Mental health,
Vitality.

The SF-6D algorithm is explained in detail by Brazier *et al.* (2002) and summarized by O'Brien *et al.* (2003). It is based on six of the eight dimensions of SF-36, each of which has a number of levels (e.g. 'limited a lot', 'limited a little'). The combination of levels over dimensions defines 18,000 unique health states. As it is impractical to measure utilities for 18,000 states a fractional factorial design was required. Hence, a general population in the UK (836 respondents) assigned values to 249 health states, using standard gamble valuation methods. Thus, from the SF-36 data, respondents can be classified on four to six levels of functioning or limitations, on the six domains, thus allowing a respondent to be classified into any of 18,000 possible unique health states (O'Brien *et al.* 2003). Regression models predicted single index scores for the health states defined by the SF-6D (Brazier *et al.* 2002, 2004; and see Brazier and Roberts 2004; Kharroubi *et al.* 2007).

The SF-6D preferences (scored from 0.0 (worst health state) to 1.0 (best health state)) can be applied to SF-36 datasets for economic evaluations (e.g. estimation of quality adjusted life years, QALYs).

An example of the physical functioning component is shown in Box 4.12.

Box 4.12 Examples from the SF-6D

Physical Functioning

Level

1 Your health does not limit you in *vigorous activities*
2 Your health limits you a little in *vigorous activities*
3 Your health limits you a little in *moderate activities*
4 Your health limits you a lot in *moderate activities*
5 Your health limits you a little in *bathing and dressing*
6 Your health limits you a lot in *bathing and dressing*

A users manual and computer programmes are available. The SF-6D is copyrighted and is available on a licence basis. A licence is available free of charge for all non-commercial applications including work funded by research councils, government agencies and charities, but a per study licence is required for commercial applications (https://www.shef.ac.uk/scharr/sections/heds/mvh/sf-6d). The SF-6D is also being used in software available from Optum Insight (https://www.optum.com). Contact information: Sheffield Health Economics Group, School of Health and Related Research, University of Sheffield, S1 4DA, UK; https://www.shef.ac.uk/scharr/sections/heds/mvh/sf-6d

---

Comparisons of the SF-6D and the Health Utilities Index mark 3 (HUI3), a widely used, valid and reliable, multi-attribute health utility scale, showed that these two instruments differed markedly in their distributions and point estimates of derived utilities (O'Brien *et al.* 2003). Brazier *et al.* (2004) compared the EQ-5D and SF-6D across seven groups of patients. They reported that the SF-6D mean index slightly exceeded the EQ-5D mean index. They pointed out that there is evidence of floor effects in the SF-6D, and ceiling effects in the EQ-5D, due to differences in their classifications of health states, and the methods used to value them.

Kuspinar and Mayo (2014) reviewed and compared the psychometric properties of four measures designed to gererate a single index value for each health state – the EQ-5D (see next section), HUI2/HUI3, the QWBS and the SF-6D; they confined their review to published studies in multiple sclerosis. They reported that the SF-6D had excellent reliability, but showed ceiling and floor effects, was not able to discriminate between moderately and severely disabled patients with multiple sclerosis, had only small to moderate correlations with instruments measuring impairments, and slightly stronger correlations against measures of activity limitations/participation restrictions and health-related QoL.

EQ-5D (EUROQoL)

The EQ-5D (EuroQoL) is a brief, generic, multidimensional health questionnaire (EuroQol Group 1990; Kind 1996). The instrument provides a simple descriptive profile, and was designed to generate a single index value for each health state. It was intended for use as a health outcome and utility measure (www.euroqol.org/about-eq-5d.html – accessed 12 October 2015), and is used in economic evaluations to calculate QALYs. Other preference based measures include the Health Utilities Index, the Quality of Well-Being Scale, and the more recently developed SF-6D. Population norms are available (Kind *et al.* 1999).

The EQ-5D consists of five items covering mobility; self-care; usual activity; pain; anxiety/depression; and a vertical 20 cm visual analogue scale (VAS) for recording an individual's rating of their health. An early version of the scale contained six dimensions as well as some design faults, which were mostly corrected in revisions. The instrument is cognitively simple, and was designed for self-completion.

While the version in widespread use has three response items (or 'levels') per dimension measured, a new five-item response version for each of the same five domains has been developed. This stemmed from a EuroQol Group task force which aimed to find ways of improving the instrument's sensitivity and reducing ceiling effects by increasing the number of severity levels. Thus the EuroQol Group launched their five-level version of the EQ-5D descriptive system, the EQ-5D-5L; this used focus groups to investigate the face and content validity of the new versions, including hypothetical health states generated from those versions. Severity labels for five levels in each dimension were identified using response scaling. The EuroQol Group coordinated a study that administered both the three-level and five-level versions of the EQ-5D, in order to develop a 'crosswalk' between the EQ-5D-3L value sets and the new EQ-5D-5L descriptive system (see http://www.euroqol.org/about-eq-5d/valuation-of-eq-5d/eq-5d-5l-value-sets.html). The calculation of its scoring can be found at http://www.euroqol.org/news-list/article/interim-scoring-for-the-eq-5d-5l-eq-5d-5l-crosswalk-index-value-calculator.html

Content

Section one consists of five single-item dimensions covering mobility, self-care, usual activities, pain/discomfort and anxiety/depression, each with a three – or the new five-point (or 'level') – response scale to indicate the level of problems. The respondent is requested to indicate their health state 'today' by ticking the box next to the response statement that applies to them. This produces a single code (number) for each dimension. One appeal of the scale is its brevity and simplicity. Section two contains a 100-point VAS – thermometer – scale on which respondents are asked to mark an X on the scale to indicate how good or bad their own health is 'today'. The anchors are 0 (worst health you can imagine) to 100 (best health you can imagine). The five domains and paraphrased summary of response categories from the EQ-5D-5L are shown in Box 4.13.

Box 4.13 The five single-item dimensions in the EQ-5D-5L English version, with paraphrased responses

Mobility: problems walking about (no problems to unable to do)

Self-care: problems washing or dressing self (no problems to unable to do)

Usual activities: problems doing usual activities (no problems to unable to do)

Pain/discomfort: degree of pain/discomfort (none to extreme)

Anxiety/depression: not anxious/depressed to extremely

Registration for use is required, licensing fees for use may apply. Contact: The EuroQol Group Association ('The EuroQol Group'), http://www.euroqol.org/, http://www.euroqol.org/register-to-use-eq-5d.html, http://www.euroqol.org/eq-5d-products/how-to-obtain-eq-5d.html, accessed 27 November 2015.

Scoring

The descriptive data from section one can be used to provide health-related QoL profiles across the five dimensions. It can also be used to generate a weighted health index, based on tables of values derived from samples of the general population. The VAS score can be used to analyse changes in health status of individuals or groups over time.

The EQ-5D health states may be converted to a single summary (EQ-5D index) by applying scores from a standard set of population values. For example, the UK EQ-5D index tariff, based on data from a population sample in the UK, links a single index value to the health states described by the EQ-5D (Dolan *et al.* 1996; Dolan 1997). Population values for a subset of health states defined by the EQ-5D are also available for several other countries.

Validity and reliability

Much of the evidence on the psychometric properties of the EQ-5D relates to previous versions. A population survey in Sweden showed that the EuroQol mean health state scores were associated with socioeconomic status in the expected direction, and discriminated between disease groups (Burström *et al.* 2001). Dorman *et al.* (1997a,

1997b) reported results from patients registered in a UK stroke trial, who were randomized to follow-up with either the EuroQol or the SF-36. Response to both instruments was about 50 per cent. Respondents to the EuroQol reported dependency in activities of daily living (ADL) significantly more often than patients responding to the SF-36. While the authors interpreted this as evidence of greater dependency among EuroQol responders, it is possible that the result might reflect the brevity of the EuroQol scale, which inevitably results in loss of information and sensitivity. Insinga and Fryback (2003) reported a lack of correspondence between the EuroQol health state descriptions and their respondents' actual health experiences, probably because the EQ-5D descriptions are too sparse to capture health states accurately. They suggested that assigning new health state levels or dimensions may improve the scale.

Luo *et al.* (2003) compared the results of the EQ-5D, the SF-36 and the Health Utilities Index mark 3 (HUI3) in patients with rheumatic diseases. They found that patients who reported no problems with mobility on the EQ-5D reported different levels of difficulty with ambulation on the HUI3. In explanation, they concluded that the instruments measure slightly different, although related, dimensions of health. It has suffered from moderate to low response rates in a number of population surveys, is highly skewed and has relatively poor sensitivity (Brazier *et al.* 1993a, 1993b), particularly in relation to disease-based outcomes research (Casellas *et al.* 2000; Selai *et al.* 2000).

Kuspinar and Mayo (2014) reviewed and compared the psychometric properties of the EQ-5D, HUI2/HUI3, the QWBS and the SF-6D in multiple sclerosis. They reported that the EQ-5D had excellent reliability, although, in contrast to the HUI3, it failed to discriminate between mildly and moderately disabled patients. The EQ-5D demonstrated small to moderate correlations with measures of impairments, and slightly stronger correlations with measures of activity limitations/participation restrictions and health-related QoL.

Test-retest reliability correlations for previous versions of the EQ-5D ranged between 0.69 and 0.94 (Uyl-de-Groot *et al.* 1994; Van Agt *et al.* 1994). Other research indicates that the instrument is highly skewed with large ceiling effects (Brazier *et al.* 1992, 1993a, 1993b). It is also possible that the length of the thermometer scale (0–100) is biasing, and the time referent is also very short ('today'). It is frequently criticized (Carr-Hill 1992; Jenkinson and McGee 1998). The EuroQol Group has recognized methodological problems with the EuroQol and has worked to improve it (Brooks 1996), although no further revisions are imminent at present.

The EuroQol is available in several languages. It is in the public domain and, on registration, can be used without charge for non-commercial research. Information about the EuroQol can be found at www.euroqol.org/about-eq-5d.html (accessed 27 November 2015).

THE DARTMOUTH COOP FUNCTION CHARTS

These charts were developed by a collaborative body of medical doctors in community settings who aimed to produce a simple, concise, valid and reliable instrument that could be used easily during doctor–patient consultations.

The original US version of the charts contains nine sections (or charts): three on functioning (social, physical and role functioning), two on symptoms (pain and emotional condition), three on perceptions (change in health, overall health and quality of life) and one on social support (Nelson *et al.* 1983, 1987, 1990a, 1990b; Nelson and Berwick 1989). The World Organization of Family Doctors (WONCA) selected the charts as an international set of approved self-administration instruments for measuring health and functional status in primary care consultations, and called them the Dartmouth COOP Functional Health Assessment Charts/WONCA (abbreviated as the COOP/WONCA charts) (Scholten and van Weel 1992; van Weel *et al.* 1995). A feasibility study was launched in seven countries by WONCA (Landgraf and Nelson 1992). The instrument was revised and comprised six, not nine, charts, and each chart was renamed: physical fitness, feelings, daily activities, social activities, change in health and overall health. The pain, QoL and social support charts were not included in the WONCA version. Other revisions were made to the question wording and response categories (van Weel and Scholten 1992). The history of the development of the charts has been summarized by Anderson *et al.* (1993). A manual is available from the developer's website (http://www.ph3c.org/4daction/w3_CatVisu/en/the-coop-/wonca-charts.html?wDocID-150).

Content

The full, original US version contains three charts on functioning (social, physical and role functioning), two on symptoms (pain and emotional condition), three on perceptions (change in health, overall health and quality of life) and one on social support. The Dartmouth Coop Project website now describes its structure as four charts on specific dimensions of function (physical endurance, emotional health, role function, social function), three on overall well-being (overall health, change in health, level of pain), and two on QoL (overall QoL, social resources/support) (see http://dartmouthcoopproject.org/coopcharts_overview.html, accessed 24 August 2015).

As mentioned earlier the WONCA version contains six, not nine, charts, and each chart was renamed: physical fitness, feelings, daily activities, social activities, change in health and overall health. Each chart contains a title, a question referring to the status of the patient, and an ordinal level five-point response scale, ranging from 'No limitation at all (1)' to 'Severely limited (5)', each illustrated with a drawing. Each item is rated on the five-point scale.

The original US charts took the last four weeks as the time reference period for each question, but the WONCA version takes two weeks (e.g. 'During the past two weeks . . . What was the hardest physical activity you could do for at least two minutes?'). Each chart has its own five-point Likert response choices (e.g. in response to the previous example of an item, the responses are: 'very heavy (for example) run, at a fast pace (1)' to 'very light (for example) walk, at a slow pace or not able to walk (5)'; 'no difficulty at all' to 'could not do'; 'much better' to 'much worse'). The problem with this particular chart is that the examples of the activities within each response item (run, jog, walk) do not all fit logically or sensibly with the response item descriptors (very heavy to very light): how does one run in a way that is 'very heavy'? How can the inability to walk logically equate with the response code 'very light'? The response codes conjure up images of strength rather than mobility. This leads to conceptual confusion. The other five charts do not suffer from this problem.

Illustrations (stick figures, faces and symbols-plus-minus and arrow signs) are included on each chart, to illustrate the response choices (Nelson *et al.* 1987). These were developed for use with the original charts to enhance the attractiveness and appeal of the scale to respondents (Nelson *et al.* 1987), and were also regarded as helpful in the WONCA version when used with populations with a high degree of illiteracy (van Weel *et al.* 1995). The charts are self-administered. The physical fitness question (WONCA version) is shown in Box 4.14.

Box 4.14 Examples from the Dartmouth COOP charts

Physical fitness chart:

During the past two weeks . . .

What was the hardest physical activity you could do for at least two minutes?

Very heavy (for example) run, at a fast pace

Heavy (for example) jog, at a slow pace

Moderate (for example) walk, at a fast pace

Light (for example) walk, at a medium pace

Very light (for example) walk, at a slow pace or not able to walk

© 2012-2013 Dartmouth CO-OP Project. All Rights Reserved. Source: Dartmouth COOP Functional Health Assessment Charts/WONCA. A handbook is available. Contact information http://dartmouthcoopproject.org/coopcharts_overview.html

---

Scoring

The scoring on each chart has 1 equalling the best, and 5 equalling the worst level of functioning. Each chart represents a distinct domain and the charts are not summed together to form an overall score (Nelson *et al.* 1990a, 1990b). The administration time for the nine charts was five minutes. The charts have been translated into 20 languages.

The developers initially advised investigators to use descriptive statistics (frequency distributions) to present results for the charts, and not to compute means, standard deviations or other statistical measures, because the charts are based on ordinal scales. However, investigators tend to assume they can be translated into interval level scales. The developers now accept this development; it is a common trend in the analysis of all health status scales.

Validity

The original Dartmouth charts were initially tested on over 1,400 patients with different groups of conditions from four medical centres in the USA (Nelson et al. 1987). Studies undertaken since, based on the Dartmouth version, have reported the charts to be suitable for use as clinical outcome measures and responsive to changes in back pain and in levels of physical fitness and ability in people aged 65 and over (Wollstadt et al. 1997; Bronfort and Bouter 1999; Aure et al. 2003).

In The Netherlands, the WONCA version was tested on over 5,000 patients, and their population norms have been published (Scholten and van Weel 1992; van Weel et al. 1995). The testing procedures for the WONCA version have been briefly summarized by van Weel and Scholten (1992) and van Weel et al. (1995). In support of the convergent validity of the WONCA version, the charts on functioning and feelings have been reported to correlate well with other measures of physical and emotional functioning respectively, such as the Barthel Index and the Zung Depression Scale (Schuling and Meyboom-de Jong 1992). The psychometric testing of the WONCA version of the scale among two populations in The Netherlands (one with an average age of 43, and the other aged 60 and over) reported that, in the younger age group, the physical fitness chart and the daily activities chart correlated moderately to moderately well with the physical mobility subscale of the Nottingham Health Profile, at 0.53 and 0.66 respectively, and with the RAND SF-36 physical functioning subscale at 0.52 and 0.55 respectively. The feelings chart correlated moderately well with Goldberg's General Health Questionnaire (0.63) and with the mental health subscale of the RAND SF-36 (0.71). The overall health chart correlated moderately well with the general health subscale of the RAND SF-36 (0.62). The results for the group aged 60 and over were weaker. Only the comparisons with the RAND SF-36 was reported for this group. The physical fitness chart and the daily activities chart correlated weakly to moderately with the physical functioning subscale of the SF-36 (0.56 and 0.31 respectively); the feelings chart correlated more strongly with the mental health subscale of the SF-36 (0.76); the overall health chart correlated moderately well with the general health subscale of the SF-36 (0.67). Responsiveness to change was investigated using data from four longitudinal Dutch studies. These showed that the charts differ in responsiveness to change by diagnosis (van Weel et al. 1995). The evidence on responsiveness to change is limited, although studies have indicated that the charts are responsive to improvements in elderly patients with a range of conditions (van Weel et al. 1995).

The performance of single charts is less precise in detecting differences in functional status than multi-item health status scales, although the full set of charts perform well together in comparison with the RAND Medical Outcomes Study short form measures (Meyboom-de Jong and Smith 1990), and show higher levels of sensitivity than Hunt et al.'s (1986) Nottingham Health Profile (Coates and Wilkin 1992). The influence of the illustrations in increasing sensitivity, rather than biasing respondents in some way, particularly in different cultural settings, is uncertain (McHorney *et al.* 1992). Jenkinson *et al.* (2002) reported that the illustrations had no impact on survey response rates.

Reliability

Test-retest correlations at four weeks in a German study were reported to be modest at 0.42–0.62 (van de Lisdonk and van Weel 1992). These results echo the low test-retest correlations reported for the original charts (Meyboom-de Jong and Smith 1990). In a Dutch study, with an interval of three weeks, they were stronger at 0.67–0.82, with a kappa of 0.49–0.59; and over one year they were 0.36–0.72, with a kappa of 0.31–0.38 (Meyboom-de Jong and Smith 1990).

The inter-chart correlations for the WONCA version range between 0.15 and 0.66 (van Weel *et al.* 1995). Multi-trait multi-method analysis has reported that the physical and role functioning charts are highly correlated, suggesting a common domain, while the emotional status and social support charts are more independent, suggesting that they are measuring different domains of functioning (Landgraf *et al.* 1990).

Despite their popularity in studies based in general practice (Harvey *et al.* 1998), the charts have not yet been satisfactorily tested for their psychometric properties, and details of the research design on which the testing has been based are often lacking (see review by Anderson *et al.* 1993). The deliberate omission of pain, social support and QoL from the short WONCA version, in the interests of brevity, is regrettable, particularly in view of the current emphasis on including a specific self-assessment of QoL in broader health status scales. The charts also suffer from the same disadvantage as single-item measures: they are limited in content and therefore potentially in their sensitivity. Anderson *et al.* (1993) concluded that the content validity of the physical fitness chart, for example, is too restricted in scope to be sensitive to disability in older people.

The psychometric testing of the adapted charts is a constant process under the umbrella of WONCA (van Weel *et al.* 1995). The charts are available in over 20 languages. The COOP/WONCA charts may be used for research and clinical care. Permission to use the COOP/WONCA charts specifically excludes the right to distribute, reproduce or share them in any form for commercial purposes.

THE McGILL PAIN QUESTIONNAIRE (MPQ)

Pain comprises an important, and often neglected, domain of health status measurement, and thus the MPQ is included here. Apart from various single-item VAS, in which horizontal or vertical lines, anchored at each end by descriptors, such as 'No pain' to 'Pain as bad as can be' are presented to people to mark the level of their pain, or numeric rating scales (a numbered version of the VAS, where people select a number to represent their pain) (see Hawker *et al.* 2011 for overview), the MPQ is the most frequently used and most tested measure of pain. It is commonly used to evaluate the effectiveness of pain interventions.

The MPQ was designed to measure present, perceived pain in adults, specifically the sensory, affective and evaluative dimensions of pain and intensity in adults with chronic pain. The MPQ consists principally of lists of terms describing the quality and intensity of pain. Melzack and Torgerson (1971) selected 102 words describing pain from the literature and sorted them into the categories of sensory, affective and evaluative words describing intensity; the results were then checked by 20 reviewers. Further testing among 140 students, 20 physicians and 20 patients led to the current 78-item format of the scale and the scale values. The MPQ comprises four subscales measuring sensory, affective, evaluative and other miscellaneous aspects of pain. These form the Pain Rating Index, which contains 78 words describing pain categorized into 20 sub-categories. Each includes two to six words within sensory, affective, evaluative and miscellaneous pain. There is an additional pain intensity scale item.

The completion of the full-length scale takes up to 15–20 minutes, depending on the familiarity of the patients with the words. The scale is interviewer administered in order to define the words.

Content

Examples of some of the words respondents are asked to choose from to describe their pain are shown in Box 4.15.

Box 4.15 Examples from the MPQ

Pain descriptors

Flickering
Quivering
Pulsing
Throbbing
Beating
Pounding

MPQ © Ronald Melzack, 1975. All rights reserved. Melzack R. (1975) The McGill Pain Questionnaire: major properties and scoring methods. *Pain*, 1: 277–99. With permission of Mapi Research Trust and the author. Contact information and permission to use: Mapi Research Trust, Lyon, France. E-mail: PROinformation@mapi-trust.org; https://eprovide.mapi-trust.org/, accessed 21 July 2016.

In addition to descriptors of pain, course over time is included, and the location of the pain is assessed with a drawing of a body with the words 'external' and 'internal' added.

Scoring

Each description carries a weight corresponding to the severity of the pain, according to evaluations of appropriate ordinal rankings by panels of doctors, patients and students.

People then receive pain scores according to the number of descriptive items they select to describe their pain and their assigned weights (0 = no pain; 1 = mild pain; 2 = discomforting; 3 = distressing; 4 = horrible; 5 = excruciating). The scores then generate the four subscales which were differentiated by factor analysis. These include sensory and evaluative subscales to designate perception of pain, an affective subscale to denote emotional response to pain, and the fourth miscellaneous subscale. These four subscales result in four scores. The four scores add up to a total score (the pain rating index).

There are four possible and distinct scoring methods ranging from the number of words chosen to the sum of the scale values (based on the scale weights) for all the words selected in a given category or across all categories (Melzack 1975). Full details of the scale were published by Melzack and Katz (1992).

Validity

Dubuisson and Melzack (1976) reported that the MPQ was able to correctly classify 77 per cent of 95 patients with eight pain syndromes into diagnostic groups on the basis of their verbal description of pain. Other research on patients with facial pain has shown that the scale can correctly predict diagnosis for 90 per cent of patients (Melzack *et al.* 1986). Correlations between MPQ score and visual analogue ratings for 40 patients ranged from 0.50 to 0.65 (Melzack 1975). The specificity of the measure was demonstrated by Greenwald (1987) in a study of 536 cancer patients.

The short version correlates consistently highly with the long version of the MPQ (Melzack 1987). It has also been shown to be sensitive to treatment for pain among patients with sciatic pain (Eisenberg *et al.* 2003), and was selected as one of the most psychometrically sound measures of pain in a review of instruments by Nemeth *et al.* (2003).

There is support from results of principal components analysis for the distinction between affective and sensory dimensions of pain, but less for a distinctive evaluative component (Reading 1979; Prieto and Geisinger 1983). Lowe *et al.* (1991) supported the basic three-factor structure of the scale, using more sophisticated analytic procedures and a large sample.

Reliability

Melzack (1975) reported a test-retest study, based on just 10 patients who completed the scale three times at intervals of three to seven days between each. The average consistency of response was reported to be 70.3 per cent. The test-retest reliability for the 20 categories of pain descriptors, the three specific subscales and the total score have been reported to range from weak to moderately good (Reading *et al.* 1982; Love *et al.* 1989).

The measure is the leading measure of pain. Cross-cultural applications of the full scale have been reviewed by Naughton and Wiklund (1993). It has been translated into several languages (Melzack and Katz 1992). It is more often used for the measurement of chronic, rather than acute, pain, as it is generally believed that most single-item VAS work adequately for acute pain (McQuay 1990). There is some evidence supporting its ability to detect change in post-operative pain (Jenkinson *et al.* 1995).

SHORT-FORM McGILL PAIN QUESTIONNAIRE (SF-MPQ)

Several versions of the MPQ scale exist, including a short version which consists of 15 items, and takes two to five minutes to complete (Melzack 1987), and is also interviewer administered. It was developed as a multidimensional measure of perceived pain in adults.

The SF-MPQ includes 15 items from the full MPQ: throbbing, shooting, stabbing, sharp, cramping, gnawing, hot-burning, aching, heavy, tender, splitting, tiring-exhausting, sickening, fearful, punishing-cruel. The 15 words included in the scale were chosen by more than one-third of patients with different types of pain (Melzack 1975).

They form a sensory subscale (11 words) and affective sub-scale (four words). They are rated on a four-point intensity scale: 0 (none), 1 (mild), 2 (moderate), 3 (severe). The SF-MPQ includes a present pain intensity item, and a VAS scale item to rate average pain.

Internal consistency is acceptable, although test-retest reliability correlations have varied from 0.45 to over 0.90 (with higher correlations achieved at shorter test-retest intervals) (Grafton *et al.* 2005; Strand *et al.* 2008; and see overview in Hawker *et al.* 2011). There is evidence of its responsiveness to clinically important changes after rehabilitation and surgery in a Norwegian version (Strand *et al.* 2008). More evidence on its reliability and validity is still needed. It has been translated into several languages (see Hawker *et al.* 2011).

In 2009 the measure was revised (SF-MPQ-2) for use with neuropathic and non-neuropathic pain patients (Dworkin *et al.* 2009). It included seven further condition-specific symptoms, with a total of 22 items, and 0–10 numeric response choices. Further psychometric evaluation is still needed.

EXAMPLE

An example of the use of measures of health status is shown in Box 4.16.

Box 4.16 Example of comparative study using health status measures

Riazi *et al.* (2003b) aimed to examine the relative impact of multiple sclerosis and Parkinson's disease on health status.

Their sample included 638 people with multiple sclerosis and 227 patients with Parkinson's disease. Health status was measured with the Medical Outcomes Study

36-item Short Form Survey (now known as the RAND SF-36) with population norms for the UK.

Scores for the eight health domains of this SF-36 were compared between patient groups after controlling for age, sex, disease duration, mobility, social class, ethnicity, education, marital status and employment status.

They reported that people with multiple sclerosis and those with Parkinson's disease had significantly worse health status than the general population on each of the eight domains.

While the relative impact of both conditions was similar, multiple sclerosis resulted in poorer physical functioning scores and better mental health scores compared with the other group of patients. They also reported that patients with mild multiple sclerosis, and who walked without an aid, had worse scores on all dimensions than the general UK population.

They concluded cautiously that, while generic measures are applicable across different disease groups, they may fail to address clinically important aspects of the impacts of specific disorders.

CHAPTER 5

MEASURING PSYCHOLOGICAL ILL-BEING AND DISTRESS

CHAPTER COVERAGE

PSYCHOLOGICAL ILL-BEING AND DISTRESS

In previous editions of this book, this chapter was called 'Measures of psychological well-being'. However, the measures included were negative in focus (depression, anxiety, psychological morbidity and mental confusion) – in effect measuring psychological ill-being and distress. In response to feedback, this chapter has been relabelled to reflect the more negative content of these measures, and, for greater consistency, the focus is only on measures of depression, anxiety and general psychological disorder.

There have been calls in the area of psychological, or mental, well-being for a greater focus on measurement of positive psychological states, and not solely psychological distress (Winefield *et al.* 2012). The positive states often suggested in the literature (Ryff and Singer 1996) are included within the concept of subjective well-being, and are presented separately in Chapter 7 ('Measuring the dimensions of subjective well-being'). It should be noted that they are not the polar opposites of the concepts and measures included in this chapter.

There are numerous scales of psychological ill-being and distress, in particular those which are aimed specifically at detecting more common conditions such as anxiety and depression. The reliability of the classifications of many such scales has been questioned.

Gold standards for diagnostic categorization have been developed over the years, including the revised *Diagnostic and Statistical Manual* (DSM-V) of the American Psychiatric Association (2013) and the *International Classification of Diseases* (10th revision) (World Health Organization 2004), and some highly regarded diagnostic instruments such as the Present State Examination (revised) and the Research Diagnostic Criteria (Wing *et al.* 1974; Spitzer *et al.* 1978; Wing 1991). However, these still fail to account realistically for features of personality or physical illness which may intervene.

The following sections review the most popular and easily administered scales of common psychiatric disorders in current use: anxiety, depression and general psychological disorder.

Some of the broader health status scales also include sections or batteries on mental health, for example the RAND Batteries (depression screener) and the SF-36 mental functioning dimension and summary scale (see Chapter 4). It should be noted that because of culture-specific concepts and values, for such measures to have cross-cultural applicability careful translations (including back-translations), assessments for cultural equivalence, adaptations and repeated psychometric testing are required.

DEPRESSION

The term 'depression' is generally used to cover a wider range of psychological disturbances. There is little confusion about the recognition of a severe state, sometimes called a psychosis, but milder degrees of the condition lack definition. Sometimes the term 'depressive neurosis' is used but a variety of concepts are associated with this term. Wing *et al.* (1974) have provided the most succinct definitions of psychopathological terms, and in an attempt to clarify the issues of terminology their definitions of depressive states relate to depressed mood, recent loss of interest, self-depreciation, hopelessness and observed depression. There are a number of additional definitions provided for neglect due to brooding, subjective anergia, slowness and under-activity, inefficient thinking, poor concentration, suicidal plans or acts, morning depression, social withdrawal, guilt and other related symptoms.

Wide discrepancies in the early literature on estimates of the prevalence of mental illness in different communities were largely the consequence of the use of different diagnostic criteria. The development and use of standardized research instruments linked to clearly stated diagnostic criteria led to less variation between studies. However, considerable differences still exist between measures with the implication that comparisons between studies can be made only if two studies have utilized the same basic measurement scale.

Many research studies have based the definition of a 'case' of depression on a certain score having been attained on one of the large number of depression rating scales. The different construction of these scales and the different individual items they include create major difficulties in comparing studies, unless they have been developed in relation to clear criteria such as the DSM-V (American Psychiatric Association 2013).

The majority of depression rating scales contain a diverse collection of symptoms, attitudes and feelings and will produce high prevalence rates and a large proportion of false positives if case detection relies upon them (Snaith 1987). Kutner *et al.* (1985), who studied depression and anxiety in dialysis patients, found that scales containing disease-related items yielded exaggerated scores.

ZUNG'S SELF-RATING DEPRESSION SCALE (ZSDS)

This scale was developed by Zung (1965). It was constructed on the basis of the clinical diagnostic criteria most commonly used to characterize depressive disorders. It aims to screen for affective, psychological and somatic symptoms of depression. Factor-analysis-derived symptom clusters led to the selection of 20 items covering 'pervasive affect', 'physiological equivalents or concomitants' and 'psychological concomitants'. The scale is simple to complete and takes about 10 minutes.

Content

The scale contains 20 statements; 10 are worded symptomatically positive and 10 are worded symptomatically negative. Respondents are asked how the listed statements apply to them. Administration is by self-completion and completion time is 'a few minutes' (Zung *et al.* 1965). Examples are shown in Box 5.1.

Box 5.1 Examples from the ZSDS

I have trouble sleeping at night.
I eat as much as I used to.
I notice I am losing weight.
I have trouble with constipation.
My heart beats faster than usual.
I feel hopeful about the future.
I find it easy to make decisions.

There are four choices of response category, with numerical values of 1–4 respectively: none or a little of the time; some of the time; a good part of the time; most of the time.

Scoring

Each item scores 1–4. The score values for the 20 items are summed. An index is derived by dividing the sum of the raw scores by the maximum possible score of 80, converted to a decimal and multiplied by 100 (Zung et al. 1965). The need to transform the scores has been questioned by Gurtman (1985).

The interpretation of scores is based on norms, which are given in the scale's manual. Below 50 = normal, 50–59 = minimal to mild depression, 60–69 = moderate to marked depression, 69+ = severe to extreme depression. The norms for these scores were based on adults aged 20–64 and may not be appropriate for younger or older people. The cut-off points are not agreed, and investigators have adopted a range of cut-offs from 50 to 60.

Zung et al. (1965) reported that the mean score on the ZSDS for outpatients diagnosed as depressive reaction was 64. Zung (1965) reported that the mean score for hospitalized inpatients diagnosed with depressive disorders was 74. Hagg et al. (2003), on the basis of a clinical trial of treatment and a study of the clinical meaning of score changes, estimated the minimal clinically important difference of Zung scores to be 8 units, not exceeding the tolerance interval of 8–9 units. They concluded that the Zung might therefore require an increase in scores in order to exceed the 95 per cent tolerance interval when used in clinical decision-making, and for the calculation of statistical power when estimating sample size.

Altogether over half of the items of this widely used depression scale are composed of feelings or symptoms which do not necessarily indicate the presence of a psychological disorder, and Kutner et al. (1985) found that these disease items led to an exaggerated score.

Validity

Zung et al. (1965) tested the scale for validity using the Minnesota Multiphasic Personality Inventory as a gold standard. They administered the scale to new psychiatric outpatients at Duke University (number not specified). The correlations between their instrument and three subscales of the Minnesota Inventory were: 0.70, 0.68 and 0.13. The authors commented that the latter correlation was 'unexpectedly low'. Brown and Zung (1972) tested the scale against the Hamilton Depression Scale and reported a correlation of 0.79. The convergent validity of the Zung scale, when tested against with physicians' judgements, was lower than that achieved by the Comprehensive Assessment and Referral Evaluation (CARE), 0.65 (kappa 0.29), in comparison with 0.73 (kappa 0.46) (Toner et al. 1988).

Davies et al. (1975) reported a correlation between the Zung and Hamilton Scale of $r = 0.62$, between the Zung and the Beck Depression Scale of $r = 0.73$, and between the Zung and a visual analogue scale (VAS) of $r = 0.62$. Biggs et al. (1978) reported a correlation between the Zung and the Hamilton of $r = 0.80$, although the correlation was lowest at greatest severity levels. In comparison with clinical ratings of severity,

Biggs *et al.* (1978) reported a correlation with the Zung of 0.69, with differences at higher severity. Toner *et al.* (1988) reported a similar correlation against psychiatric judgements at r = 0.65. The scale is also able to distinguish between patients with a confirmed diagnosis of a depressive state and patients with an initial diagnosis of depression, but subsequently reviewed and given another psychiatric diagnosis (Zung 1965, 1967). Zung *et al.* (1965) reported the scale was able to distinguish reliably between patients with psychoneurotic depression and those with an anxiety reaction and found the instrument sensitive to clinical change. Gallegos-Orozco *et al.* (2003) also reported that patients categorized as depressed had poorer scores on the Short Form-36 questionnaire (a measure of broader health status), thus supporting its construct validity.

Toner *et al.* (1988) reported that the convergent validity of the Zung scale, when tested against physicians' judgements, was lower than that of the well-tested CARE scale, 0.65 (kappa 0.29) in comparison with 0.73 (kappa 0.46). Also, Carroll *et al.* (1973) assessed patients known to have varying degrees of depression and reported that the Zung scale was unable to distinguish between the groups; they reported a correlation of 0.41 between interview-based and Zung ratings. Carroll *et al.* (1973) blame the self-report method rather than the Zung scale, as the former adopts a different perspective to a psychiatric interview. Other studies have found the ZSDS to be unresponsive to changes in treatment patterns (Hamilton 1976). Arfwidsson *et al.* (1974) cast doubt on the validity of the scale, and argued that doctors' ratings are more valid (i.e. unbiased) as a means of assessing the degree and quality of depressive symptoms.

The instrument was designed to be unidimensional, although a factor analysis by Morris *et al.* (1975) confirmed two dimensions: agitation and self-satisfaction. Blumenthal's (1975) factor analysis of the scale yielded four subscales: a well-being index, a depressed mood index, an optimism index and a somatic symptoms index. Cross-cultural applications have been reviewed by Naughton and Wiklund (1993).

Romera *et al.* (2008) analysed the factor structure of the scale in a large primary care patient sample (total 1,049) across Spain. Confirmatory factor analysis yielded a clinically interpretable four-factor solution: a *core depressive* factor; a *cognitive* factor; an *anxiety* factor; and a *somatic* factor, accounting for 36.9 per cent of the variance on the ZSDS; this four-factor structure was further validated. In contrast, Fountoulakis *et al.* (2001) examined the properties of the ZDRS in 40 depressed people and 120 normal comparison participants in Greece, and reported that factor analysis revealed five factors: anxiety-depression, thought content, somatic symptoms, irritability and social-interpersonal functioning. Further analysis of factor structure is required.

Reliability

Zung (1986) reported split half correlations of 0.92. Knight *et al.* (1983) reported a coefficient of 0.79. The scale has been used successfully with clustering techniques by Byrne (1978). Kaszmak and Allender (1985) suggest that it is unsuitable for use with elderly people because of the large number of somatic items. Also, response rates for self-completed scales may be lower than for administered scales. A comparative study of Zung's scale with the short version of CARE showed a response rate of 65 per cent for

Zung and 100 per cent for CARE. Among the reasons for non-response were visual problems (28 per cent), illiteracy (9 per cent) and lack of motivation (34 per cent) (Toner *et al.* 1988). These response difficulties apply to all self-rating scales.

Fountoulakis *et al.*'s (2001) study of the sensitivity, specificity and reliability of the Greek version of the ZSDS, included test-retesting at one to two days. They reported that the calculation of sensitivity and specificity at various cut-off levels was satisfactory (both exceeded 90.00 at cut-off levels 44/45), test-retest reliability was good for the total score (r = 0.92) and internal consistency was high (total score, Cronbach's alpha = 0.09).

The scale is popular because it is short and easy to complete. Zung (1972) developed an observer-rated scale to complement the Zung, although Thompson (1989), in line with most reviewers of the scale, reported that it has no advantages.

MONTGOMERY-ASBERG DEPRESSION RATING SCALE (MADRS)

Observer rating scales are often used in medical treatment trials for depression for patient selection and clinical assessment of outcome (Demyttenaere and Fruyt 2003). The MADRS is used for assessing the severity of depression, and changes during medical treatment for depression.

The original MADRS did not list any questions for clinicians to use when rating items. The MADRS was developed by Montgomery and Asberg (1979) on the basis of 54 English and 52 Swedish patients who completed a 65-item psychopathology scale. Analysis identified the 17 most commonly occurring symptoms in depressive illness in the sample. Subsequent analyses, using 64 patients on different types of antidepressive drugs, were then used to create a 10-item depression rating scale which consisted of those items showing the greatest changes with treatment.

This scale is oriented towards psychic symptoms and covers apparent sadness, reported sadness, inability to feel, difficulty in concentration, inner tension, pessimistic thoughts, suicidal thoughts, lassitude, reduced sleep and reduced appetite. The scale's advantage lies in its brevity and ease of use by raters.

Content

The scale's 10 items encompass the most commonly occurring symptoms of depressive illness which change in response to treatment (see above). Examples are shown in Box 5.2.

Box 5.2 Examples from the MADRS

Apparent sadness: representing despondency, gloom and despair (more than just ordinary transient low spirits), reflected in speech, facial expression and posture. Rate by depth and inability to brighten up:

0 No sadness.
1
2 Looks dispirited but does brighten up without difficulty.

3

4   Appears sad and unhappy most of the time.

5

6   Looks miserable all the time. Extremely despondent.

Pessimistic thoughts: representing thoughts of guilt, inferiority, self-reproach, sinfulness, remorse and ruin.

0   No pessimistic thoughts.

1

2   Fluctuating ideas of failure, self-reproach or self-depreciation.

3

4   Persistent self-accusation, or definite but still rational ideas of guilt or sin. Increasingly pessimistic about the future.

5

6   Delusions of ruin, remorse or unredeemable sin. Self-accusations which are absurd and unshakeable.

With permission of the developer and the Royal College of Psychiatrists. © 1979 The Royal College of Psychiatrists. Montgomery, S.A. and Åsberg, M. (1979) A new depression scale designed to be sensitive to change. *British Journal of Psychiatry*, 134: 382–9. Written permission must be obtained from the Royal College of Psychiatrists for copying and distribution to others or for republication (in print, online or by any other medium). Private clinical use does not require permission. Permission for use in research protocols should be sought from Professor Stuart Montgomery at stuart@samontgomery.co.uk. The MADRS is downloadable at: https://outcometracker.org/scales_library.php. See scale information at: https://eprovide.mapi-trust.org/ accessed 21 July 2016.

Scoring

Scoring involves computing of scale items. The procedure involves arriving at a definition of a case by adding up numbers derived from a severity-grade score of a number of symptoms.

Zimmerman *et al.* (2004) pointed out that various cut-offs have been employed in antidepressant efficacy trials to define remission, although little empirical work has been carried out to determine the validity of various thresholds. They suggested that a valid cut-off score for defining remission could be established by determining whether a person's level of symptoms fell within the normal range of values after treatment. They reviewed the relevant literature, although as they pointed out it was of variable quality, and across all studies included in their review the mean (+/− SD) weighted MADRS score, adjusting for sample size, was 4.0 (5.8) (95 per cent confidence interval 3.5–4.5). They concluded this result is consistent with their research indicating the validity of different cut-offs to define remission with the MADRS. Based on a narrow definition of remission (a complete absence of clinically significant symptoms of depression) the optimal MADRS cut-off was < or = 4, while based on a broader definition, the optimal cut-off was < or = 9.

Validity

Montgomery and Asberg (1979) tested scale scores against psychiatrists' judgements, using 18 patients who responded to treatment and 17 who did not. The scale was able to discriminate between the two groups. The scale was also tested against the Hamilton Depression Scale with a reported correlation of 0.70. Kearns *et al.* (1982) reported that the scale was able to distinguish between different levels of severity, and performed as well as the Hamilton Depression Scale. Snaith and Taylor (1985) reported a high correlation between the scale and the depression scale of their self-rated Hospital Anxiety and Depression (HAD) scale (0.81), although the correlation with the anxiety scale of the HAD was low (0.37). Cooper and Fairburn (1986) found that a group of bulimic and a group of depressed patients had similar scores on the MADRS but different symptoms, or scale items, contributed strongly to the overall score in the two groups. However, 30 per cent of the total score is apparently accounted for by three items which all commonly occur in physical illnesses and states of distress other than depression (Williams 1984; Cooper and Fairburn 1986).

Khan *et al.* (2002) reported the use of the MADRS and the Hamilton Depression Scale, in a retrospective record review of over 200 adults with depression who had been participants in clinical trials, and assigned to antidepressant or placebo treatment. The effect size of the MADRS was 0.53, which was similar to the Hamilton's effect size. The authors concluded that the scales were similar in terms of sensitivity, regardless of type of treatment.

Parker *et al.* (2003) analysed the factor structure of the MADRS with a sample of older patients with depression, and reported that all 10 items loaded <0.60 on a domain. There were three interpretable MADRS factors which reflected geriatric depression dimensions: dysphoric apathy/retardation which comprised five items (apparent sadness, reported sadness, lassitude, reduced concentration, inability to feel); psychic anxiety comprised three items (inner tension, pessimistic thoughts, suicidal thoughts); and vegetative symptoms comprised two items (sleep and appetite). They concluded that the scale may be useable for monitoring treatment outcomes among geriatric patients with depression.

Reliability

Good results for reliability have been reported by the authors and the scale was found to be robust when used by different professionals in a variety of health care settings (GPs, nurses, psychologists, psychiatrists) and high inter-rater correlations were produced. Comparisons between two English raters, two Swedish raters and one English and one Swedish rater, rating 11 to 30 patients, produced correlations of between 0.89 and 0.97 (Montgomery *et al.* 1978).

The MADRS has been used less often for rating depression than the Hamilton, although it is easy to use and Khan *et al.* (2002) recommended it as a desirable rating tool in large-scale clinical trials of treatment for depression. The advantage of observer rating scales, over patients' self-ratings, in treatment trials for depression is that the measure is not biased by the patient's optimism–pessimism or other biases (e.g. people in lower spirits tend to perceive other aspects of life in more negative terms than people in higher spirits). However, there is also a danger in assuming that clinical ratings are unbiased; the MADRS scores might be more accurately interpreted as clinical impressions of depression and change (Mulder *et al.* 2003). Demyttenaere and Fruyt (2003) pointed out that the MADRS and the Hamilton Depression Scale were both developed to evaluate medical therapy (e.g. antidepressant medication) rather than psychotherapy (where patient self-rating scales may be used more often). They also reported that where scales exist in observer and patient rating formats, differences in ratings are found.

Structured and semi-structured interview guides potentially improve the reliability of the MADRS compared with other scales. Thus, Williams and Kobak (2008) assessed the test-retest reliability of a structured interview guide for the MADRS (SIGMA), based on 162 test-retest interviews, conducted by 81 rater pairs. Each patient was interviewed twice, once by each rater conducting an independent interview. They reported that the intraclass correlation for total score between raters using the SIGMA was $r = 0.93$, $P < 0.0001$. All 10 items had good to excellent inter-rater reliability, suggesting the need for further research with this method.

HAMILTON DEPRESSION RATING SCALE

This measure is also referred to as the Hamilton Depression Scale. It has long been the most widely used observer rating scale for depression, and changes after medical treatment. It has been referred to as the gold standard in the assessment of depression, although this status has been questioned by Bagby *et al.* (2004), in their review of 70 studies, due to its variable psychometric properties.

The scale includes assessment of cognitive and behavioural components of depression and is particularly thorough in the assessment of the somatic aspects (Hamilton 1967). Like many depression scales, the Hamilton Depression Scale cannot be used to establish a diagnosis of depression, but only to assess severity once depression has already been diagnosed. It is administered in a semi-structured clinical interview, which requires about 30 minutes (no interview guide is included, although guides have been developed by others and tested with good results – Freedland *et al.* 2002). Interviewer training is required.

Content

The current version of the Hamilton Depression Scale (Hamilton 1959, 1967) consists of 17 items: depressed mood, feelings of guilt, suicidal ideation, work and activities, insight, retardation, agitation, insomnia (early, middle and late), psychic anxiety, somatic anxiety, gastrointestinal symptoms, general somatic symptoms, genital symptoms (loss of libido or menstrual disturbances), hypochondriases and loss of weight. The earlier version of the scale, which is still in use, contained 21 items. Other versions containing 23 and 24 items were also developed. Examples of scale items are shown in Box 5.3.

Box 5.3 Examples from the Hamilton Depression Scale

Depressed mood: 0–4

Gloomy attitude, pessimism about the future
Feeling of sadness
Tendency to weep:
      sadness and/or mild depression
      occasional weeping and/or moderate depression
      frequent weeping and/or severe depression
      extreme symptoms

Anxiety, psychic: 0–4

Tension and irritability
Worrying about minor matters
Apprehensive attitude
Fears

Somatic symptoms, gastrointestinal: 0–2

Loss of appetite
Heavy feelings in abdomen
Constipation

Insight: 0–2

Loss of insight
Partial or doubtful loss
No loss

Source: Hamilton, M. (1960) A rating scale for depression. *Journal of Neurology, Neurosurgery, and Psychiatry*, 23(1): 56–62 – see Appendix II, page 62. With permission. The Hamilton is downloadable at: https://outcometracker.org/scales_library.php, accessed 15 October 2015.

The somatic categories of the scale have been used alone, in conjunction with other depression rating scales. The somatic items relate to muscular, sensory systems and to cardiovascular, respiratory, gastrointestinal, genito-urinary and autonomic symptoms. For example Martin (1987) used these items without the Hamilton depression (psychosomatic) items together with the MADRS.

Scoring

Some items are scored 0–4 and others are scored 0–2. Scale items marked 0–4 have the response choices for the rater of absent (0), mild or trivial (1), moderate (2–3), severe (4); and scale items marked 0–2 have the choice of absent (0), slight or doubtful (1), clearly present (2). Four items, which provide more details of the characteristics of depression, are not included in the original scoring scheme, although some users include them. The interpretation of categories is described by Hamilton (1967) and reproduced by Williams

(1984). The total is the simple sum of responses. The total scores range from 0–100 (representing the sum of two raters' scores or double the score for one rater). Some studies report total scores with a maximum of 50. Hamilton did not provide advice on score cut-offs, although most users use scores of <7 to indicate an absence of depression, 7<17 to indicate mild depression, 18<24 moderate depression, and 25+ severe depression. Variations exist (Bech *et al.* 1986).

Validity

The scale is reported to have high concurrent validity with good agreement with other scales, particularly the Beck, with correlations reported of over 0.70 (Hamilton 1976). Schwab *et al.* (1967) compared the Hamilton with the Beck scale on 153 medical inpatients. The correlation between these two scales was 0.75. Knesevich *et al.* (1977) reported the Hamilton scale correlated 0.68 with a change in global rating on a 10-point scale. Hamer *et al.* (1991) reported that a threshold score of 8 gave a sensitivity of 88 per cent and a positive predictive value of 80 per cent in comparison with diagnoses made with the DSM. Silverstone *et al.* (2002) reported that two items from the 17-item scale – depressed mood (item 1) and psychic anxiety (item 10) – were predictive of treatment response, differentiated between treatment groups, and predicted remission rates in clinical trials of depression.

Tamaklo *et al.* (1992) reported that it correlated highly with the MADRS. However, Montgomery and Asberg (1979) reported the scale to be less sensitive than their own, especially at the severe end, a finding confirmed by Knesevich *et al.* (1977). Carroll *et al.* (1973) reported that the Hamilton scale was better able than the Beck Depression Inventory to distinguish between groups of patients known to have varying degrees of depression. They argued that self-report scales, such as the Beck, overweight subjective scores. The Hamilton scale has also been reported to have a greater effect size for change than the Beck Depression Inventory (Sayer *et al.* 1993), and is frequently reported to be sensitive to treatment (Tollefson and Holman 1993). Hamilton (1967) reported that the scale discriminated between men and women; women generally are more likely to have higher depression scores than men.

However, six of the scale items are symptoms of somatic disturbance and account for 31 per cent of the possible total score; if the insomnia items which so often rate highly in physical illness are included, then 42 per cent of the total is accounted for (Williams 1984). An updated review of 70 studies using the scale by Bagby *et al.* (2004) concluded that its convergent and discriminant validity were adequate, although its content validity was poor.

Although initial factor analyses gave poor results (Hamilton 1960), other factor analyses were more satisfactory (Hamilton 1967; Mowbray 1972; Bech 1981). Dozois (2003) analysed the factor structure of the 17- and a 23-item version of the scale with a sample of undergraduate students. Both versions yielded four factors. A review of factor analyses of the scale showed that it produced between three and seven factors (Berrios and Bulbena-Villarasa 1990). Subsequent factor analysis of the scale yielded a five-dimensional solution, although only the first factor (comprising depressed mood, guilt, suicide, work and interests, agitation, psychic anxiety, somatic anxiety and loss of libido) was well defined and clinically interpretable (Gibbons *et al.* 1993). The updated review of 70 studies using the scale by Bagby *et al.* (2004) reported that, while its factor structure was multidimensional, it had poor replication across samples.

Reliability

Its inter-rater reliability is reported to be good: correlations are high ranging from 0.84 to 0.98 (Hamilton 1976; Knesevich *et al.* 1977; Rehm 1981). Muller and Dragicevic (2003) tested the inter-rater reliability with clinically inexperienced raters, after three standardized training sessions, and reported moderately high rates (kappa = 0.57–0.73) for the total and for the items.

Results for the internal consistency of the scale have been variable (Bech 1981). Schwab *et al.* (1967), on the basis of a study of 153 medical inpatients, reported that it had higher internal consistency than the Beck Depression Inventory. However, Potts *et al.* (1990) reported research which showed that the scale has a high degree of scale reliability. However, they did point out that it has been criticized for its lower item reliability and its heavy reliance on the expertise of the interviewer. Bagby *et al.* (2004), on the basis of their updated review of the scale, concluded that it had poor inter-rater and test-retest reliability.

The Hamilton scale is the most consistently used measure by raters (Freemantle *et al.* 1993), and has been translated into many languages. However, the scale has been criticized for its narrowness, its focus on behaviour, and neglect of other pertinent areas, including cognitive and affective symptoms (Raskin 1986). Bagby *et al.* (2004), on the basis of their updated review of the scale, concluded that the measure is psychometrically and conceptually flawed, and should no longer be regarded as a gold standard for the assessment of depression.

Modified versions

Although the scale is one of the most widely used in psychiatric research (Freemantle *et al.* 1993), many investigators have modified it (Paykel 1985). For example, Potts *et al.* (1990) developed a fully structured interview version (suitable for use with lay interviewers) of the 17-item scale for use in the RAND Medical Outcomes Study. They reported that inter-rater reliability with two psychiatrists rating 20 subjects was good (Pearson's r = 0.96), a finding confirmed by other studies (Korner *et al.* 1990). The alpha correlations for internal consistency were 0.82 to 0.83. The test-retest correlations were high at 0.65 for the total score, although the item correlations were variable at –0.04 to 0.77 (15-day retest). They omitted the items with low retest results and drew up a 14-item to replace the 17-item version.

THE BECK DEPRESSION INVENTORY (BDI)

If the researcher is interested only in depression, and not more generally in both anxiety and depression, then it is reasonable to use a specially designed scale. The BDI (amended and revised) is such a specific scale, and is the most widely used instrument for detecting depression. It was designed by Beck *et al.* (1961) because other widely used scales (e.g. the Minnesota Multiphasic Personality Inventory) were not specifically designed for the measurement of depression or were based on old psychiatric nomenclature. It was developed on the basis of the authors' observations of two samples of 226 and 183 depressed patients' attitudes and symptoms while undergoing psychotherapy, and clinical consensus regarding the symptoms of depressed patients. These observations led to the creation of a 21-item inventory; each category describes a specific behavioural manifestation of depression and consists of a series of self-evaluation items which are graded and ranked according to severity (neutral to maximum). A short 13-item version of the BDI was developed although this has been less often used (Beck and Beck 1972; Beck *et al.* 1974; Reynolds and Gould 1981). A version for children and adolescents was developed (Kovacs and Beck 1977). A new edition of the BDI (BDI-II) has been developed, also consisting of 21 items to assess the intensity of depression (Beck *et al.* 1996a).

The original amended and revised BDI was generally regarded as better than the Minnesota Multiphasic Personality Inventory, and better than similar scales such as the Zung scale (Hammen 1981). Originally developed to be interviewer administered, it is now a self-rating scale. A large proportion of items relate to somatic disturbance, and this has led to some controversy. It cannot be used to diagnose depression in the absence of a prior diagnosis, and is only a measure of severity once the clinical diagnosis has been made. This is to exclude people being diagnosed as depressed when they have high BDI scores for situational reasons (e.g. bereavement). It has been reported to have acceptable levels of reliability for use as a research screening instrument with an elderly population (Gallagher *et al.* 1982). It takes 10–15 minutes to complete, and can be self- or interviewer-administered.

Content

The BDI amended and revised scale and the BDI-II consist of 21 items which stress cognitive symptoms of depression. Each has four response choices, in the form of statements, ranked in order of severity, from which the respondent selects one that best fits the way he or she feels at 'this moment'. The symptoms and attitudes which the BDI aims to measure are sadness, pessimism/discouragement, sense of failure, dissatisfaction, guilt, expectation of punishment, self-dislike, self-accusation, suicidal ideation, crying, irritability, social withdrawal, indecisiveness, body-image distortion, work retardation, insomnia, fatigability, anorexia, weight loss, somatic preoccupation and loss of libido. Each of the 21 items on the new BDI-II also consists of a list of four statements about a symptom for depression, in order of increasing severity. New items on the scale replace the previous items on symptoms of weight loss, changes in body image and somatic preoccupation. The original item on work difficulty was revised to examine loss of energy. The items on sleep loss and appetite loss were also revised in order to assess increases and decreases in these areas. In order to comply with DSM guidelines which require assessing symptoms of depression over the past two weeks, the time frame was changed from one week (original BDI) to two weeks in BDI-II.

Examples of items are shown in Box 5.4.

Box 5.4 BDI® BDI-II® simulated items

Unhappiness
0   I do not feel unhappy.
1   I feel unhappy.
2   I am unhappy.
3   I am so unhappy that I can't stand it.

Changes in activity level
0   I have not experienced any change in activity level.
1a   I am somewhat more active than usual.
1b   I am somewhat less active than usual.
2a   I am a lot more active than usual.
2b   I am a lot less active than usual.
3a   I am not active most of the day.
3b   I am active all of the day.

These simulated items provided by the publisher are similar to those in the BDI-II. Copyright © 1996 Aaron T. Beck. Reproduced with permission of the publisher, NCS Pearson, Inc. All rights reserved. 'Beck Depression Inventory' and 'BDI' are registered trademarks, in the US and/or other countries, of Pearson Education, Inc. or its affiliate(s). Information concerning the BDI-II is available from: Pearson Assessment, 80 Strand, London, WC2R 0RL, UK, info@psychcorp.co.uk and info@pearsonclinical.co.uk. The following link is to the BDI-II product page in their online catalogue: http://www.pearsonclinical.co.uk/Psychology/AdultMentalHealth/AdultMentalHealth/BeckDepressionInventory-II(BDI-II)/BeckDepressionInventory-II(BDI-II).aspx, accessed 10 June 2015.

Scoring

The BDI is based on a Guttman scale. The original amended and revised scale permitted selections of four to seven responses which were given a weight of 0 to 3. Revisions to the original scale were made in 1974 and in 1978, standardizing the response choices to four for each item; each still carries a weight of 0 to 3.

The numerical values of 0 (low) to 3 (high) which are assigned to each statement indicate the degree of severity. In some categories two alternative statements (2a and 2b) are presented at a given level but are assigned the same weight. In the revised version there is one alternative score for each level (so no statement is assigned the same weight). Items are scored, with a maximum total of 63. The ability to analyse scores as continuous data makes it preferable to critics of cut-off points who argue that they are artificial (Steer *et al.* 1986). Several, slightly different, scoring guides exist. Generally, however, normative data suggest the following categories of severity level: normal 0–9; mild 10–15; mild–moderate 16–19; moderate–severe 20–29; severe >29+. Steer *et al.* (1986) proposed a slightly different scoring scheme. The scale is available in a format suitable for computer scoring from National Computer Systems, Minneapolis. The value of the scale is that it can be analysed as continuous data, without artificial cut-off points.

Validity

A comprehensive review of the literature on the reliability and validity of the original amended and revised scale was published by Beck *et al.* (1988). Tests to date indicate that this has moderate to good levels of validity and reliability, although most testing has been conducted on psychiatric populations. The scale correlated well with clinicians' ratings of severity of depression and with other depression scales. Investigators have generally reported correlations between the Beck and global severity scores of $r = 0.62$ to 0.77 (Metcalfe and Goldman 1965; Crawford-Little and McPhail 1973; Bech *et al.* 1975). However, Kearns *et al.* (1982) have reported the Beck to be weak in differentiating moderate from severe depression. Beck *et al.* (1961), on the basis of 226 hospital outpatients and admissions, and 183 patients in a replication group, tested the BDI against independent psychiatric diagnoses made by four psychiatrists. Their agreement with the scale was 56 per cent; and agreement within one degree of specificity was achieved in 97 per cent of cases. The authors reported that the scale was able to discriminate between depth-of-depression categories based on clinical ratings for both original and replication groups, the correlations ranging from 0.59 to 0.68. Correlations of 0.66 were obtained between the Beck and Depression Adjective Check Lists and of 0.75 with the Beck and the Minnesota Multiphasic Personality Inventory (Beck 1970). It has been used successfully in clinical and general populations, although most studies have focused on psychiatric patients (Beck *et al.* 1961; Williams 1984). Against the Hamilton, correlations have been reported of 0.58 to 0.82 (Schwab *et al.* 1967; Williams *et al.* 1972; Bech *et al.* 1975; Davies *et al.* 1975). Carroll *et al.* (1973) argue that this camouflages the lack of congruence at severe levels of depression. A review of the literature from 1961 to 1986 by Beck *et al.* (1988) reported that the concurrent validities of the BDI with respect to comparisons with clinical ratings and the Hamilton scale for Depression were high. The mean correlations with the Hamilton scale and clinical ratings for psychiatric patients were over 0.70. The respective mean correlations for non-psychiatric patients were 0.74 and 0.60. The Beck was also shown to discriminate between subtypes of depression and to distinguish depression from anxiety. The literature reviewed indicated relationships with the Beck and suicidal behaviour and alcoholism. There is other support for its discriminative ability and convergent validity (Moreno *et al.* 1993). The scale has been reported to be associated with perceived social support in a study of carers for elderly confused people (those with lower BDI scores reported that they received greater social support) (Morris *et al.* 1989). Novy *et al.* (1993) reported that it was highly associated with the State–Trait Anxiety Inventory in a study of people with pain. The validity of the BDI was reviewed by Richter *et al.* (1998).

The BDI-II was compared with the original amended and revised BDI by Beck *et al.* (1996b) in a study of general psychiatric outpatients. The scale was self-administered. The mean BDI-II total score was about two points higher than with the original scale, and outpatients endorsed one more symptom on the BDI-II than with the original. The correlations of the BDI with sex, age, ethnicity, the Beck Anxiety Inventory and diagnosis of mood disorder were each within one point of the correlations of the BDI-II with the same variables. The BDI-II has been shown to be able to discriminate between outpatients with a major depressive disorder and those with a dysthymic disorder

(Ball and Steer 2003), and outpatients with mild, moderate and severe major depressive episodes (DSM criteria) (Steer *et al.* 2001). A study of psychiatric inpatients aged 55 and over suggested that the BDI-II can be used with clinically depressed geriatric inpatients (Steer *et al.* 2000). A study in primary care by Arnau *et al.* (2001) showed that the BDI-II was associated with the Short Form-36 questionnaire for measuring broader health status (including a mental health dimension), supporting its convergent validity. They reported that a receiver operating characteristic analysis demonstrated criterion-related validity: BDI scores predicted a standardized primary care diagnosis of major depressive disorder, and indicated that it can also be used in primary care settings. Krefetz *et al.* (2002) used the BDI-II in adolescent psychiatric inpatients and reported that it correlated significantly with the Reynolds Adolescent Depression Scale (RADS): r = 0.84, supporting its convergent validity with this group. The areas under the receiver operating characteristic (ROC) curves for the BDI-II and the RADS were 0.78 and 0.76 respectively. Wang and Gorenstein (2013) conducted a systematic review of the use of the revised BDI-II, and on the basis of 70 included studies reported that the BDI-II had good levels of correlation with measures of depression and anxiety, supporting its construct validity.

The early literature reviewed by Beck *et al.* (1988) suggested that the amended and revised BDI represented one underlying general syndrome of depression, comprising three highly intercorrelated factors: negative attitudes to self or suicide, performance impairment and somatic disturbance. When second-order factors are extracted, a single overall depression factor emerges (Beck *et al.* 1988; Shaver and Brennan 1991). Another factor analysis indicated that it measures depressive severity in almost a unidimensional manner, relying heavily on cognitive symptoms (Louks *et al.* 1989). Factor analyses of the BDI-II with adult outpatients with clinical depression and general psychiatric outpatients showed that two factors were represented: somatic-affective and cognitive dimensions (Beck *et al.* 1996a; Steer *et al.* 1999). A subsequent confirmatory factor analysis supported a model in which the BDI-II was composed of one underlying second-order dimension of self-reported depression, which was composed of the two first-order factors representing cognitive and non-cognitive symptoms (Steer *et al.* 1999). These results were confirmed in a study of primary care patients by Arnau *et al.* (2001).

Reliability

Reliability for the original BDI was tested by the developers on 226 hospital outpatients and admissions and 183 patients in a replication group (all adults). Internal consistency was tested using 200 of the cases. The score for each of the 21 items was tested with the total BDI score for each person; all were associated at the p <0.0001 level. Split-half reliability was tested using 97 of the cases, the correlation between the two halves of the scale was 0.86. Split-half reliability was also assessed using a group of adults by Weckowicz *et al.* (1967); these authors reported a lower figure of 0.53. Alternate forms of reliability were demonstrated by testing the original 21-item version with the 13-item short form; correlations have ranged between 0.89 and 0.97, suggesting that the short form can be substituted for the longer version (Beck *et al.* 1974), although it should be cautioned that short form versions are usually less consistent. Smith *et al.* (2000) caution against short versions of scales.

Beck *et al.* (1961) did not recommend conventional test-retest methods in case people remembered their scores and biased the retest result (short periods) or there were genuine changes in the intensity of depression over time (long period). Thus they carried out test-retest correlations, along with repeated psychiatric ratings in case people remembered their scores or genuinely changed between testings. Consistent relationships between the instrument and clinical ratings were reported, using 38 cases, at two- to five-week intervals. Reliability coefficients were above 0.90 (Beck *et al.* 1961; Beck 1970). Test-retest correlations at 6 and 21 days apart were also carried out by Gallagher *et al.* (1982) on a sample of 159 patients and volunteers from a 'senior centre' in Los Angeles. Test-retest correlations for the total sample, the normal sub-sample and the depressed sub-sample were: 0.90, 0.86 and 0.79 respectively. Groth-Marnat (1990) reported test-retest reliability ranged from 0.48 to 0.86 depending on the time interval used.

Gallagher *et al.* (1982) also carried out tests for the internal consistency of the scale and reported coefficient alphas of 0.91, 0.76 and 0.73 for these three groups respectively, indicating high internal consistency. The extensive review of the literature by Beck *et al.* (1988) reported that a meta-analysis of the BDI's internal consistency estimates yielded a mean coefficient alpha of 0.86 for psychiatric patients and 0.81 for non-psychiatric respondents. Lower item inter-correlations of 0.32 to 0.62 were reported by Schwab *et al.* (1967) on the basis of a study of 153 medical in-patients.

The developers of BDI-II tested the new items on 500 patients, and compared the item-option characteristic curves. The BDI-II showed improved clinical sensitivity and the BDI-II had higher internal consistency than the original BDI (BDI-II: coefficient alpha = 0.92) (Beck *et al.* 1996a). In Beck *et al.*'s (1996b) comparative study, the coefficient alphas of the original and the BDI-II were 0.89 and 0.91 respectively. Krefetz *et al.* (2002) used the BDI-II in adolescent psychiatric inpatients and reported that the Cronbach's alpha for BDI-II was 0.92. Wang and Gorenstein's (2013) systematic review of the use of the revised BDI-II reported that the BDI-II had high reliability.

The BDI has long been regarded as the scale of choice for researchers in the selection of depressed subjects from a larger population, although, as with most scales, its accuracy depends on people's motivation to report their emotional state accurately (Stehouwer 1985). Reynolds and Gould (1981) reported a correlation of 0.26 between the BDI and the Crowne and Marlowe Social Desirability Scale, suggesting that it suffers from modest social desirability bias. This is likely to be the case with self-report instruments in general. It has been used across the world, and the psychometric properties of the translated BDI-II are being reported (e.g. in Spanish, by Penley *et al.* 2003). Wang and Gorenstein (2013) concluded, on the basis of their systematic review of the BDI-II, that it stands as a valid DSM-based instrument, applicable for routine screening for depression, and in specialized medical clinics.

HOSPITAL ANXIETY AND DEPRESSION SCALE (HADS)

The HADS was developed by Zigmond and Snaith (1983). It is a brief assessment of anxiety and depression, consisting of 14 items divided into two subscales for anxiety and depression, in which the patient rates each item on a four-point scale.

As with all self-assessment instruments, it is useful for screening, not definitive diagnostic, purposes. The term 'hospital' in the title is misleading as many studies have confirmed that it is valid when used in community settings and primary health care (Snaith 2003).

Two common problems with questionnaires for the detection of mood disorders are that scores are affected by the physical illness of the patient, and that there is insufficient distinction between one mood disorder and another. Zigmond and Snaith developed the HADS in partial response to this. The scale measures anhedonic depression which the authors take as the best indicator of hypomelancholia and advised the prescription of antidepressants for those with a high score. Snaith (1987) also recommends the use of a combined researcher-administered and self-assessment scale.

The authors purposefully excluded all items relating to both emotional and physical disorder (e.g. dizziness, headaches), and the items included in the HADS were based solely on the psychic symptoms of neurosis. They also aimed to distinguish between the concepts of anxiety and depression. The seven items comprising the depression subscale were based on the anhedonic state. The authors justified this by reference to the evidence that this is probably the central psychopathological feature of that form of depression which responds well to antidepressant drug treatment and is therefore clinically useful information. The seven items comprising the anxiety subscale were selected after study of the Present State Examination and analysis of the psychic manifestations of anxiety neurosis. Severity scales were developed, with ratings from 0 to 3.

Content

Unlike most other scales, the HADS is not derived from factor analysis but from clinical experience. It consists of two sections, with four-point response scales. One section contains the seven items on depression and the other contains the seven items on anxiety. The scale assesses emotional state over the 'past week'. Examples of the scale are shown in Box 5.5.

Box 5.5 Examples from the HADS

I feel tense or 'wound up':

Most of the time
A lot of the time
From time to time, occasionally
Not at all

Worrying thoughts go through my mind:

A great deal of the time
A lot of the time
Not too often
Very little

I feel as if I am slowed down:

Nearly all the time
Very often
Sometimes
Not at all

I get sudden feelings of panic:

Very often indeed
Quite often
Not very often
Not at all

Scoring

Individual items are scored from 0–3 to 3–0, depending on the direction of the item wording. The item scores represent the degree of distress: none = 0, a little = 1, a lot = 2, unbearably = 3. Items are summed. The higher scores indicate the presence of problems. Using psychiatric diagnoses as a gold standard, HAD ratings of 7 or less were considered to be non-cases; scores of 8–10 were considered doubtful cases; and scores of 11+ implies definite cases. Various cut-offs have been used by investigators, but the cut-off of 11+ appears to be preferable in sorting cases from non-cases (Carroll *et al.* 1993).

Validity

The scales were tested by the developers for validity on over 100 psychiatric outpatients and hospital staff, with good results (Zigmond and Snaith 1983). Tests on 50 patients reported that the severity ratings correlated highly with psychiatric assessments ($r = 0.70$ for depression and $r = 0.74$ for anxiety) (Zigmond and Snaith 1983; and see Snaith and Taylor 1985). There was evidence that the anxiety and depression items were tapping different dimensions. It was easily understood and acceptable to patients. Fallowfield *et al.* (1987) reported a good level of acceptability among general medical patients. Aylard *et al.* (1987) reported correlations with other well-known depression and anxiety scales ranging from 0.67 to 0.77 (Aylard *et al.* 1987). It has been reported to perform better than the General Health Questionnaire (Goldberg 1978) in identifying cases against the criterion of a psychiatric assessment (Wilkinson and Barczak 1988). Bjelland et al. (2002) reviewed 747 papers on the HADS and reported that correlations between the HADS and other measures of anxiety and depression were between 0.49 and 0.83, supporting its construct validity.

The HADS appears to be equal to the General Health Questionnaire in ability to detect cases of minor psychiatric disorder (Lewis and Wessely 1990). As a screening instrument, it has a sensitivity of 88 per cent (at a threshold score of 8), when compared with the Structural Clinical Interview for the DSM (Hamer et al. 1991). It was sensitive to change in a study of treatment of patients with neurotic disorders (Tyrer et al. 1988). Further tests by Zigmond and Snaith (1983) showed that physically ill patients, who were not assessed as having mood disorder, had similar scores to the normal sample and scale scores were judged not to be affected by physical illness. In further support of its construct validity, it has successfully discriminated between people with and without epilepsy (Trueman and Duthie 1998) and between patients with primary Sjögrens syndrome and arthritis patient controls (Valtysdottir et al. 2000). It was sensitive to patients' improvements in a randomized controlled trial (RCT) of behaviour therapy (Evans et al. 1999). Le Fevre et al. (1999) compared the HADS with the GHQ and reported that a combined score cut-off of 20 had a sensitivity of 0.77 and a specificity of 0.85, with a positive prediction value of 0.48. He also suggested that the anxiety and depression subscales should be scored separately. Lloyd-Williams et al.'s (2001) study of palliative care patients reported that the HAD scales had low efficiency when used singly as a screening tool. They reported an optimum cut-off of 19, which achieved a sensitivity of 0.68 and a specificity of 0.67, with a positive prediction value of 0.36.

A factor analysis of the scale by Andersson (1993) reported that a two-factor solution did not split the items in the way originally intended, and a four-factor solution with three interpreted factors gave a better solution. However, factor analyses by Moorey et al. (1991) and Michopoulos et al. (2008) did confirm the two-factor structure of the scale. Martin et al. (2003) conducted a factor analysis of the scale with coronary care patients. They reported that the underlying factor structure of the HADS comprised three distinct factors: anhedonia, psychic anxiety and psychomotor agitation. However, a review of 747 papers on the HADS by Bjelland et al. (2002) concluded that most factor analyses demonstrated a two-factor solution, confirming the HADS anxiety and depression subscales.

The depression subscale has been reported to have a reasonable specificity and sensitivity in the Urdu language among Asian people living in Britain (Nayani 1989), although the scale was simply translated for this study and not suitably modified for the Asian subjects (see critique by Chaturvedi 1990). Research has tested the translated scale's conceptual equivalence and reported it to be satisfactory (Mumford et al. 1991). The scale has been used in several countries, including The Netherlands, Sweden and Spain, with good results for reliability and validity (Berglund et al. 2003; Kuijpers et al. 2003; Quintana et al. 2003).

Reliability

Attempts were made to overcome response bias in the scale by alternating the order of responses so that at one item the first response indicates maximum severity and at another item the last response indicates maximum severity. Four possible responses were chosen to prevent people from opting for a middle grade. It was easily understood and completed by patients.

The developers tested internal consistency of the scale, using data from 50 patients. The correlations for the anxiety items ranged from 0.41 to 0.76. The analysis of the depression items revealed one weak item which was removed from the scale ('I am awake before I need to get up'), along with the weakest of the anxiety items. The remaining depression items had correlations ranging from 0.30 to 0.60. Higher correlations were reported by Moorey *et al.* (1991). The criteria were then tested for reliability with a further 50 patients and results judged to be satisfactory (the false positive/negative rates were between 1 and 5 per cent). The review of 747 papers on the HADS by Bjelland *et al.* (2002) reported that correlations between the anxiety and depression subscales ranged from 0.40 to 0.74 (mean 0.56); and Cronbach's alphas (internal consistency) ranged from just below the threshold for acceptability to very good – between 0.67 and 0.93 – for the subscales. They reported that the sensitivity and specificity for both HADS subscales were about 0.80, and similar to the General Health Questionnaire. In sum, their review concluded that the HADS performed well in screening for anxiety and depression, and it had similar psychometric properties across populations (general population, primary care, psychiatric patients).

GOLDBERG'S GENERAL HEALTH QUESTIONNAIRE (GHQ)

The GHQ is the most widely applied self-completion measure of psychiatric disturbance in the UK and also has numerous worldwide applications. A major advantage for potential users of the GHQ is the existence of periodically updated handbooks containing its method, a comprehensive review of applications, and studies of reliability and validity (Goldberg 1978; Goldberg and Williams 1988).

The GHQ was developed in London during the 1960s and 1970s and was intended for use in general practice settings. It was derived from various scales, including the Cornell Medical Index. In the construction of the GHQ the concept of psychiatric disorder was thought to be appropriate to general practice settings.

The GHQ is a screening questionnaire for detecting independently verifiable forms of psychiatric illness and does not make clinical diagnoses. If these are necessary, a two-stage strategy must be employed. It is not suitable for the assessment of long-stage (chronic) problems, as it does not detect them. It is a pure state measure, assessing present state in relation to usual state (this question wording is not distortive as most people see their usual state as a normal state) (Goldberg and Williams 1988).

The advantage of the GHQ is that it concentrates on broader components of psychiatric morbidity (particularly anxiety and depression) and is designed to be self-administered. It does not attempt to detect mental subnormality, senile dementia or mania (most of the people within these categories would not be able to complete the questionnaire). It was not intended to be used for the detection of functional psychoses (schizophrenia or psychotic depression), although these conditions are in fact detected. A study of 111 acute geriatric medical inpatients by O'Riordan *et al.* (1990) showed that there were no significant differences on the GHQ when dementia was the variable (e.g. between normal depressed patients and demented depressed patients), although threshold scores did require increasing.

One further advantage of using the GHQ is that several short-item versions exist (12, 20, 28, 30), in addition to the 60-item GHQ, which, although slightly less valid and sensitive than the long version, are more suitable than the long version for use with older frail people. The 28-item version has an additional advantage over the other versions in that it also permits analysis by sub-categories; it was developed mainly for research purposes (Goldberg and Hillier 1979).

There have been numerous applications of the GHQ in survey research and in clinical settings (e.g. GPs' surgeries). It has been used among 662 people aged 85 and over living in London and was found to be acceptable to respondents, although some required assistance with completion due to poor sight and stiff finger joints (Bowling 1990). The GHQ-30 is popularly used in large social surveys and epidemiological research in the UK (Huppert and Garcia 1991; Stansfeld and Marmot 1992).

Although it has been used extensively in the UK, there have also been many applications of the scale in other countries, particularly in the USA. The 30-item version, for example, was used in a psychological morbidity survey of 1,649 new adult enrollers in a Health Maintenance Organization in the USA (Berwick et al. 1987). Although the GHQ is culture specific in development, it works well in other settings – for example, among both white and black residents in Philadelphia, in Calcutta, China, rural Iceland, Brazil and Australia (Tennant 1977; Marl and Williams 1985; for review see Goldberg and Williams 1988). It has been translated into at least 38 languages.

Content

The original version of the GHQ consists of 60 items; and the shorter versions comprise 30, 28, 20 and 12 items. The 12-item version is apparently as efficient as the 30-item version as a case detector. The GHQ-12 is a quick screening instrument for survey use; the GHQ-28 provides four scores: for somatic symptoms, anxiety and insomnia, social dysfunction and severe depression; the GHQ-30 is a screening instrument without the physical elements; the GHQ-60 is the full instrument, designed to identify cases for more thorough assessment.

Examples of questions, which all appear both in the GHQ-30 and the GHQ-60, each of which relate to the past few weeks, are shown in Box 5.6.

Box 5.6 Examples from the GHQ-30 and GHQ-60

Have you recently:

Been able to concentrate on whatever you're doing?
Better than usual, same as usual, less than usual, much less than usual.

Spent much time chatting with people?
More time than usual, about the same as usual, less time than usual, much less than usual.

Felt on the whole you were doing things well?
Better than usual, about the same, less well than usual, much less well.

Been feeling unhappy and depressed?
Not at all, no more than usual, rather more than usual, much more than usual.

Felt that life isn't worth living?
Not at all, no more than usual, rather more than usual, much more than usual.

Scoring

The GHQ consists of a checklist of statements asking respondents to compare their recent experience to their usual state on a four-point scale of severity. The scoring scale consists of 0 or 1 (the 0–0–1–1 scoring scale, the scores following the sequence of response categories across the page from left to right, is the most commonly used). Some items are negative, others are positive. The overall GHQ is the sum of the item scores. The 0–0–1–1 scoring scale is simply a count of the symptoms and is the simplest and also avoids the problems of middle-user response bias. An alternative is a Likert-type severity scoring system.

Because of the nature of its response scale, the GHQ is likely to miss very long-standing disorders, since respondents answer 'same as usual' (and thus score zero) for symptoms they are experiencing and have been experiencing for a long time. However, Goldberg and Williams (1988) point out that the loss of cases is minimal as many people cling to a concept of their 'usual self' as being without symptoms. They suggest including questions on medication taking and whether the person thinks he or she has a nervous illness to detect chronic patients. Goodchild and Duncan Jones (1985) argued that the response 'no more than usual' to an item describing pathology should be treated as an indicator of chronic illness rather than good health as is conventional. They reported data showing that scoring revised to reflect this (0–1–1–1) provided a better prediction of caseness, measured with the Present State Examination, than conventional scoring, and was more stable in repeated testing. This consists of dividing the GHQ questions up into items detecting caseness (negative, e.g. feeling constantly under strain) and those indicating health (positive, e.g. enjoying day-to-day activities). This method assigns a score to those replying 'same as usual' to any of the negative items (so the score for negative items becomes 0111, and for positive items 0011). A further advantage is that the scores are more normally distributed and the scale is a more sensitive indicator when used over time. Given the recent development of this method, Goldberg and Williams suggest that it should be used in addition to previous methods, rather than instead of. Surtees (1987) tested both methods of scoring in their longitudinal study of psychiatric disorder in women. They reported that ROC analysis revealed that both scoring methods discriminated affective conditions from others, and there was no significant difference in their ability to do so. Goldberg and Williams (1988) demonstrated that very similar results are obtained with the different scoring methods in existence, and little is gained by a Likert severity score.

Threshold scores are defined as equivalent to the concept of 'caseness' that corresponds to the average patient referred to psychiatrists. If the results of a population of GHQ scores are compared with independent psychiatric assessment, it is possible to state the number of symptoms where the probability that an individual will be thought to be a case exceeds 0.5. This is called a threshold score. The proportion of respondents with scores above this threshold is the probable prevalence of illness. Finlay Jones and Murphy (1979) have shown that in order to identify 'cases' that correspond to standards derived from the Present State Examination, it is necessary to raise the threshold score.

It is possible to compare the amount of psychiatric disturbance in two populations by comparison of the central tendency (mean, median) and dispersion (SD, inter-quartile range) of scores in each population. Also a given population can be tested on different occasions to assess the changes in psychiatric disturbance over time.

Since physically ill people score highly on the GHQ, it is not surprising that they are overrepresented among false positives. Goldberg and Williams suggest raising the thresholds for use with severe physical illnesses. Goldberg (1978), in the initial manual for the administration of the GHQ, pointed to the necessity of manipulating the threshold score to enhance discrimination in different populations.

Validity

The principal components and item analysis used during the development of the GHQ ensured that it has content validity; its construct validity was demonstrated in the principal components analysis which showed that there was a large general factor found in all the analyses reported. There is good evidence that assessments of the severity of psychiatric illness are directly proportional to the number of symptoms reported on the GHQ (Goldberg and Huxley 1980). The predictive validity of the GHQ in comparison with other well-known scaling tests of depression is also good (Goldberg 1985; Williams 1987).

Over 50 validity studies have been conducted of the GHQ. Vieweg and Hedlund (1983) reviewed many of the earlier studies. Although not perfect, it correlates well with psychiatric diagnoses of morbidity and depression (Finlay Jones and Murphy 1979; Williams 1987). The GHQ-30 has been the most widely validated. For example, 29 such studies were reported by Goldberg and Williams (1988). Correlations with other gold standards have established the criterion validity of the GHQ. Using standardized psychiatric interviews as a gold standard, reported sensitivities range between 0.55 and 0.92, and specificities between 0.80 and 0.99, depending on the choice of threshold score (Vieweg and Hedlund 1983). Comparisons of GHQ scores with a structured clinical interview (e.g. the Present State Examination or the Clinical Interview Schedule) report correlations from 0.45 to 0.83. The GHQ-60 had the highest correlations and the GHQ-30 the poorest (see Goldberg and Williams 1988 for review).

Also a study in the USA found a correlation of 0.72 between the Beck Depression Index and the GHQ-30 (Cavanaugh 1983), and an Australian study reported a correlation of 0.57 between the Zung depression scales and the 30-item GHQ (Henderson *et al.* 1981b). Bowling and Browne (1991), on the basis of surveys with 662 people aged 85 and over and almost 800 aged 65 and over, living at home in London and in Essex, reported correlations with the GHQ-28 and Neugarten's Life Satisfaction Scale A of 0.47 in each case. This is a moderate correlation, reflecting the different dimensions of emotional well-being tapped by these two scales. Functional ability was also predictive of changes in GHQ-28 score in a follow-up study by this research team, supporting the scale's discriminative ability (Bowling *et al.* 1992). In further support of the discriminative ability of the GHQ, Bowling *et al.* (2002), on the basis of a population survey of almost 1,000 people aged 65 and over, reported that the GHQ-12 was a significant independent predictor of self-rated quality of life (QoL). In support of its convergent validity, Watson and Evans (1986), in their study of the health of a multi-cultural sample of mothers with young children in London's East End, reported that mothers' GHQ scores correlated well with interviewers' ratings of the mothers' distress. The 30-item GHQ and the Nottingham Health Profile were administered to people suffering from either migraine or arthritis by Jenkinson *et al.* (1988). Correlations between the emotional-reactions subsection of the Nottingham Health Profile and the GHQ were moderate (0.49) for both groups of patients.

Although the GHQ was not developed as a predictive tool, some studies have reported findings demonstrating predictive validity, although two studies have reported negative results. Criterion validity was established using health services as the criterion. Those with the highest GHQ scores have been reported to have the highest use of services (e.g. general practitioner services) (Goldberg and Williams 1988). Berwick *et al.* (1987) provided further evidence of the predictive validity of the GHQ: elevations of GHQ scores, over two administrations at seven-month intervals, were strongly associated with the probability of both mental health and non-mental health care within 12 months of enrolment.

The GHQ is sensitive for transient disorders, detecting symptoms of at least two weeks' duration. It is as sensitive to depression disorders as any of the specially designed depression scales (such as the Beck or HAD) and detects anxiety disorders as well, so it is suitable for use when the researcher wants a broader measure. Numerous surveys indicate that the GHQ is suitable for use with younger and older men and women in community and primary health care settings (Sims and Salmons 1975; Tarnopolsky *et al.* 1979; Benjamin *et al.* 1982; Cleary *et al.* 1982; Banks 1983; Hobbs *et al.* 1983, 1984; Goldberg and Williams 1988).

Watson and Evans (1986) used the GHQ with a multi-cultural sample of mothers with young children. While they found that mothers' GHQ scores correlated well with interviewers' ratings of the mothers' distress, an analysis of the translation of the questionnaire into Bengali for the Bengali mothers did reveal some problems. The questionnaire was back-translated by an independent translator. There was a high level of agreement between one translation and the original, with the exception of the item: 'Have you recently been feeling nervous and strung-up all the time?' which was translated as 'Did you suffer from mental breakdown and mental anxiety?' The other translation had problems with the item 'Have you recently been finding life a struggle all the time?' which was translated as 'Are you thinking yourself a struggler?' They also found that not all items were suitable for assessing psychiatric disturbance in mothers with young babies, for example, 'Have you recently been having restless disturbed nights?', 'Have you been getting out of the house as much as usual?', 'Have you spent much time chatting with people?' Because young mothers are more likely to have false positive scores with these items, the authors recommended raising the threshold score, using the 30-item version, from 4 or 5 to 8. There can be other problems in administration which may affect reliability. Very elderly people with failing eyesight and arthritic fingers may have difficulty completing the GHQ independently and will require varying degrees of assistance from an interviewer (e.g. reading out the items or recording responses) (Bowling 1990).

Berwick *et al.* (1987) carried out a further factor analysis of responses to the GHQ which disclosed six factors (anxiety/strain, confidence, depression, energy, social function and insomnia) and a strong tendency for items of similar wording (positive phrasing) to cluster together. Ohta *et al.* (1995) tested the factor structure of the GHQ-30 in a population survey of 1,216 people in Japan. They identified eight factors: depression, anxiety and tension, anergia, interpersonal dysfunction, difficulty in coping, insomnia, anhedonia and social avoidance. Huppert *et al.* (1989) also tested the factor structure of the GHQ-30 in a population survey of 6,317 people in Britain, using 10 random samples of 600 adults each and 12 age–sex groupings. They reported that the factor structure was highly consistent, and represented fewer (five) distinct factors: anxiety, feelings of incompetence, depression, difficulty in coping and social dysfunction. Hankins (2008), using simple exploratory factor analysis, examined the structure of the shorter GHQ-12 in a cohort of the Health Survey for England (3,705 respondents) and reported a two-factor solution. He reported that this result is consistent with previous studies, which report the factor structure of the GHQ-12 as two- or three-dimensional. His confirmatory factor analysis then indicated that the model was not a good fit for the data, and suggested a unidimensional model. This, as he stated, is in accord with the intended use of the GHQ-12 as a unidimensional, non-specific measure of psychiatric morbidity. He concluded that two- or three-dimensional models are due to spurious results resulting from the neglect of response bias on the negatively worded items on mood – which can also affect internal consistency (Cronbach's alpha results).

Reliability

Split-half and test-retest correlations have been carried out on the GHQ with good results. Split-half reliability has been carried out with 853 completed questionnaires, and the correlation achieved was 0.95. Internal consistency, using Cronbach's alpha, has been reported in a range of studies with correlations ranging from 0.77 to –0.93. Bowling and Gabriel (2004) reported that Cronbach's alpha, based on their national sample of people aged 65 and over, was 0.83. Test-retest reliability correlations have been reported ranging from 0.51 to 0.90, the correlations being higher with clinically defined groups with a high prevalence of disorder (Goldberg and Williams 1988). The internal consistency of the Polish version of the GHQ-12 was tested by Makowska and Merecz (2000) in over 2,500 employees and the GHQ-28 was tested in over 1,000 employees. The Cronbach alphas of both were high and comparable to the results of the early studies of the GHQ's internal consistency (0.859 and 0.934 respectively). The correlation for test-retest reliability was 0.70. A problem posed by test-retest reliability is one of distinguishing between true change and unreliability. Goldberg and Williams state that the definitive test-retest reliability study of the GHQ remains to be done.

STATE–TRAIT ANXIETY INVENTORY (STAI)

The STAI was developed in the 1960s, and revised in 1983 (Spielberger *et al.* 1983). It measures inbuilt tendency to anxious response and current feelings of anxiety. It enables the investigator to distinguish between the two forms of anxiety: state (temporary or transitory feelings of fear or worry) and trait (dispositional or long-standing tendency to respond anxiously to stressful situations, or proneness) (Chaplin 1984).

The pre-1983 versions of the STAI are known as Y1 and Y2 and the revised 1983 versions are known as X1 and X2. The STAI was developed from an item pool of 177 questions taken from existing anxiety scales. These were subjected to various tests to ensure acceptable levels of consistency and content. This was repeated in order to develop the items for 'state' and the items for 'trait'. Extensive testing of items was carried out, largely on college students (n = 5,000). The final version was subjected to item and factor analyses. The essential qualities measured by the STAI are feelings of apprehension, tension, nervousness and worry.

Content

The STAI consists of 20 items for measuring trait anxiety and 20 items for measuring state anxiety (Spielberger *et al.* 1970, 1983). The STAI is printed on a single sheet, with the state-anxiety scale on one side and the trait-anxiety scale on the other. Each state item is rated on a four-point intensity scale, from 'not at all' to 'very much so'. Respondents are asked to blacken the circle of the appropriate response to indicate how they feel 'right now'. Each trait item is rated on a four-point frequency scale, from 'almost never' to 'almost always'. The instrument is self-administered, and takes less than 10 minutes to complete. The state-anxiety scale should be administered first to avoid bias from the anxiety arising from test conditions.

Scoring

The STAI has two scores. One score reflects the current level of state anxiety with scores between 20 and 80; the other score indicates the current level of trait anxiety, and also ranges from 20 to 80. High scores reflect greater levels of, or more, anxiety. The items are simply summed to obtain the scores, although the coding of some items requires prior reversal. A manual is available for purchase, and this includes a computer program for analysis written in Statistical Analysis Systems (SAS).

Examples from the STAI are shown in Box 5.7.

Box 5.7 Examples from the STAI

Form Y1

I feel calm
I am tense

Not at all (1) / somewhat (2) / moderately so (3) / very much so (4)

Form Y2

I feel pleasant
I feel satisfied with myself

Almost never (1) / sometimes (2) / often (3) / almost always (4)

© Charles D. Spielberger, 1968, 1977. The STAI can be obtained from the publisher. Licence and manual fees are charged. Contact information: Mind Garden, 855 Oak Grove Avenue, Suite 215, Menlo Park, CA 94025, USA. Website: http://mindgarden.com, accessed 16 October, 2015. Reproduction by special permission of the Publisher, Mind Garden, Inc., www.mindgarden.com from the State-Trait Anxiety Inventory for Adults by Charles D. Spielberger. Copyright © 1968, 1977. Further Reproduction is prohibited without the publisher's written consent. Website: http://www.mindgarden.com/index.htm, accessed 8 October 2015; http://www.mindgarden.com/145-state-trait-anxiety-inventory-for-adults, accessed 27 August 2015; http://www.mindgarden.com/146-state-trait-anxiety-inventory-for-children, accessed 27 August 2015.

Validity

Testing of the original scale for construct validity against other anxiety scales produced correlations of between 0.52 and 0.80. It has been successfully used in many clinical studies, and it has been reported to correlate well with other tests of personality. The scale is able to distinguish between normal adults and different groups of psychiatric patients (e.g. schizophrenia, anxiety reaction); and, in support of its construct validity, the STAI-state showed higher mean values in stressful situations than in neutral or relaxed situations (Spielberger *et al.* 1983; Chaplin 1984). Novy *et al.* (1993), in a study of 285 people in anxiety-provoking and stressful situations associated with pain, reported that the STAI correlated strongly with different depression scales, including the Beck Depression Inventory (Beck *et al.* 1961).

In a study of 180 randomly sampled people living in Stockholm, Forsberg and Bjorvell (1993) reported that the STAI-state was significantly and negatively associated with reported health symptoms and the RAND Health Perceptions Battery. As would be expected, the better the health and perceptions of health, the lower the rated anxiety.

In a review of the scale evidence, Chaplin (1984) concludes that the measure of state anxiety is stronger (in terms of validity) than the measure of trait anxiety. It has been reported to have poor discriminant validity in older psychiatric patients, and failed to discriminate between people with and without anxiety disorders (Kabacoff et al. 1997). Kvaal et al. (2001) warned against its use with very elderly patients, as their study of geriatric inpatients showed that a high STAI-state subscore was biased in this population due to confounding by reduced well-being.

Reliability

The alpha coefficient has been reported to be high for both state (r = 0.93) and trait (r = 0.90) anxiety, indicating internal consistency. Test-retest correlations with college students at intervals from one hour to 104 days showed stability for the trait scale (0.65–0.86), but less so for the state scale (0.16–0.62), although lower repeatability of the state scale would be expected as it measures responses to transient situations (Spielberger et al. 1983). The developers reported that factor analyses with 2,000 students and Air Force recruits confirmed the scale's homogeneity.

The STAI is one of the most widely used measures of anxiety in psychological and clinical research. It was reviewed by Andrews et al. (1994) and Julian (2011). It can be previewed briefly before deciding to purchase on http://www.mindgarden.com

Other forms of the STAI

Short STAI

Marteau and Bekker (1992) developed a six-item state scale of the STAI which performed as well as the longer version (Chlan et al. 2003; Kaipper et al. 2010).

A different six-item version was developed by Chlan et al. (2003). Tluczek et al. (2009) assessed the reliability and validity of these two versions of the six-item STAI with 288 parents of infants at three time points. They reported that both short forms were highly correlated with the 20-item STAI score, and all internal consistency reliabilities were greater than 0.90. They concluded that the version developed by Marteau and Bekker (1992) containing items 1, 3, 6, 15, 16, and 17 of the state-anxiety scale was the most reliable and valid instrument for this study sample. It had better internal consistency, and a better fitting model across the three time points than the version containing items 5, 9, 10, 12, 17, and 20.

Children's STAI (STAIC)

There is a version of the STAI for children, which is regarded as one of the best available for research purposes (Walker and Kaufman 1984). It has the same 20:20 item format for trait and state as the adult version, and has good results for reliability and validity, although it does depend on reading ability (Spielberger et al. 1973, 1983; Walker and Kaufman 1984). One example of a state scale item involves asking children about the presence of feeling upset ('I feel . . . very upset/upset/not upset'), and an example of a trait scale item is the indication of frequency of occurrence of behaviours such as sweaty hands ('My hands get sweaty') and worry ('I worry about school').

THE GERIATRIC DEPRESSION SCALE (GDS)

The GDS was developed as a screening instrument in a clinical setting to facilitate assessment of depression in older adults (Yesavage et al. 1983; Sheikh et al. 1991). Scales for assessing depression in younger people are not necessarily suitable for use with older people because some symptoms indicative of depression may occur as a result of physical illness, resulting in false positive cases if they are included. The GDS does not include somatic symptoms.

It is suitable for assessing severity, and therefore for monitoring the outcome of treatment. A short form was also developed (Sheikh and Yesavage 1986). It can be used in clinical and normal populations, and in community, hospital and residential settings. It is a self-rating scale but is recommended by the developers to be administered orally by an interviewer on the grounds that cognitive problems can affect the accuracy of self-reported problems. It is simple to administer, and takes about 10 minutes.

Content

The GDS was developed from a pool of 100 items generated by clinicians and researchers. The 30 items which formed the original GDS were selected on grounds of their high item-total correlations. The GDS has a dichotomous yes/no response choice for each item. Later versions retained the most powerful items. The most commonly used version contains 15 items (GDS-15). The time frame is feelings over the past week. Examples of items in the 15-item version are shown in Box 5.8.

Box 5.8 Examples from the 15-item GDS

Are you basically satisfied with your life?
Do you feel happy most of the time?
Do you feel that your life is empty?
Do you often get bored?
Do you often feel helpless?
Do you feel that your situation is hopeless?

Reproduced with permission of the developer. The scale is in the public domain and is free to use; free iPhone and Android apps of the 15-item GDS are also available on this website, provided by Dr Yesavage of VA Palo Alto Health Care System: http://www.stanford.edu/~yesavage/GDS.html. And see: http://www.stanford.edu/~yesavage (links accessed 22 September 2015).

Scoring

Responses indicating depression are scored as 1, and no depression as 0, and the 1s are summed to form a total score. Items are treated as equal in weight. The scores on the original 30-item scale are usually interpreted as 0–9 = no depression; 10–19 = mild depressive; and 20–30 = severe depressive. The scores on the short 15-item version are: 0–4 = no depression, 5–9 mild depression, 10+ severe depression. Some variations on the scale score interpretation exist (usually by one point). A confirmatory factor analysis by Adams *et al.* (2004), based on their sample of 327 people aged 65–94 living in the community in the USA, yielded a final measurement model using 26 of the items in five factors, with a goodness of fit index of 0.90: dysphoric mood, withdrawal-apathy-vigour, hopelessness, cognitive and anxiety. The authors suggested that, although their results were preliminary, the use of these five dimensions as subscales for scoring purposes might improve the precision and utility of the GDS.

Validity

It has been reported to perform comparably with the Hamilton Depression Rating Scale in discriminating between patients with different levels of depression, according to the Research Diagnostic Criteria (Yesavage *et al.* 1983). It has also been reported to correlate significantly with the Hamilton Depression Rating Scale (0.62–0.81) (Lyons *et al.* 1989), and with the Beck Depression Inventory (0.85) (Norris *et al.* 1987). The sensitivity of the GDS has generally been reported to be high, and the specificity somewhat lower, although this has varied between studies (Brink *et al.* 1983; Koenig *et al.* 1988; Agrell and Dehlin 1989).

The validity of the short version was assessed with good results against psychiatric diagnoses and against other validated scales among people living in residential care in London (Richardson and Hammond 1996); it approaches that of the original 30-item scale (Van-Marwijk *et al.* 1995). It was used in a large epidemiological survey of 14,545 people aged 75 and over in the UK and it was reported that, as would be expected, women were significantly more likely to score over all thresholds than men (Osborn *et al.* 2002). Alden *et al.* (1989) reported a correlation between the long and short versions of the GDS of 0.66, while Sheikh and Yesavage (1986) reported this correlation to be 0.84.

Reliability

Yesavage *et al.* (1983), in a study of normal and depressed older people, reported the coefficient alpha to be 0.94, although other investigators have reported slightly lower coefficients (Lesher 1986; Agrell and Dehlin 1989; Lyons *et al.* 1989). In a sample of nursing home residents, Brink *et al.* (1983) reported the test-retest reliability of the GDS to be between 0.85 and 0.98 at 10 to 12 days, and inter-rater reliability was 0.85. Richardson and Hammond (1996) also reported the test-retest reliability of the short version to be good among people living in residential care in London. Some studies have reported that the GDS is less psychometrically sound when used with cognitively impaired people (Kafonek *et al.* 1989), although Sutcliffe *et al.* (2000) reported that the internal reliability of the shorter GDS-15 was highest if three items were removed, and that the resulting 12 items were a suitable and reliable tool for use with people in long-term care homes.

The scale is in the public domain and has been translated into over 20 languages. In a friendly website on the GDS the scale developers provide the contact addresses for translated versions, but caution that they cannot vouch for their accuracy (http://www.stanford.edu/~yesavage/GDS.html). The short version is also available at http://www.jr2.ox.ac.uk/geratol/GDSdoc.htm

EXAMPLE

An example of the use of measures of anxiety and depression is shown in Box 5.9.

Box 5.9 Example of clinic study using measures of anxiety and depression

Doherty *et al.* (2013) undertook a prevalence study of anxiety and depression among their clinic patients with ankylosing spondylitis to examine outcomes.

Patients were recruited for the study in their annual review clinics, and 59 attenders completed the assessment questionnaires. The measures included the Hospital Anxiety and Depression Scores (HADS-A and HADS-D respectively).

They reported that both anxiety and depression were prevalent in this patient group. Worse patient reported outcomes were associated with the presence of anxiety or depression using the HADS. For example, reported pain was associated with HADS-A and HADS-D. They reported a significant correlation between unemployment and depression, but not with anxiety.

The authors concluded that recognizing and treating anxiety and depression is an important part of the management of this group. However, the small scale of this study should be noted, and the findings require wider verification.

CHAPTER 6

MEASURING SOCIAL NETWORKS AND SOCIAL SUPPORT

CHAPTER COVERAGE

SOCIAL NETWORK ANALYSIS

Social relationships and activities are one of the most important areas of life nominated by lay people, and a main area of quality of life (QoL) prioritized by people aged 65+ (Bowling 1995; Farquhar 1995b; Bowling and Windsor 2001; Bowling *et al.* 2003). The largest body of empirical research on the predictors of well-being has focused on the structure, functioning and supportiveness of human relationships, the social context in which people live, and their integration within society. Network models have been employed in numerous areas of social science, public health and social epidemiology. Quantitative sociologists, including those working in public health, have applied more complex methods of structural network analysis (Scott 2013). This is a set of quantitative tools for the analysis of social structures, and investigating the relational aspects of these structures (see Scott 2013).

In research on health, lack of social support, participation and contact has been associated with increased mortality risk, delayed recovery from disease, poor morale and mental health (e.g. Lowenthal and Haven 1968; Berkman and Syme 1979; Lin *et al.* 1979; Blazer 1982; House *et al.* 1982; Welin *et al.* 1985; Bowling and Charlton 1987; Cohen *et al.* 1987, 2000; Maes *et al.* 1987; Orth-Gomér and Johnson 1987a; Seeman *et al.* 1987; Kaplan *et al.* 1988; Sugisawa *et al.* 1994; Oman and Reed 1998; Holt-Lunstad *et al.* 2010). The evidence that social support is beneficial to health is considerable (Olsen 1992; Stansfeld 1999), and there is some evidence that this benefit remains influential in very old age (Grundy *et al.* 1996). The importance of social relationships to health internationally was demonstrated by Holt-Lunstad *et al.* (2010) in their systematic review and meta-analysis of social relationships and mortality risk. They included 148 studies, with 308,849 individuals, followed for an average of 7.5 years. They concluded that people with adequate social relationships had a 50 per cent greater likelihood of survival compared to those with poor or insufficient social relationships, and that the influence of social relationships on risk for mortality is comparable with well-established risk factors for mortality (e.g. smoking) and exceeds others (e.g. obesity, physical inactivity). Their later meta-analysis of 70 studies on loneliness and social isolation as risk factors for mortality also indicated that the influence of both objective and subjective social isolation on mortality risk is comparable with well-established risk factors for mortality (Holt-Lunstad *et al.* 2015). Evidence is also emerging that having complex social networks (in which relationship types vary) rather than homogeneous networks, may increase cognitive stimulation and thereby enhance cognitive function, although effects are small (Ellwardt *et al.* 2015). However, not all research is consistent (Schoenbach *et al.* 1986; and see reviews by Bowling 1991, 1994; Bowling and Grundy 1998), which may partly reflect cultural variations in the value attributes to social network connectiveness, and the lack of standardization in choice of measurement instruments.

Social networks and social support are distinct concepts. Network analysis was originally developed by sociologists and social anthropologists, although methodological developments were made by social psychologists (Mitchell and Trickett 1980), and social epidemiologists investigating the influence of social networks and social capital on health, their mechanisms and conceptual frameworks (Berkman and Glass 2000; Kawachi and Berkman 2000). Sociologists believe that the characteristics of the network have some explanatory power of the social behaviour of the people involved (Mitchell 1969). The framework most applicable to the study of social support derives from the theory of social networks. This describes transactions among individuals. Each individual is a node in the network and each exchange a link. Networks are defined as the web of identified social relationships that surrounds an individual and the characteristics of those linkages. It is the set of people with whom one maintains contact and has some form of social bond. Social contacts and relationships are important ways for the individual to influence the environment and provide pathways through which the environment influences the individual (Saronson *et al.* 1977), including their health (Berkman and Glass 2000; Holt-Lunstad *et al.* 2010, 2015). The three theoretical models underpinning most of the literature are based on: stress and coping models, similar to the stress buffering model, and holds that social support facilitates coping, which reduces the negative effects of stress on the individual; the social cognitive model which holds that a person's perception of support influences their self-esteem and self-identity, which then influences their health and well-being; and the relationship perspective which holds that the benefits of social support is in its qualities (e.g. companionship, intimacy, social skills, low conflict) and it is these qualities which influence outcomes (see review by López and Cooper 2011).

The importance of social networks, and their characteristics, is widely held to be the extent to which they fulfil members' needs. Their functions can be summarized as 'that set of personal contacts through which the individual maintains his social identity, and receives emotional support, material aid, services, information and new social contacts' (Walker *et al.* 1977). House (1981) has suggested that social support involves emotional concern (liking, love); instrumental aid (services); information (about environment); and appraisal (information for self-evaluation). One approach to defining social support proceeds from a consideration of its source, such as who provides it; the functions it serves for people (e.g. material aid); and the intimacy characteristics of the relationship (e.g. whether it is a confiding relationship) (Tolsdorf 1976). Thus social support can be defined as the interactive process in which emotional, instrumental or financial aid is obtained from one's social network. Cobb (1976) defines social support as 'information leading the subject to believe that he is cared for and loved, esteemed, and a member of a network of mutual obligations'. Thus support exists only if it leads to certain beliefs in the recipient. Thoits (1982) expanded this model to include instrumental aid. Despite several attempts to conceptualize social support, no agreement has yet been reached.

Several characteristics of networks are relevant in terms of support. First, people must have connections with other people (network) in order to receive social support, but social connections do not guarantee access to social support. Finch (1989) also stressed the importance of the type of genealogical relationship, the past pattern of social exchanges, the balance of dependence and independence in the relationship, timing in life, and the quality of the relationship. There is a need for theories of social support to incorporate such complexities (Sarason *et al.* 1994). The dimensions of social networks, and characteristics of members' ties have been summarized by several authors (e.g. Berkman and Glass 2000), and include those shown in Box 6.1 (note: the last two overlap with elements of social capital).

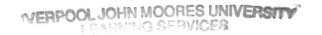

Box 6.1 Characteristics of social networks and network ties

Size: the number of people maintaining social contact in the network; this can include those who are only called on when needed.

Geographic dispersion: from those confined by a household, to those in a single neighbourhood, or more widely dispersed.

Other indicators of boundedness: extent to which people are defined by group structures (e.g. work).

Density/integration: the extent to which network members are in each other's networks.

Composition and member homogeneity: friend, neighbour, children, sibling, other relatives; similarities between members.

Frequency of contact between members: numbers of face to face and other types of contacts.

Multiplexity: numbers of types of exchanges or support between network members.

Strength of ties: degree of intimacy, reciprocity, expectation of durability, availability, emotional intensity.

Duration: length of time network members known each other.

Social participation: involvement in social, political, educational, church, other activities.

Social anchorage: years of residence in, familiarity with, neighbourhood, involvement in community.

These structural characteristics of the network will influence the availability of instrumental and emotional support, its adequacy, satisfactions with, and perceptions of the network and support/aid obtained.

Networks can thus be operationally defined in terms of size, geographic dispersion, strength of ties, density/integration, composition and member homogeneity (Mitchell 1969; Craven and Wellman 1974; Walker *et al.* 1977).

These structural characteristics are useful in calculating the number and distribution of relationships within a network and their degree of connection. The emerging patterns can then be studied in relation to the particular life situation of the individual. It can be hypothesized that different types of network structure have differing degrees of significance depending on the nature of need to be met.

'Dynamic features of the social network' refers to the positive or negative nature of network interactions. Analyses need to take account of the nature of human emotions involved. The size of the network and calculations of frequency of contact between members are of little value if these interactions are negative and stressful. It is also possible that the existence of a single confidant(e) is of greater value in terms of meeting an individual's emotional needs than a larger number of more superficial friendships. The individual's subjective 'view' of the network takes into account the meaning of relationships and the strength of affectional ties. A different but related dimension is the concept of loneliness. This can be a consequence of perceived or actual poor emotional or social support. This concept, with the measurement of loneliness, is discussed at the end of this chapter.

SOCIAL CAPITAL

There is increasing interest among health researchers and social epidemiologists in broadening social measures to include social capital in order to study its effects on health status and mortality. While the social deprivation of areas has been studied in relation to morbidity and mortality (Yen and Kaplan 1999), broader social capital is still a disputed concept. Social capital refers to the collective value of all formal and informal social networks. Investigators have used a conceptual mixture of indicators of both the structure and function of social relations (such as community memberships (structure)), and the moral resources of trust, bonding, information flows and cooperation between people, and reciprocity (function, or byproduct of the function) (Putnam 1995, 2000; Coulthard et al. 2001). The latter are influenced, and fostered, by the availability and type of societal, environmental and neighbourhood (community) facilities and resources (i.e. which enable group membership, community and civic engagement).

More specifically, social cohesion can be defined as the connectedness and solidarity between groups of people (Kawachi and Berkman 2000). A cohesive society is marked by its supportiveness, rather than forcing individuals to rely entirely on their own resources (Durkheim 1897), and is well endowed with stocks of social capital (Kawachi and Berkman 2000). The concept incorporates shared value systems and interpretations, perceptions of a common identity, a sense of belonging to the community, trust and reciprocity between individuals and towards institutions. It is typically measured with questions about feelings of commitment and trust, values and norms, and feelings of belonging.

Social capital can be defined as a subset of the concept of social cohesion: as those features of organizations and social structures which act as resources for individuals to form connections and social networks, and which lead to norms of reciprocity, trust, collective action, beneficial cooperation and organization between members (e.g. high levels of interpersonal trust and mutual aid) (Putnam 1995, 2000; Kawachi and Berkman 2000). It thus refers to the extent to which communities offer members opportunities, through active involvement in social activities, voluntary work, group membership, leisure and recreation facilities, political activism and educational facilities, to increase their personal resources (i.e. their social capital) (Coleman 1984; Putnam 1995; Brissette et al. 2000). Stocks of social capital can be cumulative, as collaborations build and extend social connections. Different types of social capital can be described in terms of different types of social networks, including *bonding social capital* which describes connections between similar people (e.g. socioeconomic status or other social groupings) and is believed to be good for coping with life's challenges; and *bridging social capital*, which describes connections between dissimilar people, which is believed to be good for progressing throughout life. *Linking social capital*, which is similar to bridging social capital, describes relationships between persons across levels of hierarchy and power (Kim et al. 2006).

High levels of social capital have been reported to be independently associated with lower mortality rates and also with better self-rated health, functional status and QoL (Kawachi et al. 1997a, 1997b, 1999; Grundy and Bowling 1999; Kawachi and Berkman 2000; Ross and Mirowsky 2001; Bowling et al. 2003; Hyyppa and Maki 2003).

A potential policy implication is that interventions aiming to improve community social capital might then improve population health (Kim *et al.* 2006). However, although there is research on the stock of social capital by the sociodemographic characteristic of individuals (Li 2003; Coulthard *et al.* 2001), relatively few investigators have explored fully the independent associations between social capital and physical health, mortality, psychological well-being or QoL (Brissette *et al.* 2000). This requires the careful controlling of sociodemographic variables, and the use of multi-level analysis. Kim *et al.* (2006) analysed the effects of community bonding and community bridging social capital on self-rated health in a sample of 24,835 people in 40 communities in the USA, surveyed by telephone, and used multi-level logistic regression analysis. Their results suggested a modest protective effect of community bonding and community bridging social capital on health.

Measures of broader social capital have included objective indicators of indices of crime, pollution, cost of living, shopping facilities, access to areas of scenic quality, cost of owner-occupied housing, education facilities, policing, employment levels, wage levels, unemployment levels, climate, access to indoor/outdoor sports, travel to work time, access to leisure facilities, quality of council housing, access to council housing and cost of private rented accommodation (in perceived order of importance to people's quality of life) (Flax 1972; Rogerson *et al.* 1989; Rogerson 1995). Other indicators have included access to convenient and affordable transport, various community resources and facilities and the general characteristics of neighbourhoods. Subjective indicators include public values, perceptions and levels of satisfaction with area of residence, its facilities, transport, travel to work time, and perceptions of neighbourliness and safety from crime (Rogerson *et al.* 1989; Cooper *et al.* 1999; Coulthard *et al.* 2001).

There has been little standardization of measures of social capital, and researchers have often devised their own items to measure this concept. The UK General Household Survey (GHS) included a set of perceived social capital questions which were developed from a review of social capital research (Cooper *et al.* 1999; Walker *et al.* 2001). They were based on Putnam's (1995) definition of social capital, and the items were subject to tests of internal consistency (co-efficient alpha) and factor analyses before being included in the final questionnaire (Coulthard *et al.* 2001). The questions cover length of residence in the area, enjoyment of the area, ratings of local services and facilities, safety, perception of power to influence neighbourhood decisions and civic engagement, crime and experience of crime, ratings of antisocial behaviour, litter, dog mess, noise, teenagers hanging around, drug problems, feelings about their immediate neighbourhood of residence (defined as their 'street or block'), including neighbourliness, trust in neighbours and social contacts. The questions are displayed in Walker *et al.* (2001), and responses and questions are displayed in Coulthard *et al.* (2001).

METHODS OF MEASUREMENT OF SOCIAL NETWORKS AND SOCIAL SUPPORT

There is no scale which comprehensively measures all or most of the main components of social networks and support, or which has been fully tested for reliability and validity. Most measures aim to measure social connectedness or embeddedness, perceived social support, and/or actual social support (López and Cooper 2011). Part of the problem stems from lack of agreement on conceptual bases, or even failure to consider these at all.

Many surveys have relied on single-item questions such as marital status, frequency of contact with others and existence of a confidant(e). Single-item measures have been found to be powerful predictors of health status and mortality but alone provide no insight into the dynamics of the network. It is important to match methodology to the empirical issue and correct disciplinary approach. Among the studies using only simple measures of social networks was the Alameda County Human Population Laboratory which provided the most convincing evidence of a link between social networks and mortality (Berkman and Syme 1979). This was modified by Lubben (1988), and labelled the Lubben Social Network Scale. If more studies used adequate and standardized measures, evidence of the links may prove to be stronger and the debate about links less controversial.

Many earlier approaches assessed social network and support by questions on marital status and household composition (see review by Hirsch 1981). Studies relying on single-item questions and crude or simplistic measures cannot be used to derive substantive implications for policy or practice. It is necessary to differentiate relationships according to their content, process and development. Failure to obtain these data precludes information on how social networks function as social support systems. Survey questions that do not separate social support from network structure do not permit identification of the social conditions under which help and support are provided. It cannot be assumed that having a daughter living nearby will necessarily lead to adequate support and help. Most attempts to measure quality of the network consist of questions asking respondents who they are close to, in contact with and if they see enough of the mentioned people. Fuller assessment of a person's perception of the social support is desirable (Adams 1967), as the perceived quality of relationships is associated with well-being, while its relationship to frequency of contact or perceived support is inconsistent (Fiore et al. 1986; Seeman and Berkman 1988).

Seeman and Berkman (1988) found that network characteristics are not so highly correlated with aspects of social support that they can be used interchangeably. Cohen et al. (1987), on the basis of their study of 155 elderly residents of midtown Manhattan single-room occupancy hotels, reported the results of a factor analysis showing that only 7 of the 19 network variables utilized had sufficient commonality to form a potential scale, suggesting that most variables are independent of each other. The authors criticized the use of scales without prior analysis of scale items and the development of scales without the use of parametric approaches such as factor analysis. As they pointed out, a possible problem with combining all network variables into one scale is the potential for premature treatment of network variables as unidimensional (i.e. representing one underlying construct). Combining variables which may be independent of each other into a simple scale may attenuate true variance and obscure differences that may be important. Much previous research has been limited to the use of bivariate statistical techniques, therefore making it impossible to control for overlap among variables or to determine the relative strength of variables. Measures of network need to be multi-faceted, taking into account structure and dynamic features of the network, as well as the individual's subjective perceptions of it.

Researchers often assume that measures of network size and frequency of social contacts are fairly 'objective' and stable in comparison with measures of the content and quality of relationships which are likely to be confounded by mental health status (House and Kahn 1985). Donald and Ware (1982) reported one-year test-retest reliability coefficients of between 0.40 and 0.60 for reports of social contacts. This lack of stability may sometimes reflect the changing nature of relationships, particularly in older populations who experience large network losses through death and illness of (also old) relatives and friends, necessitating caution in the interpretation of results (Bowling and Farquhar 1995). One problem with network scales is that visits to relatives may be routine and taken for granted – and thus unreported as formal social visits (Stueve and Lein 1979). Spouses may also be taken for granted as part of the network and unreported in network scales (Bowling et al. 1988). Feelings about the supportive nature of the network (affective component) can be influenced by psychological well-being or depression as well as by network structure and functions. Thus people with adequate support may perceive it to be inadequate because they are feeling depressed. This problem has not been resolved. Sokolovsky (1986) suggests an ethnographic approach to validate information given: participant observation, life histories, genealogies and informal interviews to probe the social support elements of social networks. An example is Francis's (1984) comparison of the Jewish elderly in Cleveland and England, using semi-structured questions about practical (transportation, shopping, money, etc.) and emotional (advice, visiting, etc.) services. Another example is Wentowski's (1982) study of an urban population in which he elicited examples of support as various events were reported by respondents (e.g. known as the critical incidents technique).

In sum, there have been relatively few attempts to test measures of social networks and support for reliability and validity (Tardy 1985; López and Cooper 2011). Existing research generally suffers from methodological problems: imprecise definitions, failure to treat social support as a multidimensional concept, and various intervening variables confounding studies. The main problem with most studies has been the inadequate conceptualization and operationalization of social support. It is common simply to itemize presence or absence of a spouse, confidant(e), household composition and social activities. Most researchers then total respondents' scores to questions about the structure of social networks and ignore the different dimensions of support. Conceptual definitions are more rarely offered, although sociologists are beginning to offer more developed conceptual statements: that the respondent believes he or she is cared for/loved/esteemed/valued and belongs to a network of significant others.

López and Cooper (2011) undertook an extensive review of social support measures, including some of those included here: the Arizona Social Support Interview (ASSIS), the Perceived Social Support Scale (from Family and Friends), the Social Support Questionnaire and the RAND Medical Outcomes Study Social Support Survey – this was one of the measures they recommended, particularly because of its strong psychometric properties, and testing in several languages. The popular RAND Social Support Scale is reviewed elsewhere, in Chapter 4, alongside other RAND scales of physical, mental and social health, functioning and perceptions.

AVAILABLE MEASURES OF SOCIAL NETWORK AND SUPPORT

Several chapters in Cohen *et al.* (2000) provide brief overviews of several measures of social networks, support and social integration; earlier reviews include those by Payne and Graham Jones (1987) and Orth-Gomér and Unden (1987b). The latter also reviewed a number of the shorter measures, consisting mainly of single-item questions with little reference to quality of, and satisfaction with, relationships, for example: Berkman's Social Network Index (Berkman and Syme 1979); House's Social Relationships and Activities Scale (House *et al.* 1982); Lin's Social Support Scale (Lin *et al.* 1979); and Orth-Gomér and Johnson's Social Network Interaction Index (1987a). Although such short items appear to be inadequate in scope and psychometric properties (Dean *et al.* 1994), they can predict mortality in longitudinal population surveys (see Holt-Lunstad *et al.*'s (2010) meta-analytic review of social relationships and mortality risk).

On the other hand, the items are insufficiently detailed to indicate precisely what dimensions of poor social support structures are most important. Moreover, there are doubts about the validity of short scales. For example, there is evidence that there is massive item bias in Berkman's Social Network Index, indicating that it cannot be used as a valid measure of social network (Dean *et al.* 1994).

A review by O'Reilly (1988) of 33 instruments purporting to measure social support reported only modest agreement on conceptual definition and frequently the concepts were not defined or were ill defined. In particular, definitional confusion between social network and social support was apparent. Variables used to operationalize these concepts reflected this conceptual confusion. For example, some of the measures he reviews define social support in terms of social network characteristics (size, source and frequency of contact). O'Reilly was less optimistic about the value of existing measures and pointed out that more rigorous standards to establish validity and reliability were required. Several scales, including some of those reviewed here, which were judged to be suitable for use with elderly people, have been briefly described by Oxman and Berkman (1990). There are also several longer scales of social support which have been designed specifically for use with people with mental health problems. For example, Lehman's (1983) Quality of Life Interview contains a sub-section on frequency and nature of social relationships and contacts, as well as social activities (rating satisfaction using the Delighted–Terrible Faces as the response scale). Bigelow *et al.*'s (1991) Quality of Life Questionnaire also includes a substantial set of questions on social relationships, support and activities including negative-positive aspects of relationships. In both scales, some of the items are specific to people with mental health problems and they are not recommended for other types of populations. The Team for the Assessment of Psychiatric Services (TAPS) have developed the Social Network Scale as part of their battery of outcome measures, but this is a semi-structured instrument and can take up to an hour to administer (Leff *et al.* 1990; Leff 1993). The full instruments were reviewed previously (Bowling 2001), and as these subscales on social support were developed for use with a specific patient population they are not included in this chapter.

A popular measure not included here, due to its more qualitative approach, and time-intensive requirement for interviewer administration, is Antonucci's (1986) network-mapping procedure, which is based on an affective approach to the dynamics of social support over one's life, and focuses on the value of a relationship to the respondents. Respondents are presented graphically with three hierarchical circles. The respondent (ego) is placed at the centre of the three circles. Individual network members are placed concentrically in three circles, depending on feelings of closeness: repondents are informed that those in the inner circle are those to whom they feel so close it is hard to imagine life without them; the middle circle is for people to whom they feel not quite that close but who are still important to them; outer circle members are those not already mentioned but who they are close to. The more central the circle, the closer and more important are the network members. It has been successfully used to distinguish network types, along with structured questions, in the Berlin Ageing Study (Fiori et al. 2007).

Some of the more general measures of health status and QoL include items on social support and activities; as these have been reviewed elsewhere in this volume, they will not be reviewed here (e.g. OARS). The RAND batteries also included two batteries on network structure (the Social Health Battery) and social support (the Social Support Scale). These were reviewed in the section on the RAND batteries in Chapter 4 and will also not be repeated here. Interested researchers are also referred to an extensive review of measures of social support published by López and Cooper (2011).

INVENTORY OF SOCIALLY SUPPORTIVE BEHAVIOURS (ISSB)

The ISSB is a measure of social support designed by Barrera et al. (1981) for use with a wide range of community populations. Social support was conceptualized as the diversity of natural helping behaviours that individuals actually receive, derived from the previous literature on social support. The authors felt that most existing scales concentrated on the structure of the network rather than what the members actually did, especially in view of noted discrepancies between actual amount of help provided and subjective perceptions of the amount of help (Liem and Liem 1978).

The ISSB is a 40-item self-report measure, designed to assess how often individuals received various forms of assistance from others during the previous month. It contains 40 items generated from the literature. It conceptualizes social support as including tangible forms of assistance (e.g. provision of goods and services), and intangible forms of assistance (e.g. guidance and expressions of esteem).

Content

The ISSB measures four types of support: emotional, instrumental, information appraisal and socializing. The index asks respondents to state how people have helped them in the last month and to respond on a five-point Likert-type scale to each of the 40 items as 'not at all', 'once or twice', 'about once a week', 'several times a week' or 'about every day'. It measures the receipt of support, but not the source. A 19-item short form ISSB has also been developed (Barrera and Baca 1990).

Examples of items are shown in Box 6.2

Box 6.2 Examples from the ISSB

During the past four weeks, how often did other people do these activities for you, or with you:

Emotional
Expressed interest and concern in your well-being.
Listened to you talk about your private feelings.
Was right there with you (physically) in a stressful situation.

Items on instrumental appraisal support
Provided you with a place where you could get away for a while.
Loaned you over $25.
Provided you with some transportation.

Informational appraisal support
Gave you some information on how to do something.
Gave you feedback on how you were doing without saying it was good or bad.
Helped you understand why you didn't do something well.

Socializing
Talked to you about some interest of yours.
Did some activity together to help you get your mind off things.

The frequency of receiving each type of support is rated on five-point Likert scales:
1 = not at all, 2 = once or twice, 3 = about once a week, 4 = several times a week, and 5 = about every day.

Reproduced in: Appendix 3.A in Barrera, M. (1981) Social support in the adjustment of pregnant adolescents: assessment issues, in B.H. Gottlieb (ed.) *Social Networks and Social Support*. Beverly Hills, CA: Sage Publications, pp. 69–96. See also: Barrera, M., Sandler, I.M. and Ramsay, T.B. (1981) Preliminary development of a scale of social support: studies on college students. *American Journal of Community Psychology*, 9: 435–46. With permission of the developer and SAGE Publications Inc. Developer contact: Professor Manuel Barrera, Department of Psychology (Clinical), College of Liberal Arts and Sciences, Arizona State University, PO Box 871104, Tempe, AZ 85287-1104, USA; manuel.barrera@asu.edu; https://psychology.clas.asu.edu/faculty/manuel-barrera, accessed 1 September 2015. The ISSB is in the public domain and can be used for research purposes without charge. It can be accessed and downloaded freely at www.performwell.org (http://www.performwell.org/index.php/find-surveyassessments/inventory-of-socially-supportive-behaviors-issb-short-form, accessed 10 September 2015); http://www.midss.org/content/inventory-socially-supportive-behaviors-issb-long-and-short-form, accessed 1 September 2015.

The average time taken to complete the questionnaire is about 10 minutes.

Scoring

The five-point ratings of each item are summed to produce a total score, with higher scores indicating greater support. The author also suggests calculating an average frequency score as this permits a global score to be produced when there is some missing data for items.

Validity

The validity of the ISSB was tested by correlating results, based on 43 students, with a measure of family relations (Family Environment Scale); the correlation, although significant, was not high: 0.35. The author speculated that this was because the two scales were measuring different dimensions of support. Construct validity was assumed by correlations of the index with a measure of life events: 0.38 to 0.41 (Barrera 1981; Sandler and Barrera 1984). Notes available from the author on the scale summarize the correlations between ISSB and measures of distress from 10 published studies. The correlations range from 0.01 to 0.50, although most were fairly weak. The ISSB has been reported to be significantly related to recovery in stroke patients (Glass and Maddox 1992), supporting its predictive ability.

There is agreement between investigators who have carried out exploratory factor analyses of the scale, and report that the ISSB yields three factors (Barrera and Ainlay 1983; Stokes and Wilson 1984; Walkey *et al.* 1987; Pretorius and Diedricks 1993). A study by Caldwell and Reinhart (1988) is also consistent with these analyses and labels the clusters as guidance, emotional support and tangible support.

Reliability

The test-retest reliability correlation coefficient, based on 71 students tested over two days, was 0.88; test-retest reliability coefficients, again using students, over a one-month period were 0.80 and 0.63 (Barrera 1981; Barrera and Ainlay 1983; Valdenegro and Barrera 1983). Internal consistency reliability coefficients of 0.92 and 0.94 were reported for the first and second administrations of the scale (Barrera 1981). Notes on the ISSB are available from the author at Arizona State University; these report that tests from five studies show the internal consistency coefficients of the scale to be above 0.90.

In sum, there are problems with interpretation of the scale. Without a distinction between available and enacted support, the scale may simply be measuring the number, type and severity of problems recently experienced by the respondent. The scale has been popular, and several investigators have adapted it for use with other cultures or with specific disease groups (e.g. Manne and Schnoll 2001).

ARIZONA SOCIAL SUPPORT INTERVIEW SCHEDULE (ASSIS)

The ISSB (above) was not designed to provide information on people who supplied resources, nor respondents' subjective appraisals of the adequacy of support. Thus

Barrera (1980, 1981) subsequently designed the ASSIS to address this gap. The ASSIS was developed as an instrument to measure several aspects of support, including procedures for identifying support network membership and subjects' satisfaction with and need for support. His conceptual definition, based on previous literature, of 'social network' relates to people who provide the functions defined as support. The scale is based on self-report and takes 15–20 minutes to complete.

Content

The scale is operationalized by asking subjects to identify individuals who provide support in the following areas: private feelings, material aid, advice, positive feedback, physical assistance and social participation. In each area, subjects are asked about such support from the named individuals in the past month, and whether the support was sufficient; ratings of satisfaction are made on a three-point scale. Examples of items are shown in Box 6.3.

Box 6.3 Examples from the ASSIS

Private feelings

1. If you wanted to talk to someone about things that are very personal and private, who would you talk to?
   Give me the first names, initials, or nicknames of the people that you would talk to about things that are very personal and private.
   Probe: Is there anyone else that you can think of?

2. During the last month, which of these people did you actually talk to about things that were personal and private?
   Probe: Ask specifically about people who were listed in response to 1 but not listed in response to 2.

3. During the last month, would you have liked:
   A lot more opportunities to talk to people about your personal and private feelings?
   A few more opportunities?
   Or was this about right?

4. During the past month, how much do you think you needed people to talk about things that were very personal and private?
   Not at all.
   A little bit.
   Quite a bit.

Social participation

1. Who are the people you get together with to have fun or relax? These could be new names or ones you listed before.
   Probe: Anyone else?

2. During the past month, which of these people did you actually get together with to have fun or relax?
   Probe: Ask about people who were named in 1 but not 2.

---

3 During the past month, would you have liked:
   A lot more opportunities to get together with people for fun and relaxation?
   A few more?
   Or was it about right?

4 How much do you think you needed to get together with other people for fun and
   relaxation during the past month?
   Not at all?
   A little bit?
   Quite a bit?

With permission of the developer and SAGE Publications Inc. Reproduced in Appendix 3.B in Barrera,
M. (1981) Social support in the adjustment of pregnant adolescents: assessment issues, in B.H.
Gottlieb (ed.) *Social Networks and Social Support*. Beverly Hills, CA: Sage Publications, pp. 69–96.
Contact: Professor Manuel Barrera, Department of Psychology (Clinical), College of Liberal Arts and
Sciences, Arizona State University, PO Box 871104, Tempe, AZ 85287-1104, USA; manuel.barrera@asu.
edu; https://psychology.clas.asu.edu/faculty/manuel-barrera, accessed 10 September 2015.

The interview schedule also includes questions concerning negative interactions, on
the basis of the psychiatric literature linking these to mental disturbance (identification of
people with whom they have had conflicts in the past month). Finally, subjects are asked
about the age, sex and ethnicity of people named.

Scoring

The data obtained allow the calculation of specified scores from the relevant items of
total available and total utilized network size, conflict network size, unconflicted network
size, amount of support satisfaction and support need. The author reported that the
support satisfaction measure suffers from an extremely skewed distribution in the
direction of high satisfaction scores (Barrera 1981). Notes which identify the item scores
which should be used in calculations are available from the author at Arizona State
University.

Validity

The ability of the instrument to discriminate between groups was tested on a sample of
86 pregnant adolescents. The ASSIS was administered along with the ISSB. Barrera
(1981) reported that conflicted network size correlated significantly with depression and
anxiety, satisfaction correlated with depression and anxiety; expressed need correlated
significantly with depression and anxiety and somatization (0.23–0.51). The reported
relationship between life events and social support was taken as evidence for the index's
construct validity (0.25–0.38), although these correlations are at best modest. The ISSB
showed a modest but significant correlation with total network size (0.32), but was not
significantly correlated with satisfaction or need on the ASSIS. It has been used
successfully in several studies of mental and physical health. Rivera *et al.* (1991) used

the ASSIS in a study of women caring for frail family members. They reported that carers who were depressed reported a higher incidence of negative interactions with others, and non-depressed carers reported greater use of social support resources. Woods *et al.* (1994), in a study of depression in young women, reported that the ASSIS was able to predict self-esteem and depression. Clinton *et al.* (1998), based on the results of their longitudinal survey of community adaptation in people with schizophrenia, reported that the perceived social support variables from the ASSIS independently accounted for most of the variance in their four measures of community adaptation.

Reliability

The instrument has been tested for test-retest reliability, and results appear moderately satisfactory to good. It was tested on 45 students and total network size produced a correlation coefficient of 0.88 over three days, and studies with a further group of students produced a test-retest correlation over one month of 0.70 (Barrera 1980; Valdenegro and Barrera 1983). Test-retest correlations were 0.54 for size of conflicted network, 0.69 for satisfaction and 0.80 for support need. There was also modest support for predictive when construct validity (Barrera 1981).

Internal consistency correlations for support satisfaction and support need were low to moderate: 0.33 and 0.52 respectively.

A study by Barrera *et al.* (1985) of 36 mental health outpatients who agreed to supply the name of one network member showed significant kappa coefficients between subjects' and informants' reports of support. Of the 31 cases of non-agreement of ASSIS items, 24 were due to informants stating that they had provided aid when subjects indicated that they had not; and seven were due to subjects reporting that aid was provided when informants did not.

Further testing for both reliability and validity is required.

Adaptations

López and Cooper (2011) have described how the scale was modified in a study to assess the social support and strain among pregnant and parenting adolescent girls. It was reported (and renamed as the Social Support Network Questionnaire), in this and later studies, to have acceptable to good internal consistency overall (Cronbach's alphas for the areas ranged from 0.73 to 0.90, but with one missing the threshold for acceptability at 0.68) (Contreras *et al.* 1999; Gee and Rhodes 2008).

PERCEIVED SOCIAL SUPPORT FROM FAMILY AND FRIENDS

This was devised by Procidano and Heller (1983) as a measure of perceived social support. It was designed to assess the functions of social networks specified by Caplan (1974): 'the extent to which an individual perceives that his/her needs for support, information, and feedback are fulfilled by friends . . . and by family'. Thoits (1982) has criticized this definition as inadequate on the grounds that it includes the very term to be defined (support). The scale measures available and received support, especially emotional support. It takes about eight minutes to complete.

Content

It comprises two 20-item self-report measures, derived, after testing with students, from an initial pool of 84 items. One 20-item measure is for perceptions of family support and one 20-item measure is for perceptions of support from/given by friends. Responses require a simple 'yes', 'no', or 'don't know'. Examples are shown in Box 6.4.

Box 6.4 Examples from Perceived Social Support from Family and Friends

Family
I rely on my family for emotional support;
My family is sensitive to my personal needs;
My family gives me the moral support I need.

Friends
My friends enjoy hearing about what I think;
I have a deep, sharing relationship with a number of friends;
I feel that I'm on the fringe of my circle of friends.

A few items refer to support given
My friends come to me for emotional support;
Certain members of my family come to me when they have problems or need advice.

Availability: Perceived Social Support from Family and Friends was published in Procidano, M.E. and Heller, K. (1983) Measures of perceived social support from friends and from family: three validation studies. *American Journal of Community Psychology*, 11(1): 1–24. © 1983 Plenum Publishing Corporation. With permission from Springer. Free to use with the permission of the authors.

Scoring

Positive item responses are totalled and presented separately for family and friends. Some items are reverse-scored. An overall score can be produced, although is not generally calculated.

Validity

The developers reported that the scale correlated with measures of psychopathology and distress (0.85) therefore supporting its discriminative ability (Procidano and Heller 1983). A study of adolescent outpatients confirmed the early results for the validity of the scale, and reported that it could predict psychosocial maturity levels (Gavazzi 1994). It has been used successfully in clinical studies. Grummon *et al.* (1994) used the scale in a study of psychological adjustment among intravenous drugs users with AIDS, and reported that perceived social support from family (but not from friends) correlated positively with psychological adjustment. A study of diabetic patients by Lyons *et al.* (1998) indicated an association between both subscales and general well-being measures. Lin (2002) reported that perceived social support from friends subscale moderated the relationship between dysfunctional attitudes and depression in a study of Taiwanese adolescents.

Reliability

In relation to internal consistency, tests by the developers with 222 students produced correlation coefficients of 0.88 and 0.90 respectively for the items relating to family and those relating to friends. Test-retest reliability, using 222 students, was 0.83 over a one-month period (Procidano and Heller 1983). In a study investigating the reliability of the scale among students, the intercorrelations among the subscales and between the subscales and the total scales were reported to be strong and highly significant (Eskin 1993).

Although the scale has good internal reliability, test-retest reliability and predictive validity, and has been popularly used in social and clinical studies, more evidence of its psychometric properties is required.

Adaptations

Adaptations have included the use of five-point Likert response scales (e.g. Rodriguez *et al.* 2003). López and Cooper (2011) have reviewed the measure and adaptations in more detail.

SOCIAL SUPPORT QUESTIONNAIRE

This questionnaire was developed by Sarason *et al.* (1983) to measure the availability of, and satisfaction with, social support. The conceptual definition of support was derived from Colby's theory of attachment and is based on the existence or availability of people who can be relied upon, who care about, love and value the recipient.

In the construction of the scale, which is based on self-report, 61 items were written to sample the situations in which social support might be important to people. They were administered to 602 students who were asked to list people who provided them with such support. Items that showed low correlations with other items were deleted. Scoring methods were also piloted. The scoring method selected was the simplest – a count of supportive persons. The availability index selected was the number of persons listed divided by the number of items.

Most of the items are concerned with emotional support, so this scale is appropriate for measurement of emotional support only. The scale takes an average of 15 minutes to complete. Short three-item and six-item versions were developed by Sarason *et al.* (1987b).

Content

The instrument comprises 27 items which ask the subjects (a) to list all the people to whom they can turn in specific situations and (b) to indicate their satisfaction with each of these identified supports on a scale ranging from very satisfied to very dissatisfied. The scale was published in full in Sarason *et al.* (1983). Examples are shown in Box 6.5.

Box 6.5 Examples from the Social Support Questionnaire

Whom can you really count on to listen to you when you need to talk?
Whom could you really count on to help you out in a crisis situation, even though they would have to go out of their way to do so?
With whom can you totally be yourself?
Whom can you really count on to be dependable when you need help?
Who do you feel really appreciates you as a person?
Whom can you count on to console you when you are very upset?

Table 1, p. 129, from Sarason, I.G., Levine, H.M., Basham, R.B. and Sarason, B.R. (1983) Assessing social support: the Social Support Questionnaire. *Journal of Personality and Social Psychology*, 44: 127–39, http://dx.doi.org/10.1037/0022-3514.44.1.127. Published by the American Psychological Association. Copyright © 1983 by the American Psychological Association. Reproduced with permission from the American Psychological Association and the developers. The SSQ instructions, questionnaire items, and scoring information were published in Sarason *et al.* (1983), and are accessible in PDF format at: http://web.psych.washington.edu/research/sarason/files/SocialSupportQuestionnaire.pdf, accessed 10 September 2015. Developers: Irwin and Barbara Sarason and their associates: Sarason *et al.* (1983). The measure is free to access and use. The developers' University of Washington website states that they grant permission to researchers to use these instruments at no charge; the developers would appreciate information about the findings of studies in which they are used. Contact details: Dr Irwin Sarason, isarason@u.washington.edu; Dr Barbara Sarason, bsarason@u.washington.edu; http://web.psych.washington.edu/psych.php?p=161, accessed 22 September 2015. Department of Psychology, Guthrie Hall, Room 119A, UW Box 351525, Seattle, WA, 98195; tel.: 206 543 2640.

Scoring

Each item is scored (number of persons listed); the satisfaction score ranges from 1 to 6 (very satisfied to not very satisfied). Two scores are computed by dividing the sum of each of the two scores (number of people; overall satisfaction) by the 27 items: average (per item) number of people, and average level of satisfaction with support.

Validity

Sarason *et al.* (1983) tested the measure in a study of 227 students who were administered the scale along with personality scales (extraversion and neuroticism). The correlations with the Social Support Questionnaire were weak to moderate: –0.02 and –0.43 for availability and satisfaction with support. Another study they reported with 295 students showed an association between positive life events and number of social supports. And a study with 440 students showed that people with more social supports had more positive self-concepts. In addition, students who were high in social support were rated as more attractive and skilled socially (Sarason *et al.* 1983, 1985). Also in further support of its construct validity, Swindells *et al.* (1999), based on a study of patients with HIV, reported significant correlation between the Social Support Questionnaire and the Short Form-36 measure of broader health status. The developers have published the results of several similar studies supporting the construct validity of the scale (Sarason *et al.* 1987a, 1987b). Predictive validity was judged to be satisfactory on the basis of correlations with depression (the correlations for 100 men and 127 women for each dimension were from −0.22 to −0.43). Sinha *et al.* (2002) supported the construct validity of the scale in their study of older people in India. Their prediction that social support, as measured by the scale, would have a modifying effect on positive attitudes to life and perceived control over life was supported. Separate factor analyses were performed by the developers for each of the two scores. Each analysis showed a very strong first (unrotated) factor. The first factor accounted for 82 per cent of the common variance for the availability score, and 72 per cent for the satisfaction with support score.

All factor loadings exceeded 0.60 and 0.30 for each score respectively. There appeared to be good evidence that one strong factor underlies each score and that they represent different dimensions of the concept. Pretorius and Diedricks (1993) also carried out exploratory factor analysis and confirmed that the Social Support Questionnaire contained one factor that represented the structure of the scale.

Reliability

Test-retest reliability over a four-week period, using 602 students, was 0.90 for the availability of support items, and 0.83 for satisfaction with support, using 105 students. The alpha coefficients for internal reliability were 0.97 for availability and 0.94 for satisfaction with support, using 602 university students. Inter-item correlations ranged from 0.37 to −0.71 for availability, and from 0.21 to −0.74 for satisfaction with support. A second study of 227 students showed a correlation between the availability and satisfaction with support scores of 0.31 for men and 0.21 for women (Sarason *et al.* 1983).

A validated German version exists (Franke *et al.* 2003). This research led the authors to emphasize the importance of perceived support, rather than network size per se, as the most relevant variable (Sarason *et al.* 1987a), and they subsequently developed the Quality of Relationship Index (published in full by Pierce *et al.* 1991). This is not reviewed here and interested readers are referred to the latter reference. A Spanish version has also been developed and tested (see López and Cooper 2011 for reviews).

In sum, it is a viable measure of support, with good results for internal reliability and some support for its construct and predictive validity.

Short version

Sarason *et al.* (1987b) also developed a six-item version, using item and factor analysis to identify the items for inclusion. Based on their studies of three samples of college students, they reported that the Cronbach's alphas of internal consistency were consistent with those for the full scale at 0.90 to 0.93 for both subscales. The full and short versions of the measure were reported to be associated with measures of anxiety, depression, loneliness and social skills (Sarason *et al.* 1987b; Boury *et al.* 2004).

INTERVIEW SCHEDULE FOR SOCIAL INTERACTION (ISSI)

This index was developed by Henderson *et al.* (1980, 1981a). The conceptual definition of support was based on the theory that social relations are based on attachment, social integration, nurturance, reassurance of personal worth, sense of reliability, help and guidance. The scale was developed over a year in pilot studies of 130 people in health centres, outpatient departments in a club for the elderly, and in a general population sample in Canberra. It was reported to be acceptable to both healthy and psychiatrically disturbed respondents.

The scale takes approximately 30 minutes to complete, although reports of 60 minutes have also been published. A short version of the scale has been developed by Unden and Orth-Gomer (1989), with similar levels of reliability, validity and discriminative ability as the full scale.

Content

The scale comprises 52 questions asking about the availability and adequacy of people in specific roles: attachment, provided by close affectional relationships; social integration, provided by membership of a network of persons having shared interests and values; the opportunity for nurturing others; reassurance of personal worth; a sense of reliable alliance; and obtaining help and guidance from informal advisers in times of difficulty. It does not adequately measure the availability and adequacy of attachment and social integration.

A question about the availability of provision is immediately followed by a question on adequacy. Examples are shown in Box 6.6.

Box 6.6 Examples from the ISSI

How many friends do you have whom you could visit at any time, without waiting for an invitation? You could arrive without being expected and still be sure you would be welcome.

Would you like to have more or fewer friends like this, or is it about right for you?

Three items ask about negative interactions. One example is:

How many people whom you have to see regularly do you dislike?

Reproduced in Henderson, S., Byrne, D.G. and Duncan-Jones, P. (1981) *Neurosis and the Social Environment*, Appendix, p. 214. Sydney: Academic Press. Copyright Elsevier. With permission. There is no charge for the use of this scale – see http://www.incamresearch.ca/content/interview-schedule-social-interaction, accessed 16 September 2015.

Scoring

The four principal indices yield four scores: availability of attachment, perceived adequacy of attachment, availability of social integration and perceived adequacy of social integration. The following indices are created:

AVAT: the availability of affectionally close relationships (attachments).

ADAT: the perceived adequacy of what comprises these close relationships, expressed as a percentage of what is available.

NONDAT: those who lack close relationships might not be unhappy with their situation. The NONDAT index is a measure of such satisfaction despite the absence of attachment.

ATTROWN: the number of attachment persons with whom the respondent has been having rows in the last month.

AVSI: the availability of more diffuse relationships, as with friends, work associates and acquaintances (social integration).

ADSI: the perceived adequacy of these more diffuse relationships.

The scoring and computing instructions have been published by Henderson et al. (1981a).

Validity

The authors judged the scale to have face validity and stated that the items effectively tap the constructs of availability and adequacy of attachment in adulthood and social integration. Henderson et al. (1980) established the validity of the scale by analysing its four dimensions in relation to personality assessments (neuroticism and introversion–extraversion as measured by the Eysenck Personality Inventory). The sample comprised 225 members of the general population. The authors hypothesized that a neurotic person would have problems in forming and maintaining social relationships and would consequently be dissatisfied with those relationships. Inverse relationships with availability and satisfaction measures and neuroticism were reported (–0.18 to –0.31). Results were less consistent with extraversion. The construct validity of the scale was also supported by findings reported by Magne et al. (1992). They found that, of their sample of inpatients who had attempted suicide, social support was associated with marital status and economic activity in the expected directions.

Predictive validity was reported by Henderson et al. (1980) on the basis of a study of neurosis on 756 residents of Canberra, Australia. The measure was associated with Zung's Self-Rating Depression Scale and Goldberg's General Health Questionnaire (–0.15 to –0.96) (Henderson 1981a). The study, which was based on baseline data collection from 756 residents in Canberra, with three follow-up interviews with a sub-sample over 12 months, reported that deficiencies in social relationships had an effect on the early development of neurotic symptoms. As both availability and adequacy items correlated significantly and negatively with psychiatric disorder and depression, predictive validity was judged to be satisfactory. The scale was also able to discriminate between new migrants to Canberra and those who had been living there for seven months or more. The strength of this study was that it was carried out on a representative sample of the population and was prospective, not cross-sectional; thus the measures of social ties were less likely to be contaminated by already established neurotic symptoms. The correlations between respondents' ISSI scores and those of someone who was nominated as well informed about their social relationships were weak to moderate, although significant, ranging between 0.26 and 0.59 for the items. This may be an indicator of the difference between actual and perceived support. Persson and Orbaek (2003) also reported that the ISSI was sensitive to differences in trait anxiety levels in a group of healthy women, as defined by the STAI-Y.

A short version of the ISSI was tested by Eklund *et al.* (2007), for construct and discriminant validity and dimensionality, among in- and outpatient psychiatric samples. The measure was associated with psychosocial functioning and life domains characterized by social interaction, supporting construct validity, although only three of the four subscales discriminated between the samples. The authors concluded that, overall, as similar results were obtained in all three samples, their study strongly supported the validity of the ISSI.

Eklund *et al.*'s (2007) study also showed that the ISSI was a unidimensional construct, and the subscales relating to attachment constituted less stable factors, suggesting that the subscales are used cautiously.

Reliability

Test-retest reliability scores for the scale indices over an 18-day period using 51 people from the general population ranged from 0.71 to 0.76; using 756 adults from a general population over an 18-day period, scores ranged from 0.66 to 0.85, and over a 12-month period ranged from 0.66 to 0.85. The problem with this long time period is that support structures might have changed and thus a lower correlation may reflect this rather than the reliability of the measure. Internal consistency reliability coefficients range from 0.67 to 0.81 for the indices.

In sum, once again more testing is required.

THE SOCIAL NETWORK SCALE (SNS)

The SNS was adapted by Stokes (1983), based on Hirsch's (1980) work on social support. This work was based on just 20 recent young widows and 14 older women recently re-entering college studies. Stokes (1983) based the SNS on four dimensions of network that he judged to be important: network size, number of people the respondent feels close to, number of relatives in the network and network density.

A supplement to the SNS is an eight-item scale which asks people to rate their total social networks, and their networks of friends, on four dimensions: general satisfaction with the network, amount of desired change in the network, satisfaction with assistance in daily activities, and satisfaction with emotional support. The eight ratings are summed to provide a measure of satisfaction.

Content

Hirsch's (1980) conceptual definition of support was based on interaction that affects coping ability: guidance, social reinforcement, aid, socializing and emotional support.

The social support dimension of the scale was operationalized by asking respondents to specify the amount of interaction with network members in five areas of supportive activity, and their degree of satisfaction with the interaction.

The social network dimension of the scale conceptualized social network as a natural support system, based on significant others. This is operationalized by asking people to list in a matrix 'the initials of up to 20 people who are significant in your life and with whom you have contact at least once a month'. People then put an X in those boxes of the matrix that connect people who are significant in each other's lives and who have contact with each other at least once a month. They also indicate which persons in their lists are relatives, and which persons they can 'confide in or turn to for help in an emergency'. This is probably more important in terms of providing effective, satisfying support than network size (Brown *et al.* 1975; Conner *et al.* 1979; Stokes 1983). This yields information on the domains shown in Box 6.7.

Box 6.7 Information collected by the SNS

1 Network size, defining network as people who are significant in the respondent's life and with whom the respondent interacts regularly.
2 The number of people in the network who the respondent feels close to – how many one can confide in or turn to for help in an emergency.
3 The number of relatives in the network.
4 Network density (degree to which network members are themselves interconnected).

The SNS is free to use and is in the public domain. Developer: Professor Joseph Stokes, Professor Emeritus, University of Illinois at Chicago; http://stokes.socialpsychology.org – accessed 1-9-2015.

Scoring

Scoring consists of totalling the number of network members, relatives and confidant(e)s. Scoring could also identify the overlap between these categories (e.g. between relatives and confidant(e)s).

A larger number of variables (see Box 6.8) can be computed and scored from the grid.

Box 6.8 Variables that can be derived from the SNS

(i)   Network size: number of people listed
(ii)   Relatives: number of relatives listed
(iii)   Friends: number of people listed who are not relatives
(iv)   Confidant(e)s: number of people respondents said they could confide in or turn to for help in an emergency
(v)   Relative confidant(e)s: number of confidant(e)s who are relatives
(vi)   Friend confidant(e)s: number of confidant(e)s who are not relatives
(vii)   Percentage relatives: proportion of the network who are relatives (relatives/size)

(viii) Percentage confidant(e)s: proportion of the network members who are confidant(e)s (confidant(e)s/size)
 (ix) Percentage relative confidant(e)s: proportion of confidant(e)s who are relatives (relative confidant(e)s/confidant(e)s)
  (x) Density: proportion of the total possible number of relationships which actually exist among members of a social network, excluding the respondent
 (xi) Relative density: density of the relatives in the social network list
(xii) Friend density: density of the friends in the social network list
(xiii) Relative–friend density: number of relationships between relatives and friends as a proportion of the total possible number of such relationships.

Reproduced in Stokes, J.P. (1983) Predicting satisfaction with social support from social network structure. *American Journal of Community Psychology*, 11: 141–52. With permission of the developer.

Validity and reliability

Although the scale has been judged to have face validity, it has not been tested fully for reliability and validity. It is also limited in scope; Stokes has himself supplemented the use of the SNS with other scales measuring the frequency of receipt of support (e.g. the Inventory of Socially Supportive Behaviours (Stokes 1985)). Stokes (1983), on the basis of administering the SNS to 82 students, submitted these dimensions to a principal components analysis and four factors emerged which accounted for over 80 per cent of the variance in the original matrix: size, with emphasis on the number of friends in the network; presence of confidant(e)s; dominance of relatives in the network; and density. Stokes (1983) also reported that the number of confidant(e)s in the social network was predictive of perceived support satisfaction.

It is not clear what the basis is for limiting social network members to 20. Also, a flaw with calculating the percentage of relatives, confidant(e)s or friends in the network is that this does not take account of size in the presentation: for example, a network composed of 50 per cent relatives could be a network of just two members, one of whom is a relative, or it could be a network size of 20, 10 of whom are relatives. This does not appear to be a satisfactory basis for making comparisons between respondents.

Other main problems with this scale are that it does not have an index of geographical proximity, or frequency of contact, of network members, and it does not distinguish between types of relative (e.g. sons and daughters are not distinguishable) or the nature of the contact (supportive, instrumental, etc.).

The value of the scale is the conciseness of the grid, which saves pages of questions, and it is easily supplemented with other structural items and questions on support (Bowling and Farquhar 1995). The structural network features measured by the grid have been reported to have little predictive value in longitudinal studies of psychological morbidity or life satisfaction (Bowling et al. 1992, 1993). Moreover, the author's own experience with the scale is that respondents tend to omit their spouses from the network scale – their significance and contact being taken for granted – hence instructions need to ask them to include them where appropriate (Bowling et al. 1988).

The social support part of the scale has been little tested but was judged to have face reliability; the correlation between respondent and interviewer ratings of satisfaction and support was 0.53 and was judged to be reliable. Inter-item correlations, testing for reliability, ranged from 0.22 to 0.51 (Hirsch 1980).

The sensitivity of the scale is unknown. Generally, it will require supplementation with other items.

THE LUBBEN SOCIAL NETWORK SCALE (LSNS)

The LSNS was developed for use among elderly populations (Lubben 1985, 1988). It was a modification of the well-known Berkman-Syme Social Network Index, which successfully distinguished between survivors and non-survivors in their longitudinal general population survey in Alameda County (Berkman and Syme 1979). The LSNS attempted to take into account many of the criticisms levelled at existing social network measures. These included the need to measure more than household composition (as most older people live alone, this is an inadequate indicator of social isolation or need); the need to distinguish between social support and social networks (to facilitate attempts to distinguish between lack of available support and lack of need for support), and between family, friend and peer interactions and networks (given the literature on the superiority of friendship over family networks for psychological well-being); the need to measure network size, the existence of a confidant(e) relationship, and the existence of reciprocal relationships (given their theoretical importance for the timely provision of help and support when required, and their contribution to psychological well-being); the unwieldy nature of existing instruments (most were too long).

The original Berkman and Syme indicator consisted of a simple index based on four main components: marital status, nature of relationships with relatives and friends, church membership, and membership of other organizations and clubs. It was able to predict risk of mortality among members of their longitudinal survey. However, Lubben noted that there was little variation among samples of elderly people in relation to the indicators of organizational participation and marital status and therefore deleted these items. However, this decision needs revising in view of the increasing participation of the current generation of people aged 65 and over in community and voluntary activities and associations between marital status and health, well-being and mortality. Lubben also simplified the original scoring system.

Content

The LSNS is a composite measure of social networks and the original version consists of 10 items within three dimensions:

(i) family networks: composed of three areas: size of active family network, size of intimate family network, and frequency of contact with a family member. These are covered by questions on the number seen monthly, number feels close to, and frequency of social contact;

(ii) friends networks: composed of three similar areas, and covered by questions on the number feels close to, number seen monthly, and frequency of social contact;

(iii) interdependent social supports: composed of interdependent relationships covered by four questions on existence of a confidant, is a confidant, relies upon and helps others, living arrangements.

An additional question covers living arrangements (lives alone, with spouse, other relatives or friends, unrelated individuals or lives alone). A copy of the scale can be found in Lubben (1988). Revised, 18-item and six-item versions are available.

Examples are shown in Box 6.9.

Box 6.9 Examples from the LSNS

Confidant relationships

When you have an important decision to make, do you have someone you can talk to about it?

5 = always/4 = very often/3 = often/2 = sometimes/1 = seldom/0 = never

When other people you know have an important decision to make, do they talk to you about it?

5 = always/4 = very often/3 = often/2 = sometimes/1 = seldom/0 = never

Helping others

Does anybody rely on you to do something for them each day? For example: shopping, cooking dinner, doing repairs, cleaning house, providing child care, etc.

No/Yes

If No: Do you help anybody with things like shopping, filling out forms, doing repairs, providing child care, etc.?

4 = very often/3 = often/2 = sometimes/1 = seldom/0 = never

© Lubben (1984, 1988). Reprinted with permission of the developer. Access: the LSNS, 18-item and six-item versions are downloadable at: https://www.bc.edu/schools/gssw/lubben.html. Permission to use the measures can be requested at: https://www.bc.edu/schools/gssw/lubben/permission_to_usescales.html, accessed 16 September 2015.

Scoring

The LSNS score is obtained from an equally weighted sum of the 10 items, each of which ranges from 0 to 5. The total score can therefore range from 0 to 50.

Validity

There is support for the discriminative ability of the scale. Lubben (1988) tested the LSNS with non-institutionalized members of the California Senior Survey, a random sample of elderly Medicaid recipients from eight communities within California. The LSNS correlated significantly with a life satisfaction index, inpatient hospital admissions for six or more days within the last 12 months, and health behaviours. Rutledge *et al.* (2003), in their follow-up study of osteoporosis among women aged 65 and over, reported that the LSNS scores were a robust predictor of mortality. Chou and Chi (2001), in their study of a cross-section of elderly people in Hong Kong, also reported that the LSNS mediated the association between everyday competence and depression. Low LSNS scores have been correlated with mortality, all-cause hospitalization and depression (Lubben and Gironda 2004).

Reliability

All 10 items of social networks were reported to inter-correlate highly, with a Cronbach's alpha of 0.70, indicating high internal consistency (Lubben 1988). Chou and Chi (2001), in their study of a cross-section of elderly people in Hong Kong, reported a slightly higher Cronbach's alpha of 0.76.

In sum, the scale has been popular due to its simplicity (Chou and Chi 1999, 2001), and its derivation from the well-known Alameda County social network measure, although more evidence of its psychometric properties is needed.

Abbreviated Lubben Social Network Scale (LSNS-6)

A brief six-item form of the measure has also been developed (Lubben *et al.* 2006; Crooks *et al.* 2008). The LSNS-6 is a self-reported scale to assess social isolation in older adults by measuring perceived social support received from family and friends. It assesses the size of the respondent's active social network (i.e. relatives or friends seen or heard from ≥1 times/month), perceived support (i.e. close relatives or friends who could be called on for help), perceived confidants (i.e. relatives or friends to whom the respondent could talk about private matters), and contacts with friends and neighbours. The six questions are divided into three on the size of three different areas of social network attributable to family ties, and three on friendship ties. See Box 6.10 for examples.

Box 6.10 Examples from the LSNS-6

1. How many relatives or family members do you see or hear from at least once a month?
   (Note: include spouse, in-laws, and any other relatives)
5. How many friends/neighbours do you feel close to that you can call on for help?

© Lubben *et al.* 2006. Reprinted with permission of the developer. Access: the LSNS, 18-item and six-item versions are downloadable at: https://www.bc.edu/schools/gssw/lubben.html. Permission to use the measures can be requested at: https://www.bc.edu/schools/gssw/lubben/permission_to_usescales.html, accessed 16 September 2015.

Each question is scored on a scale of 0 to 5. The total score is an equally weighted sum of these six questions; scores ranging from 0 to 30. Subscale scores for family and friends can be scored (0 to 15) (Lubben *et al.* 2003). Higher scores indicate larger social networks. A cut-off point of 12 is reported to carry optimal sensitivity. A validation study, conducted in three European cities, with 7,432 elderly men and women, reported an overall Cronbach's alpha of 0.83 that was consistent across all cities (Lubben *et al.* 2006).

Crooks *et al.* (2008), in their study of older people in health maintenance organizations in the US, reported that their factor analysis showed structures similar to those reported by Lubben *et al.*, and factors from the two subscales mirrored those reported in that study (2006). Crooks *et al.*'s (2008) Cronbach alpha values for the measure were 0.84 for the LSNS-6, 0.86 for the family subscale, and 0.82 for the friend subscale, also consistent with earlier research (Lubben 1988). It is a popular, low-burden measure, also used in intervention studies (e.g. Iliffe *et al.* 2014)

THE SOCIAL SUPPORT APPRAISALS SCALE (SS-A) AND THE SOCIAL SUPPORT BEHAVIOURS SCALE (SS-B)

The SS-A was developed by Vaux *et al.* (1986a, 1986b). The concept of social support employed was based on Cobb's (1976) definition of social support and was designed to tap the extent to which individuals believe that they are loved by, esteemed by and involved with family, friends and others. One of the authors has reported a relationship between type of network orientation (e.g. positive or negative) and respondents indicating either secure or anxious attachment styles (Wallace and Vaux 1993). One main advantage is the brevity of the scale.

Content: SS-A

The SS-A is a 23-item scale consisting of a list of statements about relationships with family and friends. Eight items relate to family relationships, seven to relationships with friends and eight to 'others' in a general way. Respondents have four response choices: 'strongly agree', 'agree', 'disagree' or 'strongly disagree'. There is no middle value. Examples are shown in Box 6.11.

Box 6.11 Examples from the SS-A

My friends respect me
My family cares for me very much
I am not important to others
I am well liked
I feel a strong bond with my friends
If I died tomorrow very few people would miss me
I feel close to members of my family
My friends and I have done a lot for one another

(Strongly agree/agree/disagree/strongly disagree)

Source: the SS-A is reproduced in the Appendix of: Vaux, A., Phillips, J., Holly, L. *et al.* (1986) The social support appraisals (SS-A) scale: studies of reliability and validity. *American Journal of Community Psychology*, 14: 195–219. Reprinted with permission from Springer. The SS-A is in the public domain and is free to use without charge. See www.incamresearch.ca/content/social-support-appraisals-scale, accessed 1 September 2015.

Scoring

Three scores can be computed: SS-A, which is the sum of all 23 items; SS-A (family) which is the sum of the eight family items; and SS-A (friends) which is the sum of the seven friends' items. The limitation of the scale is that it provides no information about the numbers of people involved in providing supportive behaviour, nor of who they are (e.g. spouse, sister, son, etc.).

Validity

Convergent and divergent validity was tested in relation to five samples of students and five community samples (the total number of respondents was around 1,000). It was tested against other measures of social support (the Perceived Social Support Scale; the Family Relations Index; the Social Support Questionnaire and two other less well-known scales; and three single-item questions on satisfaction with friends). The authors also employed two further scales developed by themselves. One of these was the Social Support Resources Scale. This was designed to tap many aspects of the individual's social support network. Respondents were asked to list up to 10 people who provided them with five types of support: emotional support, practical assistance, financial assistance, socializing and advice/guidance. Respondents provided satisfaction ratings for the five types of assessed support. Respondents were asked further questions about the characteristics of the people identified and the nature of the relationship (e.g. spouse, friend). Mean scores were computed for each variable. The final scale tested against the SS-A was the Social Support Behaviours Scale, also developed by the authors (see below). The authors also tested the SS-A against six personality and depression inventories, including the Affect-Balance Scale, and the UCLA Revised Loneliness Scale (see later). The authors provided evidence of convergent validity with a variety of the support measures. The vast number of correlation coefficients presented by the authors is too extensive to reproduce here. However, none of the correlations with other support or personality measures were very strong (ranging from 0.03 to –0.51, with one correlation coefficient achieving –0.72). This is not surprising given the very different theoretical concepts underlying the different scales. Also in support of the discriminative ability of the SS-A, Coen *et al.* (1997) reported, on the basis of their study of the burden on carers of patients with Alzheimer's disease, that the carer burden was independently associated with the SS-A.

Reliability

There is no published evidence of reliability. In sum, the validity of the scale remains questionable, and evidence of reliability is also required.

Content: SS-B

The SS-B was developed by Vaux *et al.* (1987) to tap five modes of supportive behaviour. It is similar to Barrera *et al.*'s ISSB (1985: 94) but does not suffer from the limitation of asking solely about actual rather than potential support (which may simply reflect number of problems). This lists 45 specific supportive behaviours, in five subscales, tapping the five modes of support listed in their Social Support Resources scale: emotional support, socializing, practical assistance, financial assistance and advice/guidance. Respondents indicate how likely their family and friends would be to engage in each of the behaviours in time of need. Examples are shown in Box 6.12.

Box 6.12 Examples from the SS-B

Would suggest doing something, just to take my mind off my problems.
Would visit with me, or invite me over.
Would give me a ride if I needed one.
Would have lunch or dinner with me.
Would loan me a car if I needed one.
Would go to a movie or concert with me.

(No one would do this/someone might do this/some family member/friends would probably do this/some family member/friend would certainly do this/most family members/friends would certainly do this.)

SS-B is reproduced in the Appendix of: Vaux, A., Riedel, S. and Stewart, D. (1987) Modes of social support: the social support behaviours (SS-B) scale. *American Journal of Community Psychology*, 15: 209–337. Reprinted with permission from Springer. SS-B is in the public domain and is free to use without charge. See http://www.incamresearch.ca/content/social-support-behaviour-scale, accessed 1 September 2015.

A problem with such scales is that the assumptions made about social values and norms, i.e. that respondents all equally value 'a movie or concert', and that other people are in a financial position to, for example, 'loan a car'.

Scoring

The choice of five responses for each type of behaviour itemized ranges from 'no one would do this' to 'most family members/friends would certainly do this' (see above). Items are scored 0 (no one) to 5 (certainly) and summed.

Validity

The predictive validity of the SS-B has been demonstrated in relation to psychological distress and it correlates moderately with other support measures (including SS-A) (Vaux and Wood 1985; Vaux *et al.* 1986a, 1986b). In addition, five methods were used to test the validity of the SS-B as a measure of support: the classification of items by judges; an analogue (role-playing) simulation of samples deficient in each mode of support; tests against a related measure of supportive behaviour (ISSB); an examination of levels of each type of support provided for different problems and confirmatory factor analysis (Vaux *et al.* 1987). The classification of items according to their content by judges (students) provided some evidence of the content validity of the SS-B. The percentage of items correctly classified by judges ranged from 13 to 100 per cent; in most cases it was over 60 per cent. The unique role-playing exercise with students showed deficits in available support corresponding to their enacted role, providing evidence of subscale sensitivity. However, the correlations were weak with the ISSB. This may be because the two measures are based on different concepts of social support – available and enacted respectively.

The factor analysis conducted by the developers demonstrated that the pattern of item convergence and divergence was highly consistent with predictions and confirmed that the SS-B taps the five modes of support conceptualized very well (Vaux *et al.* 1987). Further psychometric testing of the SS-B by Corcoran *et al.* (1998) showed that their factor analyses on separate subscales showed loadings which were more consistent for 'family' than 'friends'. They also found the SS-B to be a poor discriminator between adolescents in different ethnic groups who were attending pregnancy prevention programmes, and concluded that the scale needs further development to enhance its sensitivity among people with varying ethnic and socioeconomic backgrounds.

Reliability

Excellent internal consistency was obtained for the SS-B items (the lowest alpha was 0.82). In sum, the SS-A and SS-B scales are promising but have been little tested for reliability and validity.

INTERPERSONAL SUPPORT EVALUATION LIST (ISEL)

The ISEL was developed by Cohen *et al.* (1985), on the basis of the theoretical assumption that the buffering effect of social support is cognitively mediated. The testing of this theoretical assumption required an instrument which aimed to measure the perceived availability of support. The items were developed on theoretical grounds to cover the domain of social support that could facilitate coping with stress. It was designed to assess perceived availability of support in four distinct areas: material aid (tangible subscale); someone to talk to about one's problems (appraisal subscale); comparisons of self with others (self-esteem subscale); people to share activities with (belonging subscale).

Content

The ISEL consists of a list of 40 (48 in the version for students) statements about the perceived availability of potential social resources. The items are balanced: half the statements comprising the scale contain positive items about social relationships, and half contain negative items.

Respondents are asked to indicate whether each statement is 'probably true' or 'probably false'. Examples of the items are shown in Box 6.13.

Box 6.13 Examples from the ISEL

There is at least one person I know whose advice I really trust.

There are very few people I trust to help solve my problems.

If I decide on a Friday afternoon that I would like to go to a movie that evening, I could find someone to go with me.

Most people I know don't enjoy the same things that I do.

If I were sick and needed someone to drive me to the doctor, I would have trouble finding someone.

If I had to mail an important letter at the post office by 5.00 and couldn't make it, there is someone who could do it for me.

In general people don't have much confidence in me.

Most people I know think highly of me.

Reproduced from: Cohen, S., Mermelstein, R., Karmack, T., and Hoberman, H.M. (1985) Measuring the functional components of social support, in I.S. Saronson and B.R. Saronson (eds) *Social Support: Theory, Research and Applications*. Boston, MA: Martinus Nijhoff, pp. 73–94. Reprinted with permission from the developer. ISEL and the scoring information are in the public domain and can be used without charge. See Appendix in Cohen *et al.* (1985) for the scale. Website: http://www. psy.cmu.edu/~scohen/scales.html, accessed 16 September 2015. The website states that permission for the use of Dr Cohen's scales is not necessary in relation to non-profit academic research or non-profit education. For other uses the contact is commoncoldproject@andrew.cmu.edu.

Scoring

The ISEL is scored by counting the number of responses indicating support. There is no information on the validity of this method. Factor analyses, based on data from 133 college students, by Brookings and Bolton (1988) recommended that ISEL subscale scores should be analysed and that a total should not be calculated which results in loss of unique information.

Validity

Cohen *et al.* (1985) reviewed the evidence on the reliability and validity of the scale, most of which was previously unpublished. The scale was tested on over 500 students in Oregon; over 100 students at Carnegie-Mellon University; almost 100 students at Delaware University; over 100 students at Guelph University; and over 100 students at Arizona State University. Four studies were also carried out on the version of the scale for the general population using student samples at the University of California, Carnegie-Mellon University and the University of Oregon (total: over 200 students), and a general population sample participating in the Oregon Smoking Cessation Program (over 60 adults).

The ISEL student scale was found to correlate moderately with other social support scales: 0.46 with Barrera's ISSB; 0.30 with the total score of the Moos Family Environment Scale; 0.39 with reported network size; 0.46 with number of close friends reported; and 0.42 with number of close relatives reported. The scale for the general population correlated 0.31 with a scale measuring the quality of relationships with partner/spouse. It was expected that the scale would be associated with self-esteem, as this is influenced by feedback from others; the correlation with the Rosenberg Self-Esteem Scale was 0.74. The scale was reported to be significantly associated with depression; social anxiety was controlled to eliminate the possibility that the social support concept was not merely a proxy measure of personality (e.g. social anxiety or social skills). Longitudinal analyses of the groups in the studies showed that the scale was able to predict changes in depressive symptomatology. The latter association indicated that the scale was not simply measuring symptomatology. There was a small but significant association with physical symptomatology and changes in these symptoms. The scale was reported to be a good predictor of smoking cessation and was associated with measures of stress in the direction suggestive of the buffering effects of social support. These data suggest the importance of appraisal support as a protector against the pathogenic effects of stressful life events. Espwall and Olofsson (2002) also reported that patients with musculo-skeletal disorders reported less emotional support on a condensed version of the scale, supporting its construct validity.

Factor analyses, based on data from 133 college students, by Brookings and Bolton (1988) confirmed a four-factor model, which provided a reasonable fit for the data, although the high correlations between the four factors suggested a general second-order social support factor.

Reliability

Adequate internal and test-retest reliability was reported by the authors. With the scale for students, the internal-reliability alpha coefficient was 0.86, ranging from 0.60 to 0.92 for each subscale. The alpha coefficients for the general population scale ranged from 0.88 to 0.90. The subscale correlations ranged from 0.62 to 0.82.

The student scales were tested for test-retest reliability at four-week intervals with reported correlations of 0.87 for the total scale, and correlations of 0.71–0.87 for the subscales. The general population scale was administered twice with a two-day interval; the reported correlation for the total scale was 0.87, and the subscale correlations ranged from 0.67 to 0.84. The six-week test-retest correlations from the smoking cessation group sample were 0.70 overall, and 0.63–0.69 for the subscales. The six-month test-retest correlations for this group were 0.74 for the total scale and 0.49–0.68 for the subscales. In sum, although this is a scale which has only recently been developed, and further testing is required, it does cover a wide range of supportive relationships and results of testing for reliability and validity are fairly good. One limitation is that the scale does appear to be orientated towards an active population group (e.g. questions on advice over job changes, sexual problems and availability of people to give lifts to the airport). The scale has been used successfully with psychiatric patients living in the community, and the scale was able to discriminate between those who lived independently and those who lived with their families or in group homes (Pomeroy *et al.* 1992). It has been translated into several languages with good results for internal consistency and construct validity (Wills and Filer 2006). A 12-item version is available (http://www.psy.cmu.edu/~scohen/scales.html, accessed 16 September 2015).

THE NETWORK TYPOLOGY: THE NETWORK ASSESSMENT INSTRUMENT

Because support can be predictive of outcomes in a range of areas of life, knowing a person's network type can be valuable to health and social services professionals. Also, the aim of social service providers is to develop a care plan for people which supplements, rather than supplants, the care they receive from members of their social network. Therefore, several investigators have attempted to develop frameworks for the assessment of the network for care plans (Kaufman 1990). One of the more successful attempts has been that of Wenger (1989, 1992, 1994, 1995) in relation to elderly people.

As a result of qualitative, more anthropological, research with elderly people, Wenger was able to identify different types of social networks and she constructed a typology of support networks (Wenger 1989, 1994; Wenger and Shahtahmasebi 1991). The typology is based on the theory that the experience of ageing is mediated through, and determined by, the capacity of the support network to respond to change and the nature of the resulting change (Wenger and Shahtahmasebi 1991). The support network was defined as those involved with the person in a significant way: as a member of the household, in providing or receiving companionship, emotional support, instrumental help, advice or personal care.

The Network Typology is developed from the data collected by a questionnaire – the Network Assessment Instrument identifes the availability and proximity of family and other 'support ties', the degree of involvement demonstrated by respondents with family, friends, neighbours and community, network density (how many network members know each other), and the size and content of the larger social network. The distinguishing factors between the different types of network are the availability of local close kin, the level of involvement of family, friends and neighbours, and the level of interaction with the community and voluntary groups. The collection of this data enabled the investigators to identify five types of support network in relation to the lifestyle and relationship of the elderly person to their network:

Local family-dependent support network: This network is mainly focused on close local family ties, with few peripheral friends and neighbours; it is often based on a shared household with, or close to, an adult child, usually a daughter. Nearly all support needs are met by the family. Community involvement is low. The network is small, and the person is more likely to be widowed, older and in poorer health than people with other types of network.

The most numerous members of this network are relatives living within one mile, followed by household members and neighbours.

Locally integrated support network: This includes close relationships with local family, friends and neighbours (the latter two often overlap). These are based on long-term residence and active community involvement in religious/voluntary organizations currently, or in the recent past. These networks are larger than others.

These networks have the highest numbers of neighbours, who are also likely to be friends.

Local self-contained support network: This is characterized by 'arm's-length' relationships or infrequent contact with at least one relative living in the same or adjacent community (usually a sibling, niece or nephew). Childlessness is common. Reliance is mainly on neighbours, and the lifestyle is focused on the household. Community involvement, if any, is low key. Networks are smaller than average.

These networks also have more neighbours than other network categories, and the network is predominantly local.

Wider community focused support network: This network is typified by active relationships with distant relatives, usually children, and high salience of friends and neighbours. The distinction between friends and neighbours is maintained and there is engagement in community or voluntary organizations. There has frequently been retirement migration, absence of local kin, and networks are larger than average. This network is commonly a middle-class or skilled working-class adaptation.

The most numerous membership of these networks are friends who live within a one-mile radius, followed by relatives who live more than 50 miles away, and then equal numbers of friends at one to five miles away and neighbours. This membership reflects the absence of local kin.

Private restricted support network: This network is associated with absence of local kin, although a high proportion are married. Contacts with neighbours are minimal, there are few friends nearby and there is a low level of community contacts or involvements. There are two sub-types included in this network: independent married couples and dependent elderly people who have withdrawn or become isolated from local involvement. A low level of social contact often represents a lifelong adaptation. Networks are smaller than average.

The most numerous members of this type of network are relatives who live more than 50 miles away, followed by members of the household or relatives who live 15–50 miles away, reflecting the absence of local kin.

Wenger (1994) reported that most networks can be categorized into one of these types, and that local self-contained and private restricted networks are less robust than other network types, and more vulnerable in the face of ill health or a crisis. The different lifestyles and social characteristics of people represented by the different network types were described.

Content

The Network Assessment Instrument is used in conjunction with the appropriate training package developed by Wenger. This is because the identification of the network is the planning aid and is no substitute for professional training on appropriate interventions. A video-based training and resource pack for practitioners and service providers was produced (Wenger 1995). The use of the typology has been piloted with a number of social services teams, and a guide has been published (Wenger 1994).

The Instrument contains eight questions, each with one of three types of 1–3 (coded A, B, C) or 1–6 (coded A–F) point response categories, relating to distance of residence of network member or frequency of interaction/activity (e.g. No relatives (A) to (lives) 50+ miles (F); Never/no friends (A) to (chat/do something) Less often (F); Yes, regularly (A) to No (C)). The questionnaire also contains the information for the interviewer to be able to code (A–F) immediately the type of network from each response code. Examples of the questions are shown in Box 6.14.

Box 6.14 Examples from the Wenger Network Assessment Instrument

How far away, in distance, does your nearest child or other relative live? (Do not include spouse.)

If you have any friends in this community/neighbourhood, how often do you have a chat or do something with one of your friends?

Do you attend meetings of any community/neighbourhood or social groups, such as old people's clubs, lectures or anything like that?

Sources: Wenger, G.C. (1994) *Support Networks of Older People: A Guide for Practitioners*. Bangor: Centre for Social Policy Research and Development, University of Wales. ISBN 0 904567 14 1; Wenger, G.C. (1995) *Practitioner Assessment of Network Type (PANT). Training and Resource Pack*. Brighton: Pavilion Press. Reprinted with permission Pavilion Publishing and Media. Developer Professor Claire Wenger gives permission for anyone to use the instrument if they cite it in the following way: This form should only be used in conjunction with the appropriate training package devised by Dr G. Clare Wenger, Centre for Social Policy Research and Development, University of Wales, Bangor. Source reference: Wenger, G.C. (1994) Support network of older people: a guide for practitioners. CSRPD, University of Wales Bangor, ISBN 0 904567 14 1. Access: e-copies of the guide for practitioners, and the official syntax for calculating network types that should be used by researchers, are available from: Professor Vanessa Burholt FacSS, director: Centre for Innovative Ageing, College of Human Sciences & Health Sciences, Rm 20, Haldane, Swansea University, Singleton Park, Swansea, Wales, SA2 8PP; email: v.burholt@swansea.ac.uk

---

Scoring

Each item is analysed independently, and the network typology is constructed on the computer, using the response codes and the network type coded by interviewers on the questionnaires.

Validity and reliability

While much descriptive data has been published based on the Network Typology and the Network Assessment Instrument, little information on its reliability and validity has been published to date. It was piloted with social services practitioners, and Wenger (1994) reported that most of her sample members were able to be classified by the typology. Network type was associated, as predicted, with levels of dependency, reliance on services, informal help, emotional support and social interaction, and survival of respondents over an eight-year follow-up period (Wenger and Shahtahmasebi 1991). These associations suggest that the instrument has construct and predictive validity. Despite changes over time in the network sizes of respondents, the overall frequency distribution of the network type of the sample remained constant (Wenger and Shahtahmasebi 1991), suggesting that the instrument is robust.

Kirby et al. (2000) used the measure in a study of over 1,000 elderly people living at home. They reported associations between cognitive impairment and network type in the expected direction: those with cognitive impairment had a lower proportion of locally integrated and a higher proportion of private restricted networks. Late-life depression was also associated with low levels of community integration. Golden et al. (2009) interviewed over 1,000 people aged 65+ in their homes, recruited from primary care practices in Dublin. They also assessed social networks with Wenger's Network Typology, and depression. In support of the construct validity of Wenger's measure, indicators of well-being, depressed mood and hopelessness were all independently associated with non-integrated social networks, as well as loneliness.

Litwin and Shiovitz-Ezra (2011) used cluster analysis to derive social network type with a sub-sample of almost 1,500 people aged 65+ from the first wave of the US National Social Life, Health, and Aging Project. They reported that respondents embedded in network types characterized by greater social capital tended to exhibit better well-being in terms of less loneliness, less anxiety and greater happiness. The five network types they distinguished were: diverse, friend focused, congregant, family focused, and restricted network types – four of these were consistent with Litwin's (2001) previous research findings in Israel (which yielded diverse, friend, family and restricted networks). However, in the US sample, a fifth network grouping also emerged: the congregant network, because its main feature was social exchanges with other people at a place of worship (these members had high relative frequency of attendance at religious services, and minimal attendance at other types of organized group meetings). While they did not use Wenger's measure, the associations reported are consistent with the latter's findings, and with the conclusions of Wenger that assessment of social network type can be useful in risk assessments of older people.

The measure is presented here in view of its popularity among service providers in risk assessment of older people.

LONELINESS

A relevant concept in research on social networks and support is loneliness. Loneliness is distinct from social isolation and can be defined as an unwelcome feeling of lack or loss of companionship. De Jong Gierveld and Van Tilburg (2006) defined loneliness as pertaining to the feeling of missing an intimate relationship (emotional loneliness) or missing a wider social network (social loneliness). Russell et al. (2012) tested the cognitive discrepancy model, which holds that loneliness is experienced when people perceive a difference between their desired and their actual levels of social involvement. In their analyses of data from students, they reported that support for the cognitive discrepancy model of loneliness was found only for social contact measures relating to close friendships. Weiss (1973) distinguished between situational and personality theories of loneliness. The former emphasize environmental factors as causes of loneliness – for example, death of a spouse, moving to a new city. Several variables have been associated with loneliness. While research across Europe has reported that loneliness was associated with age as well as area (Yang and Victor 2011), research on loneliness in relation to the actual quality of social networks is still relatively scarce (Jones *et al.* 1985; Bowling *et al.* 1989).

Various scales for the assessment of loneliness have been devised, but few have been fully tested. Scales measuring loneliness were reviewed by Russell (1982). Measures include the long and short forms of the De Jong Gierveld Loneliness Scale for overall, emotional and social loneliness, and the UCLA Loneliness Scale. The latter is the most widely used worldwide, and is reviewed here.

THE REVISED UNIVERSITY OF CALIFORNIA AT LOS ANGELES (UCLA) LONELINESS SCALE

The UCLA Loneliness Scale is the most well-known and widely used measure of loneliness. It was developed to measure subjective feelings of loneliness or social isolation, and later revised by Russell *et al.* (1978, 1980a, 1980b). The authors aimed to identify common themes that characterized the experience of loneliness for a broad spectrum of individuals. The UCLA Loneliness Scale was intended to be global.

The scale was based on statements used by people to describe their loneliness. It began with 25 items and asked individuals to rate how frequently they felt the way described, from 'never' to 'often' on a four-point scale. The scale was tested on clinic volunteers and students. The final loneliness scale consisted of 20 items; selected items all had item-total correlations above 0.50.

One problem with the original version of the scale was that all the items on the measure were worded in the same (lonely) direction. The implication is that tendencies to respond in a certain way could systematically influence loneliness scores. A second potential problem was social desirability bias, given the possible stigma associated with admissions of loneliness. Thus Russell *et al.* (1980a, 1980b) revised the scale to take account of these problems, and 10 negatively (lonely) worded and 10 positively (non-lonely) worded items were included. The revised version was tested on 162 students. Testing involved using the original scale and 19 new items, written by the authors, and anxiety and depression measures. The 10 positively and 10 negatively worded items with the highest correlations with a set of items about whether they were lonely were included in the scale. All of the item-criterion correlations were above 0.40. Further revisions led to the current version 3 (Russell *et al.* 1980a, 1980b; Russell and Cutrona 1991; Russell 1996). In the current version 3, the wording of the items and the response format were simplified to facilitate the administration of the measure to less educated populations.

Content

The scale consists of 20 statements with a Likert response scale attached to each, half of which are descriptive of feelings of loneliness and half descriptive of non-loneliness or satisfaction with relationships. A copy of the most recent version can be seen in Russell (1996). Examples of items are shown in Box 6.15.

Box 6.15 Examples from the UCLA Loneliness Scale

I lack companionship
It is difficult for me to make friends
There is no one I can turn to
I feel part of a group of friends
There are people I feel close to

There are four choices for replies: never (1), rarely (2), sometimes (3) and often (4).

© D. Russell. The measure was first published in 1978 by Russell, D., Peplau, L.A., and Ferguson, M.L. and was revised in 1980 and 1996. Reprinted with permission of the developer. The measure is freely available and can be used without charge or permissions; the developers request that users should send them a copy of all results once work is completed. Contact: Professor Daniel W. Russell, Department of Human Development and Family Studies, Iowa State University, 4380 Palmer Suite 2330, Ames, IA 50011, USA; email: drussell@iastate.edu; website: https://public.psych. iastate.edu/ccutrona/uclalone.htm, accessed 16 September 2015.

Scoring

The total score of the scale is the sum of all 20 items. Some need to be reversed before scoring (i.e. 1 = 4, 2 = 3, 3 = 2, 4 = 1); these are asterisked on the scale.

Validity

Validity was initially assessed by correlations of the scale with a single-item self-rating of loneliness measure (0.79); a comparison of the scores of two samples of participants (the mean of the clinic sample was 60.1, significantly different from the student group's mean of 39.1); and the loneliness scores were also strongly associated with depression, anxiety, dissatisfaction, unhappiness and shyness. High correlations with other measures of loneliness have been reported (ranging from 0.72 to 0.74). These have been reviewed by Russell (1982). The main limitation of this research is that it has been largely confined to samples of students, raising questions about the validity of the scale in assessing loneliness for other populations. Although there is a need for further testing of the scale on other population groups, initial results do appear encouraging.

Early evidence of the discriminative and predictive validity of the revised scale was provided by studies reporting strong relationships between the scale and measures of depression, and earlier research showed strong relationships between loneliness items and anxiety and self-esteem (Russell 1982). The scale was tested for validity on 162 students, and also using the Beck Depression Inventory. Correlations of 0.32 were obtained with an anxiety index and of 0.62 with the Beck Depression Inventory. The discriminant validity was also assessed by a study of 237 students, with the aim of assessing whether it was measuring a different dimension of well-being to the depression scales. Multivariate analysis was used for this purpose and it was reported that a loneliness index explained an additional 18 per cent of the variance in loneliness scores beyond that accounted for by the mood and personality measures. Concurrent validity was also assessed, and significant associations were reported between solitary activities, having fewer friends and loneliness scores (Russell 1982).

However, the validity of loneliness scales is difficult to assess. In terms of content and face validity, the most face-valid loneliness measures are questions simply asking 'are you lonely?' This then faces the problem of social desirability bias that could limit validity. Problems with the assessment of criterion validity also exist. Loneliness is not synonymous with isolation. There is an absence of external validity criteria for loneliness. Even ratings by others known to the person are not highly reliable.

The scale has been used in a number of studies of emotional well-being, and its validity supported. Stokes (1985) analysed social network structure and personality factors in relation to loneliness, using the earlier version of the UCLA, in a sample of 97 male and 82 female students. He reported network density to be the most strongly related to loneliness: people with interconnected networks tend to be less lonely. This may be because they feel more sense of community, of belonging to a group. Extraversion and introversion were also related to loneliness.

In further support of its construct validity, Mellor and Edelmann (1988) used the revised UCLA Loneliness Scale (version 3) in a study of loneliness in 36 people aged over 65. They found that loneliness was associated with having fewer confidant(e)s and with lack of mobility. Riggio et al. (1993) also used the scale and reported that level of social skills predicted perceptions of loneliness. Mahon et al. (1995), in a study of adolescents, reported that the construct validity of the scale was supported by its associations with theoretically relevant variables including friend solidarity and dependency. Russell (1996) also reported significant correlations with other measures of loneliness, and measures of health and well-being. Analyses of study data using the Danish version of the scale reported comparable results to its original version; reported correlations between the UCLA Loneliness Scale and measures of emotional loneliness, social loneliness, self-esteem, depression, extraversion and neuroticism supported the convergent and discriminant validity of the scale (Lasgaard 2007).

Factor structures have been reported suggesting either unidimensional or two- to three-factor structures (Cuffel and Akamatsu 1989; Mahon and Yarcheski 1990; McWhirter 1990; Mahon et al. 1995). Russell (1996) reported a confirmatory factor analysis which indicated that a model incorporating a global bipolar loneliness factor, along with a two-method factor reflecting direction of item wording, provided a good fit. The unidimensional factor structure of the measure was supported in a study of the Danish version of the scale, although the structure remains controversial (Lasgaard 2007).

Reliability

Studies of both the original version (which had a different scoring method of 0–3) by Russell *et al.* (1978) and Perlman and Peplau (1981), and the revised version, all reported good results for the validity and reliability of the scale (Russell *et al.* 1980a, 1980b; Russell 1982). Russell (1996) cited coefficient alphas ranging from 0.89 to 0.94 for the revised version 3, in support of its internal consistency.

In relation to test-retest consistency, Jones (cited in Russell *et al.* 1978) found a correlation of 0.73 over a two-month period in a student sample, and Russell (1996) reported a test-retest reliability of r = 0.73. In sum, this scale is the most extensively tested of all the loneliness scales available, and results are generally good. The study of the Danish version of the scale showed high internal consistency (Lasgaard 2007).

In sum, this is the most widely used scale of loneliness worldwide, and it has been found to predict a wide range of mental and physical health outcomes. The scale is available in Russell (1996) and while freely available for use, it is copyrighted by Russell, and the developers request that users should send them a copy of all results once work is completed.

EXAMPLE

An example of the use of measures of social network and support measures is shown in Box 6.16.

Box 6.16 Example of secondary analyses of study using social network support outcome measures

Iliffe *et al.* (2007) conducted analyses with the aim of exploring the significance of social isolation in the older population.

They undertook secondary analyses of previously collected baseline data from a randomized controlled trial (RCT) evaluating health risk appraisal. The sample was 2,641 community-dwelling, non-disabled people aged 65+ in suburban London.

Their measures included the six-item Lubben Social Network Scale.

They reported that more than 15 per cent of the older age group in this sample were at risk of social isolation. The risk of social isolation was higher in older men, older people who lived alone, and people who had mood or cognitive problems. It was not associated with greater use of services.

They concluded that awareness of social isolation should trigger further assessment in primary care, and consideration of potential interventions to reduce isolation, treat depression or ameliorate cognitive impairment.

CHAPTER 7

MEASURING THE DIMENSIONS OF SUBJECTIVE WELL-BEING

CHAPTER COVERAGE

SUBJECTIVE WELL-BEING

Research and theory on subjective well-being has developed from two conceptual perspectives – hedonic, which focuses on happiness, feeling good about life, and emotional well-being, and eudaimonic: meaning and self-realization, focusing on full functioning, living a good life (Keyes 2002).

It has been argued by some that, in the developed world where basic human needs have generally been met, quality of life (QoL) equates with perceived subjective well-being, and is the extent to which pleasure and happiness, and ultimately satisfaction with life, have been obtained (Andrews 1974). This reflects the influence of early Greek and nineteenth-century utilitarian philosophy, with their focus on emotional well-being and hedonistic aspects of life – the maximization of well-being, happiness, pleasure and satisfaction. This is also reminiscent of Bentham's ([1834] 1983) utilitarian philosophy, which regarded well-being as 'the difference in value between the sum of pleasures of all sorts and the sum of pains of all sorts which a man experienced in a given period of time', and held that society should aim for the greatest good of the greatest number. Others argue that pleasure and satisfaction are insufficient for a good QoL and that a sense of purpose or meaning, self-esteem and self-worth, among other dimensions, are crucial for good QoL, including QoL in people with dementia (Sarvimäki 1999). Others have criticized interchangeable uses of the terms and concepts of well-being and QoL, which has muddied attempts to define well-being (Dodge et al. 2012).

The concept of subjective well-being emerged in the 1950s in attempts to move beyond objective indicators of life quality in the monitoring of social change (e.g. societal levels of income, crime, housing quality), and towards more subjective measures, which more meaningfully reflected people's lives and experiences (Land 1975; Keyes et al. 2002). Influential social science models of QoL in North America were then based primarily on the related but distinct concepts of 'the good life', 'life satisfaction', 'subjective well-being', 'social well-being', 'morale', the balance between positive and negative affect, 'the social temperature', or 'happiness' (Gurin et al. 1960; Cantril 1965; Bradburn 1969; Andrews and Withey 1976; Campbell et al. 1976; Andrews 1986). Of concern, however, both theoretically and methodologically, is the interchangeable use, without justification, of these distinct concepts. For example, morale and well-being are commonly categorized as components of psychological well-being and measured using one of a number of overlapping scales of life satisfaction, well-being, or morale and affect (e.g. Kutner et al. 1956; Neugarten et al. 1961; Cantril 1965; Bradburn 1969; Wood et al. 1969; Lawton 1972, 1975; Andrews and Withey 1976; Campbell et al. 1976; Coleman 1984; Dupuy 1984; Antonovsky 1993).

The terms subjective well-being and psychological well-being are also used interchangeably, although these concepts have been distinguished by Keyes et al. (2002) who defined *subjective well-being* as the evaluation of life in terms of satisfaction and balance between positive and negative affect, and *psychological well-being*, drawing on theories of human development, as the perception of engagement with existential challenges of life. They argued that while both approaches assess well-being, they address different features of this concept: subjective well-being was said to involve more global evaluations of affect and life quality, whereas psychological well-being addressed perceived thriving in relation to the existential challenges of life (examples include the pursuit of meaningful goals, personal development, self-actualization, coping strategies, growth and mastery – especially in the face of cumulative adversity – and the development of quality social relationships). Their study of over 3,000 adult Americans provided strong empirical evidence to support their hypothesis that these are related but distinct areas. Their factor analyses confirmed the two concepts are related but distinct; and their analyses also showed that people who were younger and more educated had different combinations of them (higher psychological than subjective well-being) in comparison with respondents who were older and with less education.

However, the selection of measures is often made by investigators without any theoretical justification or any attempts to fit a predefined definition or model of 'well-being', despite the fact that, while overlapping, a scale measuring life satisfaction cannot adequately measure the other related but distinct concepts.

As the various dimensions of well-being are subjective, their measurement is also based largely on subjective self-ratings (Campbell 1976). The measurement of well-being has been enhanced by the development and use of psychometrically sound measurement scales (Andrews and Crandall 1976). However, a major methodological problem has still been the lack of consistency in the usage of the terms 'happiness', 'life satisfaction' and 'morale' and related concepts (Stones and Kozma 1980; Stull 1987). As previously indicated, these concepts are not identical, although many researchers continue to treat them as interchangeable (George and Bearon 1980). For example, while the concepts and measures of the different dimensions of well-being are related, and generally correlate highly, suggesting that they are all tapping a common underlying construct (Lohmann 1977), 'life satisfaction' and 'morale' have a more cognitive component to them, while happiness has a more affective or emotional component (Andrews and McKennel 1980). The cognitive component implies evaluation, while affect refers to the positive/negative feeling. Distinguishing between cognitive and affective components of subjective well-being is particularly useful when interpreting data. For example, elderly people often report lower levels of happiness but higher levels of life satisfaction than younger people (Campbell et al. 1976; Campbell 1981). This suggests, then, that while cognitive evaluations of life as a whole increase with age, positive affect may decline. Perhaps people become more jaded in their emotions with age, but increase their perceptions of their level of achievement, or adjust their aspirations (Andrews and Robinson 1991). While the differences could simply be due to birth cohort effects (Campbell 1981; Inglehart and Rabier 1986), the example still illustrates the value of the different concepts.

The theoretical literature on subjective well-being also divides this global concept into state (current well-being) and trait (well-being as a feature of character), and postulates self-reported well-being measures that reflect at least four factors: circumstances, aspirations, comparisons with others, and a person's baseline happiness or disposition (Warr 1999). At a different level, developments in dynamic equilibrium theory led to Headey and Wearing's (1989) suggestion that for most people subjective well-being is fairly stable most of the time, because stocks, flows and levels of subjective well-being are in dynamic equilibrium, thus well-being depends on prior equilibrium levels of well-being, on life and recent events. An extension of the theory by Cummins (2010) focused on homeostasis and the strength of the challenge to it, and how it affects subjective well-being. These models were examined in detail by Dodge *et al.* (2012).

Ryff and Singer (1996) proposed a rich, multidimensional view of well-being including components of autonomy, environmental mastery, personal growth, positive relations with others, purpose in life and self-acceptance. Some concepts and measures of well-being also include individuals' assessments of their overall past and present life. The following dimensions are defined next for conceptual clarity: happiness, life satisfaction, morale, self-esteem and self-concept, and sense of coherence. The measures that are reviewed here relate to these concepts of subjective well-being, although some of these measures also include items relating to psychological well-being as defined by Keyes *et al.* (2002), and not all authors have made their theoretical underpinning (i.e. concepts and definitions) fully explicit.

HAPPINESS

Happiness has an affective or emotional component (Andrews and McKennel 1980). In contrast to morale and life satisfaction, happiness is a short-term affect and can fluctuate on a daily basis; it is a transitory mood of 'gaiety and elation' that reflects how people feel towards their current state of affairs (Campbell *et al.* 1976). Blanchflower and Oswald (2001), following Veenhoven (1991, 1993) defined happiness as the degree to which the individual judges the overall quality of his or her life to be favourable or unfavourable. Some have argued that the achievement of happiness depends on what one has relative to a norm, although Veenhoven (1991) has criticized relativity theory and points to data that shows that happiness is associated with objective, rather than relative, improvements in one's circumstances. Heylighten and Bernheim (2000) have incorporated both arguments and define the dimensions that make up well-being and QoL, including happiness, as the sum of mainly relative subjective factors but with a small contribution from objective factors. Some investigators also define happiness in terms of life satisfaction, thus confusing the two concepts. For example, Argyle *et al.* (1989) defined happiness in their studies of the concept as the frequency of joy, the average level of satisfaction and the absence of negative feelings. Reflecting the vogue for self-empowerment and self-improvement, the term 'authentic happiness' has been coined by Seligman (2002), who claimed that happiness can be cultivated from self-knowledge and building on one's signature (positive, optimistic) characteristics by knowing one's greatest strengths and then recrafting one's life to use them. He also provided over a dozen questionnaires purporting to measure different dimensions of happiness including current happiness, general happiness, approaches to happiness, sensitive happiness, positive and negative affect, optimism, purpose in life and also Diener *et al.*'s (1985) Satisfaction with Life scale.

Happiness, like other subjective measures, is not without measurement problems. Smith (1979) has stated that there appears to be seasonal variation in the global measure of happiness, with happiness highest in the spring, declining in the summer and autumn and dropping to its lowest point in winter. There is also the possibility of positivism bias among sample members: some people may be reluctant to admit the extent of any unhappiness they may feel on the basis of the assumption that it is socially desirable to be 'happy'. However, most investigators chose relatively simple measures of happiness, which are likely to be less robust than developed scales. A long-used, simple question on happiness has been asked in the US General Social Surveys since 1946: 'Taken all together, how would you say things are these days – would you say you are very happy, pretty happy, or not too happy?' (GSS question 157, reproduced by Blanchflower and Oswald 2001; and see classic studies by Gurin *et al.* 1960 and Bradburn 1969). In contrast to life satisfaction measures which show stability over time, happiness levels using such questions have been reported to change, both within population groups and nations (Blanchflower and Oswald 2001, 2004).

LIFE SATISFACTION

Life satisfaction refers to an overall assessment of one's life, or a comparison reflecting some perceived discrepancy between one's aspirations and achievement. As well as feelings of success in achieving life goals, commonly used measures of life satisfaction usually include several factors pertaining to the present, including pleasure from everyday activities, perception of life as meaningful, positive self-image, optimistic outlook, and satisfaction with different domains of life, such as health, work, relationships, activities and standard of living (Neugarten *et al.* 1961). Some explicit or implicit comparison group is usually involved ('compared to others'). Thus, it is a long-term cognitive appraisal of past, present and overall life and is relatively stable in middle to old age (Campbell *et al.* 1976; Campbell 1981; Bowling *et al.* 1996). This is the likely explanation for overall lack of changes in life satisfaction measures when administered in longitudinal surveys. Some studies report an increase in satisfaction in older age groups; and there are no consistent associations with sex. It is uncertain whether investigators have adequately separated life satisfaction from happiness. It has been widely used as a social indicator of QoL (e.g. Andrews and Withey 1976; Campbell *et al.* 1976).

In addition to the development of measures of overall life satisfaction, some investigators have developed measures of satisfaction with illness (Hyland and Kenyon 1992) and customized measures of life satisfaction as a complement to symptom-orientated measures (Frisch *et al.* 1992). These indicators are not included here, but are a welcome development in a field dominated by negative measures of broader health and health-related QoL.

MORALE

Morale is the most poorly defined concept of these terms, despite its importance in older age (Wenger 1992). In contrast to happiness, morale (like life satisfaction) has a more cognitive component, which relates to the positive/negative feeling (Andrews and McKennel 1980). It has been suggested that it can be measured multidimensionally in relation to a person's feelings about their life, himself/herself and their relation to the world (Nydegger 1986). It is often defined in terms of a basic sense of satisfaction with oneself, a feeling that there is a place in the environment for oneself, acceptance of life, and a generalizable feeling of well-being (Lawton 1972, 1975), or more precisely, in terms of confidence and enthusiasm (George 1979; Stones and Kozma 1980). Kutner *et al.* (1956) defined morale as a mental state, or set of dispositions, which condition one's response to problems in daily life.

SELF-ESTEEM AND SELF-CONCEPT

Self-esteem is viewed as a component of mental health, as well as a component of general assessment of life (Andrews and Withey 1976), and thus satisfaction with life. Again, these concepts are distinct, while interlinked. Psychologists refer to self-esteem in relation to a sense of self-worth – a belief that one is a person of value, accepting personal strengths and weaknesses (Rosenberg 1965; Coopersmith 1967; Wells and Marwell 1976). Self-esteem is therefore a self-evaluation. There are several commonly used scales of self-esteem in adults of all ages (e.g. Fitts 1965; Rosenberg 1965; Coopersmith 1967).

Related concepts include self-regard, self-acceptance, self-concept or self-image. These are all based upon the individual's assessment and evaluation of himself or herself (Crandall 1973; Wells and Marwell 1976). Self-concept is the cognitive component of the self and consists of individuals' perceptions of themselves (i.e. what I am really like?). Self-esteem is reflected in one's self-concept, or self-image (which can be divided into ideal self (the image aspired to) and the actual self (Coopersmith 1967). Self-concept is multidimensional in that people might also view themselves as having multiple selves – for example, different self-related beliefs can emerge in different life domains (family, friends, romantic relationships, work, standard of living/material domains) (Campbell *et al.* 1976).

Available evidence suggests that positive self-esteem is an important component of general assessment of life (Andrews and Withey 1976). Self-esteem may become increasingly salient with the transition from middle to old age (Schwartz 1975). Most self-esteem theorists suggest, with some evidence, that self-esteem is developed and maintained through a successful process of personal interaction and negotiation with the environment (Rosenberg 1965; Wells and Marwell 1976). In sociology, the critical role of social interaction and the significance of others in developing self-esteem and its maintenance are generally emphasized (Wylie 1974). In relation to health and illness, negative self-image has been analysed in relation to effects on recovery from disease (Wilson-Barnett 1981). As successful negotiations are less likely in later life, self-esteem among older people is less likely to be positive. If age changes in self-esteem are to be expected, measures of the impact of a relevant intervention could become confounded with developmental changes over time.

SENSE OF COHERENCE

Antonovsky (1987) developed the salutogenic theory of a 'sense of coherence', as a global orientation to perceive the environment as comprehensible, manageable, and meaningful, arguing that the individual's perceptions of life have a positive influence on health. The theory relates to the extent to which one has a dispositional orientation, a pervasive, yet dynamic, feeling of confidence, that:

- stimuli deriving from one's internal and external environments in the course of living are structured, predictable, and explicable (comprehensibility),
- resources are available to one to meet the demands posed by these stimuli (manageability),
- demands are challenges, worthy of investment and engagement (meaningfulness).

This dispositional orientation is distinct from a personality trait or coping mechanism (Antonovsky 1993). The concept of sense of coherence has been little tested, although its inclusion within a model of QoL has been given some empirical support (Sarvimäki and Stonbock-Hult 2000).

GLOBAL MEASURES

Life satisfaction, morale and happiness are all global concepts, referring to life as a whole rather than to specific aspects of it. Global measures are of relevance in assessing well-being, although they may be of limited utility in evaluative research (George and Bearon 1980). Carp (1977) cautions against drawing policy-relevant inferences from data which do not reveal why and with what people are satisfied. Specific measures are an alternative (e.g. housing satisfaction in evaluating effect of relocation) (Andrews and Withey 1976; Campbell *et al.* 1976). Global and item-specific measures are appropriate for different research questions.

One of the advantages of using a few global items rather than global or specific scales is brevity: one or two questions rather than a whole battery. However, a positivism bias, for example, respondents' desire to be socially desirable, can be obtained with short items. Also, short items lack sensitivity and therefore are of limited predictive value in longitudinal studies. The effect of question order with such items has been relatively unexplored, although the National Opinion Research Centre found that placing a question about marital happiness immediately before a global question of happiness resulted in a more positive response on global happiness (Smith 1979). A review of the literature indicates that well-being has been measured by three major scales as well as short global items: Life Satisfaction A (Neugarten *et al.* 1961); Bradburn Affect-Balance Scales (Bradburn and Caplovitz 1965; Bradburn 1969); Philadelphia Geriatric Center Morale Scale (Lawton 1975); and global items of happiness and life satisfaction (Robinson and Shaver 1973; Campbell *et al.* 1976; Smith 1979). Other popular scales are the Delighted–Terrible Faces Scale (Andrews and Withey 1976) and the Psychological Well-Being Schedule (Dupuy 1978). These scales produce global scores of well-being (life satisfaction or morale), except the Delighted–Terrible Faces Scale which contains current life-specific items that should be analysed separately. These will be reviewed in the following sections. Popular single-item measures and batteries, asking respondents to assess their lives as a whole, are the

Ladder Scale (Cantril 1965) and the Delighted–Terrible scales (Andrews and Withey 1976) in which respondents rate themselves on a Likert category scale, mark a rung on a ladder or select a circle or a face to represent how they feel about a specified area of life. Robinson and Shaver (1973), Sauer and Warland (1982) and Andrews and Robinson (1991) have reviewed a wide range of items and measures of life satisfaction, well-being and happiness.

THE LIFE SATISFACTION INDEX A (LSIA) AND INDEX B (LSIB)

The LSIA and LSIB were developed by Neugarten *et al.* (1961) in order to produce a relatively short self-report measure of life satisfaction based on respondents' feelings. The aim of these scales is to measure general feelings of well-being in order to identify 'successful' ageing.

Several versions of the LSI exist. All were derived from the five dimensions of past and present life from life satisfaction ratings obtained by a clinical interview: zest and apathy, resolution and fortitude, congruence between desired and achieved goals, positive self-concept and mood tone.

LSIA and LSIB were first developed in 1956 on the basis of item analyses of four rounds of interviews on the subject of life satisfaction, with people aged 50–70. The samples were based on a stratified probability sample of middle- and working-class people residing in Kansas City. A second sample aged 70–90 was interviewed two years later, based on a quota sample (overall total 177).

All versions of the index are easily administered and rest on a substantial amount of empirical support. The problem with the scale is its global nature which poses uncertainty about what is being measured. Scale A has been further criticized by Liang (1984) for failing to measure transitory effects.

Content

Scales A and B differ only slightly in content but greatly in form. LSIA has a checklist of 20 items, statements with which the respondent either agrees or disagrees. LSIB has 12 open-ended questions that are given a score based upon the content of the answers. The two instruments can be used together or separately (Neugarten *et al.* 1961). Index A has been used more frequently than B, probably due to ease of administration and quantification of structured items.

The original LSIA consists of 20 items (12 positive and eight negative). A second version, adapted by Wood *et al.* (1969), contains 13 of the original 20 items. Another version uses 18 items (Adams 1969). An advantage of Scales A and B, and the shorter versions of A, is that they have positive and negative items.

A wide variety of content areas are tapped by each of these scales, for example, ranging from happiness to satisfaction with level of activity. Some items reflect back over past lives or involve comparing the present with the past, as well as assessment of the present. Examples of Scale A items are shown in Box 7.1.

Box 7.1 Examples from the LSIA

Positive items
These are the best years of my life.
The things I do today are as interesting to me as they ever were.
I am just as happy as when I was younger.

Negative items
This is the dreariest time of my life.
Most of the things I do are boring and monotonous.
Compared to other people I get down in the dumps too often.

Respondents are asked to agree or disagree with the items on Scale A; they can also classify statements as undecided with the alternative version of the scoring. Examples of the open-ended items on B are:

Positive
What are the best things about being the age you are now?
(1 = positive answer; 0 = nothing good about it.)

What is the most important thing in your life at the moment?
(2 = anything outside of self, or pleasant interpretation of future; 1 = hanging on, keeping health or job; 0 = getting out of present difficulty, or nothing now, or reference to past.)

Negative
Do you wish you could see more of your close friends than you do, or would you like more time to yourself?
(2 = OK as it is; 1 = wish could see more of friends; 0 = wish more time to self.)

How much unhappiness would you say you find in your life today?
(2 = almost none; 1 = some; 0 = a great deal.)

Availability: the scale has long been in the public domain, free to use; it can be accessed in Neugarten *et al.*'s (1961) publication. Reproduced from Neugarten B.L. *et al.* (1961). The measurement of life satisfaction, *J. Gerontol.*, 16(2): 134–43. By permission of Oxford University Press on behalf of the Gerontological Society of America. The LSI can also be viewed, on free registration, at http://www.medicalalgorithms.com/life-satisfaction-index-a-of-neugarten-et-al – link, accessed 1 September 2015.

Scoring

Scores are summed over all the items; thus ratings of each dimension are combined. The criticism of this is that the separate dimensions are confounded.

There are two scoring methods for the LSI. In the original method, a two-point agree/disagree response choice rated dissatisfaction as 0 and satisfaction as 1. Subsequent analysis of the 'undecided' responses then led to the use of a three-point scale, rating satisfaction as 2, uncertain as 1, and dissatisfaction as 0 (Wood *et al.* 1969), although this has shown little advantage over the original two-point method.

Population norms for North America have been provided for the full and 13-item versions of the scale, but they vary between studies, probably reflecting the different samples, and should be used with caution (see Harris 1975 and reviews by George and Bearon 1980 and McDowell and Newell 1996). Comparisons between studies also require caution, given the different scoring systems used.

In sum, in view of the multidimensionality of the scale, the use of a single score blurs the relationships between the items and a series of subscales should be calculated instead.

Validity

Using a sample of 177 people aged 50 and over, Neugarten *et al.* (1961) reported a correlation of 0.55 between LSIA and the original clinical life satisfaction rating instrument. The correlation of scores on LSIA with judges' ratings was 0.52, and the correlation of LSIB with judges' ratings was 0.59. Details of these were described by Neugarten *et al.* (1961).

Criterion validity was established by assessments by a clinical psychologist, although these took place 18–22 months after the fourth interview on 80 remaining sample members, and were of questionable value.

Correlations between the LSIA and the Affect-Balance Scale and the Philadelphia Geriatric Center Morale Scale have been reported as 0.66 and 0.76 respectively (Bild and Havighurst 1976; Lohmann 1977). Bowling and Browne (1991), in an interview study of 662 people aged 85 and over living at home in London, also supported the convergent validity of the scale. As hypothesized, the correlation between Neugarten's Life Satisfaction Scale A and the Delighted–Terrible Faces Scale (life satisfaction – current circumstances) was significant at r = –0.65, and with the General Health Questionnaire (which assesses mainly anxiety and depression) was –0.47 (i.e. greater life satisfaction was associated with low anxiety and depression). A similar study by the authors of almost 300 people aged 65 and over living at home in Essex, and of almost 400 people aged 65–85 living at home in London, reported correlations between Neugarten's Scale and the Delighted–Terrible Faces Scale and the General Health Questionnaire of –0.24 and –0.47 (Essex) and –0.57 and –0.41 (London) respectively (unpublished data). Although the correlations with the General Health Questionnaire were very similar for the three studies (–0.41 to –0.47), it is uncertain why the correlations with the Faces Scale vary between studies (–0.24 to –0.65), or should be weaker with the younger elderly groups. High correlations between these scales would not be expected as they tap different dimensions of well-being, although overlap would be (as is demonstrated). Scale A was reported in follow-up studies to be significantly associated with poor functioning and health, supporting the scale's discriminative ability (Bowling *et al.* 1993).

The scale was able to predict outcome of reminiscence therapy with elderly nursing home residents (Cook 1998), although it has not always been successful in distinguishing between patients with different conditions (Celiker and Borman 2001). Other inconsistencies using the scale have been reported. For example, although the original authors reported that LSIA did not correlate with demographic factors, other studies have indicated that it does. In particular, positive correlations with socioeconomic status have been reported by a number of authors. For example, Zegers Prado *et al.* (2009) in their sample of 473 adults in Chile, reported that scores varied by age, income and education level, but not sex.

Several studies using factor analysis and multiple-regression models have confirmed the multidimensional nature of the scale, and have questioned the original conceptual formulation (Hoyt and Creech 1983). Zegers Prado *et al.* (2009), with their sample of 473 adults in Chile, defined five factors, accounting for 50.62 per cent of variance.

Reliability

Cronbach's alpha internal consistency coefficients in various studies range from 0.70 to 0.76 (Dobson *et al.* 1979) to around 0.79 (Wood *et al.* 1969; Stock and Okun 1982), depending upon the version used. Zegers Prado *et al.* (2009) in their study in Chile, reported that the Cronbach's alpha was 0.80.

Inter-rater reliability was assessed with seven pairs of judges who rated descriptions of 177 cases. The coefficient of correlation between the pairs of ratings was 0.79. For the 177 cases life satisfaction scores for Scale A ranged from 8 to 25, with a mean of 17.8, and a standard deviation of 4.6. There was no significant difference with sex (Neugarten *et al.* 1961). The correlation between judges' and clinical ratings was 0.64 which was regarded as satisfactory in view of these problems. Test-retest reliability coefficients have been reported to range between 0.80 and 0.90 in patients with chronic diseases (Burchhardt *et al.* 1989).

Bowling *et al.* (1993, 1996), in their longitudinal study of people aged 85 and over in London, and aged 65 and over in Essex and London found the measure to be stable over two and a half years, but also detected problems with the scale which affect reliability (unpublished information). The final item 'In spite of what people say, the life of the average person is getting worse not better' is often received with puzzlement about a stereotyped 'average person'. This item assumes agreement over an 'average' person. Moreover, respondents' agreement with this item does not necessarily inform us about whether their own lives are getting 'worse not better'. It makes the scale too diverse in the number of different dimensions of life satisfaction covered. Two other items also require refinement: 'I feel my age but it does not bother me' is difficult for respondents to reply to if they feel their age, but it does bother them; and 'Compared to other people my age, I look smart when I am dressed to go out' is difficult to reply to in the case of respondents who are housebound or who live in institutions and do not go out. Bowling *et al.* (1993, 1996) found the alpha reliability coefficients for the scale ranged from alpha 0.73 to 0.80; and the split-half reliability coefficients ranged from 0.65 to 0.74 (unpublished data).

THE LIFE SATISFACTION INDEX Z 13-ITEM VERSION (LSIZ)

Validity and reliability

Wood *et al.* (1969) derived a 13-item version of Neugarten *et al.*'s (1961) Scale A, known as LSIZ, which is probably the most popular. The scoring for this version of the scale ranges from 0 to 26. Item scores are: satisfaction: 2; dissatisfaction: 1; don't know: 1. The 13-item LSIZ has been used extensively in the USA.

Moderate correlations were obtained between the LSIZ and a scale of social engagement (0.49) and between the LSIZ and the Symptoms of Anxiety and Depression Scale (0.49), suggesting that the scales assess some common aspect of well-being (Wood *et al.* 1969). It was used by Usui *et al.* (1985) in a community survey of people aged 60+ in Jefferson County, Kentucky. It was significantly associated with other variables in the expected direction, in support of its construct validity. The authors reported a correlation of –0.22 between the number of physical health problems and life satisfaction, and similar correlations with various social activities, income level and life satisfaction; these were confirmed by multiple regression analysis. In contrast to Morgan *et al.*'s (1987) study of over 1,500 people aged 65+ in Nottinghamshire in the UK, they reported that older respondents had higher life satisfaction scores.

The LSIZ was used by Kozma and Stones (1987), along with other measures of well-being, in a study of 150 people, aged between 50 and 82, in acute psychiatric or community psychiatric wards in Newfoundland. Correlations between the LSIZ and the Philadelphia Geriatric Center Morale Scale (PGCMS) were reported to be high (0.74). The authors reported that the LSIZ was able to correctly identify 72 per cent of the community hospital or acute ward samples, and PGCMS correctly identified 74 per cent. A scale of social desirability was also used, and the authors reported that controlling for social desirability did not enhance the construct validity of the well-being scales.

It was found to be sensitive to change in a study of participation in community programmes (Wylie 1970). Kritz-Silverstein *et al.* (2002) reported that it was able to discriminate between women who had undergone hysterectomy and those who had not, with the former group expressing significantly higher life satisfaction. A longitudinal study of menopausal transitions by Dennerstein *et al.* (2000) which used the LSIZ reported that, at six years after baseline measurement, there were no differences in life satisfaction (irrespective of menopausal status or use of hormone replacement therapy), although life satisfaction was associated with mood, earlier attitudes towards the menopause and ageing, and relationship with partner.

Wood *et al.* (1969) reported that the refined 13-item version of the index shows a split-half reliability of 0.79. Edwards and Klemmack (1973) reported an internal consistency reliability coefficient of 0.90.

Although the LSI measures are satisfactory in terms of standard tests of reliability and validity, their global and multidimensional nature poses problems. The issue is: what is being predicted? However, these scales are the most commonly used to measure well-being in gerontological research (Larson 1978; Stull 1987).

THE AFFECT-BALANCE SCALE (ABS)

Bradburn (1969) described the ABS as an indicator of happiness or general psychological well-being. Bradburn and Caplovitz (1965) hypothesized that subjective well-being could be indicated by a person's position on two independent dimensions: positive and negative affect. Well-being is expressed as the balance between these two. Research on the structure of psychological well-being supports the hypothesis that positive and negative well-being are related, although they do not form a bipolar continuum (Bradburn 1969; Ryff 1989; Ryff and Keyes 1995). Thus, a person could experience some aspects of negative well-being and other aspects of positive well-being simultaneously (Marks and Lambert 1999). Positive factors can compensate for negative feelings. The scale was developed on the basis of a sample of 2,006 adults in Illinois (Bradburn and Caplovitz 1965), and revised on the basis of a study of 2,787 adults of mixed socioeconomic and ethnic groups based on five probability random samples in Detroit, Chicago, Washington and 10 other US cities (Bradburn 1969). Respondents were reinterviewed 12 weeks apart for the latter study.

This scale has been subjected to a great deal of analysis (Knapp 1976). Originally 12 items, it is now composed of 10 items, five referring to 'positive affect', and five referring to 'negative affect'. The two subscales are independent, although both correlate with happiness (Bradburn 1969). Balance refers to the balance between positive and negative affect reflected by an individual's score on the scale (the balance is the result of an additive process). However, this scale is also complicated by items referring to activation (e.g. the item 'excited' or 'interested' in something). Additionally, some of the items also appear to measure accomplishments. The scale is self-administered.

Content

The wording of the questions appears to have varied between studies. Bradburn specified that the time referent should be 'the past few weeks' (originally 'the past week'). Others have used 'the past few months' or even no time referent. An advantage of using the scale is that some items refer to positive psychological states, reflecting the recent interest in positive health. Examples of scale items are shown in Box 7.2.

Box 7.2 Examples from the ABS

We are interested in the way people are feeling these days. During the past few weeks, did you ever feel . . . [Alternate wording: 'how often did you feel . . .']:

Positive items include
Things going your way.
Excited, interested in something.
Pleased about having accomplished something.

Negative items include
Upset because someone criticized you.
Very lonely, remote from people.
Bored.

Bradburn, N.M. (1969) *The Structure of Psychological Wellbeing*. Chicago, IL: Aldine Publishing. Reprinted with permission of the author. Not copyrighted. The measure is free to use, and can be accessed at: https://eprovide.mapi-trust.org/, accessed 21 July 2016. Also see: http://onlinelibrary. wiley.com/doi/10.1002/art.11408/full, accessed 6 October 2015.

Scoring

Replies are dichotomous (yes/no). Differential weights were tested but did not significantly alter the results and so are not used. Each yes response to the 10 items in the scale is assigned a value of 1. The five items that reflect positive affect are summed separately to the five that reflect negative affect. The difference between the scores on positive and negative affect is computed and is taken as the final score, indicating the level of psychological well-being. Bradburn (1969) suggested adding a constant (+5) to remove the negative summary scale scores.

Validity

Correlations with other measures (testing for validity) are around 0.66; this was achieved with an 18-item version of Neugarten's LSIA (Bild and Havighurst 1976). A review of the scale by George and Bearon (1980) reports inter-scale correlations with other morale scales and an 18-item version of the LSIA of between 0.61 and 0.64.

The scale was used by Berkanovic *et al.* (1988) in an interview study of distress and help-seeking among 950 respondents in Los Angeles. The authors found no relationship between distress and use of medical care, although they reported that the distressed reported more illnesses. Significant differences on scale scores by sex of respondents have been reported (Kushman and Lane 1980). Possibly the most well-known application of the scale was by Berkman (1971) in the Alameda County survey, although she only used eight of the items. She reported a correlation of 0.48 with a 20-item index of neurotic traits. Subsequent studies have reported associations in the expected direction with the ABS and extraversion and neuroticism (Charles *et al.* 2001; Cheng 2003) and social interactions (Balaswamy and Richardson 2001). It was reported to be sensitive to change (Bradburn 1969).

Maitland *et al.* (2001) tested the factor structure of the scale using data from cross-sectional and longitudinal surveys of adults aged 54+. They reported that the stability of the positive and negative affect factors was moderate over a three-year follow-up period, and reported age differences in loadings (for the 'upset' item at Time 1) and also gender differences in loadings (for items on 'feeling on top of the world' and things 'going your way'). Cherlin and Reeder (1975) argued that the two-dimensional structure is not correct. They suggested that there is a third component (activation level) included (e.g. 'particularly excited or interested in something'). Borgatta and Montgomery (1987) have also argued that some items also seem to be measuring instrumental aspects (e.g. accomplishments). Helmes *et al.* (2010) conducted confirmatory factor analyses of data from 187 older Canadian adults (mean age 69.7 years) and showed that a two-dimensional structure fitted the item data much better than the unidimensional, bipolar model suggested by the original scoring key. The two dimensions showed parallel patterns of correlations with two measures of morale and with a measure of social desirability, but these patterns differed from that of the conventional unidimensional ABS score.

Reliability

Internal consistency (inter-item) correlations range from 0.47 to 0.73 for the positive scale and from 0.48 to 0.73 for the negative scale (Cherlin and Reeder 1975; Warr 1978).

Inter-scale correlations were modest at 0.24 to 0.26 (Warr 1978). These correlations are considerably higher than the early correlations reported by Bradburn (1969).

Bradburn (1969) tested the scale for reliability and reported a test-retest correlation of 0.76 three days apart; for nine items associations exceeded 0.90 and for the item 'excited or interested' the test-retest correlation was 0.86.

In sum, it has acceptable levels of validity and reliability and has been found to be applicable for use with older people, although it was not developed specifically as a measure for them. It is easily administered. George and Bearon (1980) rate it as the best measure of affect (frequency of experienced feelings and kinds of reported feelings).

THE PHILADELPHIA GERIATRIC CENTER MORALE SCALE (PGCMS)

This scale, and its revised version, were developed on the basis of the assumption that morale is a general feeling of well-being, and which is multidimensional (Lawton 1972, 1975). Lawton viewed morale in terms of general well-being. The scale also takes into account two other properties: applicability to older, institutionalized populations, and optimal scale length, allowing reliability without respondent fatigue (Knapp 1976). A preliminary version of the scale with 41 items was tested on 300 people, with an average age of 78. The scale was reduced to 22 items, but with subsequent analyses was revised and now contains 17 (Lawton 1975; Morris and Sherwood 1975). Lawton recommended that these 17 items be referred to as the 'revised PGC Morale Scale'. It was developed for use with older people and is, therefore, appropriate for these populations. It is easily administered and can be self- or interviewer-administered.

Content

The 17 items form three major dimensions: agitation (six items), attitude towards own ageing (five items) and lonely dissatisfaction (six items). The scale consists largely of attitude statements, and respondents are asked to indicate whether they apply to them or not, plus specific questions. Examples of scale statements and questions are shown in Box 7.3.

Box 7.3 Examples from the PGCMS, items retained in revised version

How much do you feel lonely?
Things keep getting worse as I get older.
I see enough of my friends and relatives.
As I get older, things are (better, worse, same) than/as I thought they would be.
I am as happy now as when I was younger.
Life is hard for me much of the time.
How satisfied are you with your life today?

The scale is in the public domain, is free to use without permission, with acknowledgement of source. Original version: Lawton, M. (1972) The dimensions of morale, in D. Kent, R. Kastenbaum, S. Sherwood (eds) *Research Planning and Action for the Elderly: the Power and Potential of Social Science*. New York: Behavioral Publications, pp. 144–65. Items are on pp. 152–3. Revised version: Lawton M.P. (1975) The Philadelphia Geriatric Center Morale Scale: a revision. *Journal of Gerontology*, 30: 85–9. Items are on p. 78, Table 1. By permission of Oxford University Press on behalf of The Gerontological Society of America. See https://eprovide.mapi-trust.org/ accessed 21 July 2016. The scale is free to use and can be downloaded at: www.cebp.nl/vault_public/filesystem/?ID=1460. Contact: Polisher Research Institute, Madlyn and Leonard Abramson Center for Jewish Life, 1425 Horsham Road, North Wales, PA 19454-1320, USA; https://www.abramsoncenter.org/research/applications/assessment-instruments/, accessed 12 October 2015.

Scoring

Most items are dichotomously coded. One point is scored for each response indicating high morale. The range of scores is from 0 (low) to 17 (high), with higher scores indicating greater morale. The scale can be treated as three subscales or as an overall scale. The scale, descriptive statistics and details of the scoring are available from Lawton. Liang and Bollen (1983) have reviewed the various scoring methods, and recommended that three subscales should be calculated: agitation, dissatisfaction and attitudes towards one's own ageing.

Validity

Correlations testing the PGCMS for validity with Neugarten's scales (reported earlier) vary with Neugarten's various indexes from 0.57 to 0.79 (Lawton 1972; Lohmann 1977). It has been reported that the scale is able to discriminate between social groups. The PGCMS has had numerous applications. Ward *et al.* (1984) used the 17-item version and excluded two items that they were already measuring in a series of questions about social integration: 'How much do you feel lonely?' and 'I see enough of my friends and relatives'. They used the scale with a sample of people, average age 70.6, living in Albany-Schenectady-Troy, New York, and reported that morale was associated with satisfaction with frequency of contact with others, thus supporting its discriminative ability. It was also used by Noelker and Harel (1978) in their survey of 14 nursing home residents in the USA. The average age of respondents was 81. The authors reported that twice as many residents who desired to live in the homes had high morale scores (mean: 12.98; standard deviation: 4.25), compared to residents who desired to live elsewhere (mean: 10.33; standard deviation: 4.96). Morale was also best predicted by functional health status: 39 per cent of the variance in morale scores was explained by self-rated health. There is limited evidence of sensitivity to change (some reports exist by Kalson (1976) and Morris (1975)).

The content validity of the scale has been questioned by Borgatta and Montgomery (1987) because it includes measures of happiness and life satisfaction, alleged to be questionable in a scale purporting to measure 'morale'. This confusion, they argue, is made even more problematic by the use of different time referents (e.g. 'I am as happy now as when I was younger' and 'How satisfied are you with your life today?').

While early factor analyses reported that the scale formed six factors, three factors have since been confirmed for the 17-item version of the scale: agitation (six items), attitude towards one's own ageing (five items) and lonely dissatisfaction (six items) (Lawton 1975; Morris and Sherwood 1975). Most studies of the factor structure have confirmed the three-factor structure. Liang and Bollen (1985) confirmed these three first-order factors and also identified a second-order factor: global life satisfaction, linked with the three first-order factors. Ranzijn and Luszcz (2000) also confirmed that the scale contained factors of positive and negative affect.

Reliability

Lawton (1972) reported a split-half reliability coefficient of 0.74, a coefficient of internal consistency of 0.81, and test-retest reliability coefficients ranging from 0.75 (after three months) to 0.91 (after five weeks). Lawton (1975) provided alpha coefficients for internal consistency of between 0.81 and 0.85.

In sum, the scale has acceptable levels of reliability and validity and is widely believed to be the superior of the existing life satisfaction and morale scales. It has been used successfully in other cultural groups (e.g. Japanese people in the USA, Liang *et al.* (1992)). One criticism of it is that the inclusion of items measuring both happiness and satisfaction is questionable, given the earlier definition of morale (Stull 1987).

DELIGHTED–TERRIBLE FACES (D–T) SCALE

The D–T scales were developed in response to the recognition of deficiencies in other scales, and on the basis of the recognition that life satisfaction is subjective and dependent on one's evaluations of the different components of life (Andrews and Withey 1974, 1976). These authors also reported that the survey of well-being by Campbell *et al.* (1976) found that one-half to two-thirds of respondents selected one of the two most satisfied categories which were presented to them. They felt that this concentration of responses at the 'satisfied' end of the scale posed statistical and conceptual problems. Therefore, they developed their D–T scales with a broader range of response categories. For example, the inclusion of seven faces on the D–T scale was an attempt to reduce the skew of distributions and improve discrimination between respondents. In the Faces Scale, they also offered a neutral face, as they felt it was important for respondents to 'opt out' if none of the faces represented their feelings.

The faces show clear expressions and each face is represented by an alphabetical letter, ranging from A (delighted) to G (terrible), depending on its expression. This was seen as an improvement on visual analogue scales (VAS) which are laid out along a single dimension with only the end categories labelled, leaving the respondent to infer the appropriate meanings for the intermediate categories.

While the D–T Faces Scale appears to be the most popular and best tested, other D–T scales were developed and tested by the authors. These included the following.

- A D–T ladder scale. This was originally developed by Cantril (1965). There are many adaptations of this scale, usually with good psychometric properties (Andrews and Robinson 1991; Keyes *et al.* 2002). Respondents rate their life satisfaction via one of the nine ladder rungs (the top rung is labelled 'Best I could expect to have' and the bottom is labelled 'Worst I could expect to have'. They are told: 'Here is a picture of a ladder. At the bottom of this ladder is the worst situation you might reasonably expect to have. At the top is the best you might expect to have. The other rungs are in-between . . . Where on the ladder is your . . .? On which rung would you put it?'
- A D–T VAS with seven boxes at intervals along the line representing statements about life satisfaction (delighted–pleased–mostly satisfied–mixed (about equally satisfied and dissatisfied)–mostly dissatisfied–unhappy–terrible) (Andrews and Withey 1976). Respondents are told: 'We want to find out how you feel about various parts of your life, and life in this country as you see it. Please indicate the feelings you have now – taking into account what has happened in the last year and what you expect to happen in the near future . . . How do you feel about . . .?'
- A D–T circles scale consisting of nine circles, divided into eight slices containing a progressive number of either plus or negative (minus) signs, so that the extreme left-hand circle (8) contains eight plus signs in each of the eight slices and the extreme right-hand circle (0) contains eight minus signs in each slice. The middle circle contains four plus and four negative signs. Respondents are told: 'Here are some circles that we can imagine represent the lives of different people. Circle 0 has all minuses in it, to represent a person who has all bad things in his or her life. Circle 8 has all pluses in it, to represent a person who has all good things in his or her life. Other circles are in-between. Which circle comes closest to matching how you feel about . . .?'

The D–T scales all provide an affective evaluation of QoL which involves a cognitive evaluation and some degree of positive/negative feeling (affect).

Content

Respondents are shown seven faces ranging from wide smiles to turned-down mouths. They are told: 'Here are some faces expressing various feelings (delighted, pleased, mostly satisfied, mixed, mostly dissatisfied, unhappy, and terrible). Below each is a letter. Which face comes closest to expressing how you feel about . . .?' (specific items and/or 'life as a whole' are asked about). The faces are shown in Box 7.4.

Box 7.4. D–T faces

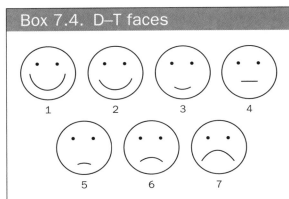

Source: Andrews and Withey (1976) *Social Indicators of Well-being: Americans' Perceptions of Life Quality.* New York: Plenum, p. 376. Reproduced with permission of Springer.

Andrews and Withey (1976) published a wide selection of topic items which could be incorporated within a scale measuring life satisfaction. Examples of items which they suggested could be included, and which were reported to explain 50–62 per cent of the variance in evaluations of life, are self-accomplishment and problem-handling, family life, income, fun and enjoyment, accommodation, family togetherness, time to do things one wants to, non-work activities, national government activities, quality of local goods and services, health status and employment.

Scoring

The seven faces are given scores from 1 (delighted) to 7 (terrible). While item responses can be summed, each item can also be analysed independently.

A study of 662 people aged 85+ in the East End of London by Bowling and Browne (1991) and Bowling *et al.* (1993) reported that the D–T Faces Scale was fairly skewed, with about a quarter of respondents choosing the terrible faces, while over half selected a delighted face. Research on stroke patients in the UK by Anderson (1988) also found the measure to be skewed, with 19 per cent of respondents choosing a terrible face and two-thirds choosing a delighted face. However, both studies reported good acceptance of the scale by respondents. Andrews and Withey (1976) had recognized this problem of a positive skew, which was their reason for increasing the response categories.

Validity and reliability

Comparisons between studies are difficult to make because investigators choose the topic item they wish to include for self-evaluation using the D–T scales. However, the authors of the scale compared the D–T scales with other similar scales and presented evidence that they were more valid measures than most other scales assessed; the exception was their more visually complex 'circles' scale. Based on multimethod-multitrait analysis, the median validity coefficients for each of their four D–T scales, in the assessment of six areas of life satisfaction, ranged from 0.70 to 0.82, and were constant when different areas of life were evaluated using the same scale (Andrews and Crandall 1976).

It was previously reported by Bowling and Browne (1991) (see section on Neugarten Life Satisfaction Scales) that, on the basis of their samples of elderly people living at home in London and Essex, the Spearman's correlations between the D–T Faces Scales used and Neugarten's Life Satisfaction Scale A fluctuated fairly widely from weak to moderate: from r = −0.24 to −0.65 (the correlations were in the expected direction – the minus sign reflects the direction of the scoring). Further analyses (unpublished) showed reliability coefficients for the D–T Faces Scale of around coefficient alpha 0.80; correlations between D–T Faces Scale items were weak to moderate, ranging from 0.30 to 0.59 (this is not unexpected as quite different areas of life were being assessed). Andrews and Withey (1976) reported average test-retest reliabilities of the D–T scales across several studies, when administered during the same interview, about 0.70.

The D–T Faces Scale, and the D–T response scale, are popular among investigators in mental health, where they have been frequently adapted and used (e.g. Baker and Intagliata 1982; Lehman 1988; Oliver et al. 1997). Elsewhere, the use of the D–T faces and the category scale as a response format on a range of topics is increasingly common. The authors have published the topic items, and suggested that investigators select relevant items for their own questionnaires. Apart from the original work by Andrews and Withey, which reported good reliability and validity, there have been relatively few published studies reporting usage of the D–T scales in their original format, as opposed to the selection of items.

SATISFACTION WITH LIFE SCALE (SWLS)

The SWLS is a short instrument which assesses a person's conscious evaluative judgement of domains of life using his or her own criteria, and weighting each domain themselves (Diener et al. 1985). The developers conceptualized subjective well-being as consisting of the emotional or affective component and the judgemental or cognitive evaluation of life (Diener et al. 2003). Most researchers focus on the former. The SWLS was developed as a judgemental component of subjective well-being (Pavot et al. 1991). It aimed to improve on existing scales which appeared to include factors other than life satisfaction and, unlike Neugarten et al.'s (1961) LSI-A, does not include related concepts such as vigour. It was designed to be appropriate for adults of all ages (Pavot et al. 1991).

Content

The SWLS comprises five items which measure global cognitive judgements about one's life. It takes about one minute to complete. The scale is reproduced in Box 7.5.

> ## Box 7.5 Examples from the SWLS
>
> Below are five statements that you may agree or disagree with. Using the 1–7 scale below indicate your agreement with each item by placing the appropriate number on the line preceding that item. Please be open and honest about your responding. The 7-point scale is as follows:
>
> 7 – Strongly agree
> 6 – Agree
> 5 – Slightly agree
> 4 – Neither agree nor disagree
> 3 – Slightly disagree
> 2 – Disagree
> 1 – Strongly disagree
>
> ___ In most ways my life is close to my ideal
> ___ The conditions of my life are excellent
> ___ I am satisfied with my life
> ___ So far I have gotten the important things I want in life
> ___ If I could live my life over, I would change almost nothing
>
> The scale is copyrighted but free to use without permission or charge (Pavot and Diener 1993) by all professionals (researchers and practitioners) as long as credit is given to the authors of the scale (see http://internal.psychology.illinois.edu/~ediener/SWLS.html, accessed 1 September 2015). Diener., E., Emmons, R.A., Larsen, R.J. and Griffin, S. (1985). The Satisfaction with Life Scale. *Journal of Personality Assessment, 49: 71–5.* Reprinted with permission of the author. Available at www.psych.uiuc.edu/_ediener, accessed 1 September 2015. Contact details: 415 Psychology Bldg., 603 E. Daniel Street, M/C 716, Champaign, IL 61820; email ediener@illinois.edu; http://www.psychology.illinois.edu/people/ediener, accessed 1 September 2015.

Scoring

Each item is scored 1–7. The items are summed, leading to a range of 5 to 35. The interpretation of scores was given as:

5–9 extremely dissatisfied,
10–14 dissatisfied,
15–19 slightly dissatisfied,
20 neutral,
21–25 slightly satisfied,
26–30 satisfied,
31–35 extremely satisfied.

Validity

A series of studies with college students by Diener *et al.* (1985) showed that scores on the SWLS correlated moderately to highly with several other measures of subjective well-being (including Andrews and Withey's D–T Scale; Bradburn's Affect-Balance Scale and Cantril's Self-Anchoring Ladder). They reported that the correlations between all the other measures and the SWLS, in two samples of college students, ranged from −0.37 to 0.68, giving support to the convergent validity of the SWLS. Pavot et al. (1991), in two studies of college students, reported further evidence of the convergent validity of the scale, with correlations between the SWLS and Neugarten et al.'s (1961) Life Satisfaction Scale A and the Philadelphia Geriatric Center Morale Scale of 0.65 and 0.81 respectively. They also reported a significant, moderate correlation between respondents' peer and family reports of life satisfaction of 0.54. Criterion validity was assessed in a further study of college students in terms of correlations of the SWBS with a life satisfaction rating made by interviewers (0.73) (Diener et al. 1985).

The psychometric properties of the scale were reviewed by Pavot and Diener (1993) who reported that the scale had good convergent validity when compared with other scales and assessments of subjective well-being, and discriminant validity when compared with measures of emotional well-being. It was also demonstrated to have sufficient sensitivity to be able to detect changes in life satisfaction after clinical interventions.

It has been reported to correlate moderately in the expected direction with personality characteristics (extraversion) (Emmons and Diener 1985). A study of adolescents and college students in Portugal and Cape Verde found that the scale was able to predict reported loneliness (Neto and Barros 2000), and a study of residents in Japan and Australia found that it could predict loneliness among Australian but not Japanese respondents (Schumaker et al. 1993). Harrington and Loffredo (2001), in a study based on college students, also reported that extraverts showed higher life satisfaction than introverts, again supporting the discriminate ability of the SWLS. Pavot and Dieners' (1993) review of the scale further concluded that the SWLS showed discriminant validity from emotional well-being measures.

Reliability

The series of studies with college students by Diener et al. (1985) demonstrated that the scale had a high level of stability on test-retest at two months (correlation coefficient: 0.82; coefficient alpha: 0.87). They reported a further study of college students which showed that the inter-item correlations for the five SWLS items were: 0.81, 0.63, 0.61, 0.75 and 0.66, supporting the internal consistency of the scale. Pavot et al.'s (1991) study of students reported average test-retest coefficients at five days of 0.83. Pavot and Diener (1993) reviewed the scale. They reported that it showed some temporal stability (e.g. from 0.89 at two weeks to 0.54 for four years); it showed sufficient sensitivity to change after clinical intervention; the test-retest correlation coefficients ranged from moderate to good: 0.54 to 0.83. Reviews by Pavot and Diener (1993) and Diener et al. (2013) reported that the Cronbach's alphas all passed the threshold of acceptability, ranging from 0.80 to 0.96.

Diener et al. (1985) reported that the scale had a single factor, in a study of college students, which confirmed 66 per cent of the variance. Pavot et al. (1991), Lewis et al. (1995), and Slocum-Gori et al. (2009) also supported a single-factor model, and thus the unidimensionality of the scale. The factor structure, convergent and discriminant validity of the scale was supported by Clark *et al.* (1995). Reviews of the properties of the scale also confirm that the SWLS measures a single underlying dimension (Pavot and Diener 1993; Diener *et al.* 2013).

The scale is relatively popular because it is short and simple, and quick for respondents to complete. The scale language needs minor adaptations to the wording for use in the UK (e.g. changing 'responding' to 'responses', 'gotten' to 'got'). The SWLS is available in several languages. It has potential for cross-cultural application, if used with caution, given reported differences between individualistic and collectivistic societies in the value attributed to emotions versus normative beliefs for life satisfaction judgements (Suh *et al.* 1998). Also, people in religious societies, compared with people in less religious societies, place greater weight on religiousity in making life satisfaction judgements (Diener *et al.* 2011).

SCALES OF PSYCHOLOGICAL WELL-BEING (PWB)

The scales of PWB were derived from theories of adult development as well as conceptions of positive psychological functioning from existential and humanistic psychology, and clinical psychology (Ryff 1989, 1995; Ryff and Essex 1991; Ryff and Keyes 1995). The scales contain both positive and negative items which cover six dimensions derived from theoretical constructs of psychological well-being (Ryff 1989).

Content

The original parent version of the PWB contains six scales, with 20 items for each of six dimensions: autonomy, environmental mastery, personal growth, positive relations with others, purpose in life and self-acceptance. There are three versions of the scales. Each of these covers all six dimensions; they vary in the number of items per dimension (14, 9 and 3 respectively). The 14-item version is used by Ryff in her own studies. The items representing each dimension are mixed on the questionnaire. The scales are self-administered. Some examples from the 14-item scale are shown in Box 7.6.

Box 7.6 Examples from PWB

Environmental mastery
In general, I feel I am in charge of the situation in which I live.
I am quite good at managing the many responsibilities of my daily life.
If I were unhappy with my living situation, I would take effective steps to change it.

Autonomy
People rarely talk me into doing things I don't want to do.
It's difficult for me to voice my own opinions on controversial matters.
I am not the kind of person who gives in to social pressures to think or act in certain ways.

Strongly disagree (1)/moderately disagree (2)/slightly disagree (3)/slightly agree (4)/ moderately agree (5)/strongly agree (6)

Reprinted with permission of the developer. The Scales of PWB are free to use without charge, with the request to send the developer a description of how the information will be used and the scale results. Developer and contact: Professor Carol D. Ryff, PhD, Pennsylvania State University, Hilldale Professor, Department of Psychology, Director, Institute on Aging, University of Wisconsin, 2245 Medical Sciences Center, 1300 University Avenue, Madison, WI 53706, USA; email: cryff@wisc. edu; http://psych.wisc.edu/faculty-ryff.htm, accessed 1 September 2015.

Scoring

The items have a six-point response format from strongly disagree (1) to strongly agree (6). Negatively phrased items are reverse coded in the scoring scales. High scores indicate high self-ratings. Definitions of high and low scorers on each scale are provided.

Validity

There is strong support for the validity of the scales indicating that they are adequate measures of psychological functioning. The results of tests for the validity of the 20-item parent scales were given by Ryff (1989). The validity of the scales is supported by the pattern of correlations between the PWB and various measures of personality in samples of the adult population show distinct associations, which also indicate that the association between psychological well-being and personality is complex (Schmutte and Ryff 1997; Ruini et al. 2003). It was reported to be negatively associated with self-consciousness in a study of college students (Harrington and Loffredo 2001). Abbott et al. (2006) analysed data from over 1,000 women in a UK birth cohort study. Consistent with previous results supporting its validity, they reported that the PWB was negatively associated with dimensions of mental health (psychological distress).

Factor analyses by Ryff and Keyes (1995) provided evidence that the best fitting model for the scales was six dimensional. Clarke et al. (2001) also reported a confirmatory factor analysis, which supported a six-factor structure. However, the factorial validity of the scales has been questioned, in particular the inclusion of several theoretical constructs. Abbott et al.'s (2006) analyses of their UK cohort data supported a single, second-order factor.

Reliability

The results of tests for the reliability of the 20-item parent scales were given by Ryff (1989). The internal consistency coefficient alphas for the scales, and their correlations with the 20-item parent scale respectively, were reported to be high: autonomy (0.83; 0.97), environmental mastery (0.86; 0.98), personal growth (0.85; 0.97), positive relations with others (0.88; 0.98), purpose in life (0.88; 0.98), and self-acceptance (0.91; 0.99) (Ryff 1989). Ruini et al. (2003) reported the Pearson coefficients for test-retest reliability of the scales at one month, based on a sample of 450 members of the population, which were judged to be satisfactory for all six scales. However, a version of the scale with 18 items achieved lower internal consistency alphas in the Canadian Study of Health and Aging (Clarke *et al.* 2001).

The results of tests for reliability and validity of the short three-item scales were presented by Ryff and Keyes (1995). They reported that the three-item scales correlated from 0.70 to 0.89 with the original scales. The three-item version has low internal consistency: autonomy (alpha = 0.43), environmental mastery (alpha = 0.57), personal growth (alpha = 0.50), positive relations with others (alpha = 0.54), purpose in life (alpha = 0.37) and self-acceptance (alpha = 0.53). Thus Ryff does not recommend them for high quality assessments of well-being. The lower internal consistency for the shorter version reflects Ryff's decision to create short versions of the scales which represented the multi-factorial structure of the full-length 20-item version, rather than aim for high internal consistency.

The scales have been used successfully in large longitudinal population studies in the USA and Canada (Marks and Lambert 1999; Clarke *et al.* 2001). They have also been translated and used successfully in other languages, including Dutch (Spruytte *et al.* 1999) and Swedish (Lindfors 2002). While more information on psychometric properties of PWB from a wider range of descriptive and outcome studies is still needed, existing studies of the reliability and validity of the full-length scales have been good. In particular, the scales make a potentially valuable contribution to research on ageing, given the emphasis in social gerontology on the theoretical importance of autonomy, self-acceptance and self-mastery for 'successful ageing' (Baltes and Baltes 1990). The PWB is freely available, although the developer requests copies of how the instrument will be used and a copy of the results.

THE PSYCHOLOGICAL GENERAL WELL-BEING SCHEDULE (PGWBS)

The PGWBS is a concise multidimensional indicator of subjective feelings of well-being and distress. It was designed by Dupuy (1973, 1974, 1978, 1984) for use in the US Health and Nutrition Examination Survey (HANES), with the aim of providing an index that could be used to measure self-reports of intrapersonal affective or emotional states reflecting a sense of subjective well-being or distress. The Psychological General Well-Being Index (PGWBI) is an overall score (index) that can be derived from the current, 22-item PGWBS. It represents overall self-perceived psychological well-being (Chassany *et al.* 2004).

The most well-known application of the measure is the modified version incorporated into the RAND Mental Health Inventory, based on a large community sample of people aged 14–60+ (Brook *et al.* 1979a, 1979b). Fifteen of the PGWBS items were retained for use in the final version of the RAND Mental Health Inventory. Brook *et al.* (1979a, 1979b) have extensively reviewed the scale.

Content

The initial draft of the instrument contained 68 items, 18 of which were used for the US HANES; these were referred to as the General Well-Being Schedule (Dupuy 1973, 1974,

1978, 1984). A 33-item version was developed and tested (Fazio 1977). The current version contains 22 items; a short six-item version has also been developed and tested (Grossi *et al.* 2006). The items include indicators of both positive and negative affect. It is a self-administered questionnaire; administration time is 12 minutes.

The PGWBS includes items for six states of being (well-being and distress). The subscales used to measure these six states contain three to five items each. The six subscales are anxiety (e.g. bothered by nervousness; generally tense; anxious, worried, upset; relaxed, at ease versus highly strung; felt under strain, stress or pressure); depressed mood (e.g. felt depressed; felt downhearted and blue; sad, discouraged, hopeless); positive well-being (e.g. general spirits; happy, satisfied with personal life; interesting daily life; felt cheerful, light-hearted); self-control (e.g. in firm control; afraid of losing control; felt emotionally stable, sure of self); general health (e.g. bothered by illness, bodily disorders, or aches and pains; healthy enough to do things; concerned, worried about health); and vitality (e.g. energy, pep; waking feeling fresh, rested; felt active, vigorous versus dull, sluggish; felt tired, worn-out, used up). The frame of reference for questions is 'during the last month'.

Examples of questions are shown in Box 7.7.

Box 7.7 Examples from the original PGWBS

How have you been feeling in general (*during the past month*)?

In excellent spirits
In very good spirits
In good spirits mostly
I have been up and down in spirits a lot
In low spirits mostly
In very low spirits

How happy, satisfied, or pleased have you been with your personal life (*during the past month*)?

Extremely happy – could not have been more satisfied or pleased
Very happy
Fairly happy
Satisfied . . . pleased
Somewhat dissatisfied
Very dissatisfied

How concerned or worried about your health have you been (*during the past month*)?

```
0    1    2    3    4    5    6    7    8    9    10
|                                                  |
```
Not concerned   Very
at all   concerned

Scoring

Six subscores can be produced to represent the six subscales. A range of different scoring algorithms have been used. Chassany *et al.* (2004) pointed out that the original scoring for each item was 0–5 (possible score range: 0–110), and the scoring is now usually on a 1–6 scale (score range: 22–132). Following the common practice in multidimensional health measurement of expressing scale scores on a 0–100 scale, Chassany *et al.* (2004) in their manual of the PGWBI linearly transformed scores to this scale.

Validity

Fazio's (1977) study of 195 students found that the PGWBS correlated moderately with interviewers' ratings of depression (0.47); the average correlation of the PGWBS and six other depression scales was 0.69, and 0.64 with three anxiety scales. Fazio (1977) and Ware *et al.* (1979) also reported criterion correlations between the PGWBS and interviewers' ratings generally ranging between 0.65 and 0.90. Nakayama *et al.* (2000) tested the Japanese version of the scale in over 1,000 adults and reported that it had good concurrent validity in comparison with five other validated scales of anxiety and depression.

Edwards *et al.* (1978) showed that the scale was sensitive enough to detect the progress over three weeks of the 21 psychiatric day patients in their study. Kammann and Flett (1983) reported a correlation of 0.74 between the PGWBS and their 96-item scale of general happiness and well-being (the Affectometer). Leonardson *et al.* (2003), in their study of 88 diabetic American Indians, reported adequate concurrent and convergent validity in relation to the PGWBS associations with measures of depression, including the Beck Depression Inventory (second edition), family adaptation, partnership, growth, affection and resolve. Taylor *et al.* (2003) examined the PGWBS in 599 African-American women who participated in a multicentre weight loss trial. They reported that their factor analysis indicated that the PGWBS is primarily unidimensional, and that the existence of the six hypothesized subscales was not supported.

The PGWBS demonstrated evidence of concurrent and construct validity when analysed in relation to measures of self-concept, depression and health behaviours.

Dupuy (1978) and Wan and Livieratos (1977) reported factor analyses of the PGWBS which showed three factors explaining 51 per cent of the variance: anxiety, tension and depression; health and energy; and positive well-being or life satisfaction. A six-factor solution was produced confirming the six subscales using multitrait and factor analysis (Ware *et al.* 1979). Studies of the factor structure of the scale in other cultures have supported the structural validity of six-factor, three-factor and four-factor models (Nakayama *et al.* 2000). Lundgren-Nilsson *et al.* (2013), in a study of 179 patients attending a stress clinic, assessed the structure of the PGWBI using modern psychometric techniques. They conducted factor analyses and Rasch analysis, and concluded that the PGWBI achieved satisfactory internal construct validity, and the total score reflected the scoring structure indicated in the manual (i.e. the six domains are summed, and then the domain totals are summed together to make the total score).

Reliability

Extensive scaling tests and tests of reliability and validity were carried out on 1,209 respondents. Internal consistency coefficients for the six subscales ranged between 0.72 and 0.88. Test-retest reliability produced good results (with the exception of a lowered test-retest coefficient of 0.50 when the interval was extended from one week to one month). Test-retest reliability coefficients ranged from 0.50 to 0.86, with a median of 0.66. These results were based on a wide range of studies from samples of students to the large sample of adults participating in the RAND Health Insurance Study. They have been reviewed by Dupuy (1984).

Test-retest reliability coefficients of 0.68 and 0.85 for two sub-samples within the US HANS were also reported by Monk (1981). It is difficult to know whether the lower correlations reflect the instability of the instrument or changes in individuals.

Monk (1981) also reported internal consistency coefficients of 0.93 on the basis of analyses of 6,913 people. Fazio (1977) reported similar internal consistency coefficients of 0.91 for males and 0.95 for females; and correlations among sub-scores ranging from 0.16 to 0.72. Ware *et al.*'s (1979) review reported three studies using the PGWBS which also found internal consistency coefficients of over 0.90. Leonardson *et al.* (2003) reported a similar Cronbach's alpha for internal consistency of 0.89 in their different population group sample of 88 diabetic American Indians. However, Edwards *et al.* (1978) reported a lower coefficient of 0.69.

This is a scale with good test results on the whole. One advantage of this scale is that it avoids reference to physical symptoms of emotional distress and so avoids problems of interpretation. Fluctuations in test-retest reliability may be problematic in assessing individuals. A major disadvantage is that most of the early validation studies of it are unpublished, although these have been thoroughly reviewed by Brook *et al.* (1979a, 1979b). The scale was adapted and tested for use in Britain, as an outcome indicator of depression, by Hunt and McKenna (1992).

SENSE OF COHERENCE SCALE (SOC)

A measure of sense of coherence, which is related to life satisfaction, is included in this section (an orientation to life questionnaire, or SOC by Antonovsky 1987, 1993). The SOC is global in content, and is increasingly popular in European studies of health outcome (to measure modifying factors). The sense of coherence was defined by Antonovsky (1987) as:

> a global orientation that expresses the extent to which one has a pervasive, enduring though dynamic feeling of confidence that (1) the stimuli deriving from one's internal and external environments in the course of living are structured, predictable, and explicable; (2) the resources are available to one to meet the demands posed by these stimuli; and (3) these demands are challenges, worthy of investment and engagement.

The development of the sense of coherence concept and the scale was based on intensive interviews with 52 respondents who had suffered major life crises. The SOC was derived from the salutogenic model designed to explain the maintenance or improvement of one's position on a health-ease/disease continuum (Antonovsky 1993).

Sense of coherence is a global orientation toward one's inner and outer environments, comprised of three interrelated components: comprehensibility, manageability and meaningfulness. It can be used as an indicator of coping capacity in stressful life situations, although the scale should not be used as a diagnostic tool. Antonovsky argued that a strong sense of coherence is necessary for the successful management of stress, and the movement towards the healthy end of the ease–disease continuum (Antonovsky 1990). Antonovsky (1993) reviewed 42 studies using the SOC. This was updated by Eriksson and Lindström (2005) in their extensive systematic review of the validity and reliability of the SOC, which included 458 scientific publications and 13 doctoral theses published between 1992–2003.

Content

The scale is a 29-item seven-point semantic differential scale, comprising 11 items on comprehensibility, 10 on manageability and eight on meaningfulness. High levels of internal consistency and construct validity were found for the scale (e.g. Antonovsky 1993; Söderhamn *et al.* 2015). A range of shorter versions have been described; of these the 13-item version is the generally accepted short version, with acceptable levels of internal consistency and test-retest reliability as well as content, predictive and construct validity (Antonovsky 1993; Langius 1995; Gana and Garnier 2001; Pallant and Lae 2002).

Examples from the 29-item version are shown in Box 7.8.

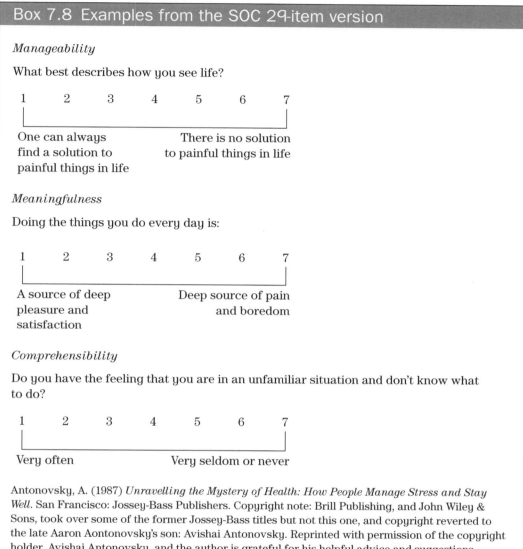

Box 7.8 Examples from the SOC 29-item version

Manageability

What best describes how you see life?

1   2   3   4   5   6   7

One can always   There is no solution
find a solution to   to painful things in life
painful things in life

Meaningfulness

Doing the things you do every day is:

1   2   3   4   5   6   7

A source of deep   Deep source of pain
pleasure and   and boredom
satisfaction

Comprehensibility

Do you have the feeling that you are in an unfamiliar situation and don't know what to do?

1   2   3   4   5   6   7

Very often   Very seldom or never

Scoring

The scale score is the sum of the item scores (some items are reversed for prevention of bias and should be recoded accordingly before summing). The higher the score, the stronger the sense of coherence. Thus, scores range from 13 to 203 (29-item) and from 13 to 91 (13-item).

Langius *et al.* (1992) reported testing the numeric semantic-differential format of the scale against the linear VAS response method, and no significant differences were found between the two scaling formats.

Validity

The validity and reliability of the SOC have been tested in several countries. It was judged to be applicable cross-culturally (Antonovsky 1993), but as it uses some culture-specific colloquialisms, care in translation and testing for meaning is required. Antonovsky (1993) presented the evidence for the scale's validity from all published studies up to 1993, and reported significant correlations between the SOC and measures of health, illness, well-being, orientation to self and stress, indicating the scale's criterion and convergent validity.

A study of the outcome of patients undergoing heart surgery by Dantas *et al.* (2002) supported the discriminative ability validity of the scale on the basis of its hypothesized independent associations with QoL ratings.

Pallant and Lae (2002) used the 13-item version alongside measures of physical and psychological health, personality and coping, and reported significant associations between these measures and the SOC in the expected directions. Eriksson *et al.* (2007), in their survey of over 1,000 adults in Finland, reported that the 13-item version of the SOC was significantly associated with self-rated health in the expected direction (higher sense of coherence was associated with better reported health, in support of its construct validity). The 13-item version of the scale is increasingly popular in clinical and social research, and it appears to have good psychometric properties. In a representative sample of more than 3,700 adults in three UK cities, Walsh *et al.* (2014) also used the 13-item version to investigate whether levels of sense of coherence differed between the cities and could be a plausible explanation for excess mortality levels. Their modelling confirmed the relationship between sense of coherence and self-assessed health status, supporting the validity of the SOC. However, they concluded from their wider findings that it was unlikely that a low sense of coherence provided any explanation for high levels of excess mortality observed in two of the cities included in the study.

Söderhamn *et al.* (2015) tested the homogeneity and construct validity of the Norwegian version of the SOC 29-item scale in a postal survey of over 2,000 people aged 65+ who lived at home in southern Norway. The construct validity of the SOC-29 was supported: it could distinguish between hypothesized groups, and the factors that could predict sense of coherence were mental health, self-care ability, feeling lonely, being active and chronic disease or handicap.

Matsuura *et al.* (2003) reported a high correlation between the Japanese version of the SOC and the Beck Depression Inventory in patients with systemic sclerosis, and multiple-regression analysis confirmed that low SOC was an independent predictor of depression. Björvell *et al.* (1994), in a study of obese patients, reported a moderate and significant correlation between the SOC and a measure of motivation, indicating that the stronger the self-rated sense of coherence, the greater the perceived self-motivation. It has also been reported to be significantly associated with measures of life satisfaction

(Anke and Fugl-Meyer 2003) and to discriminate between women with and without irritable bowel syndrome (Motzer *et al.* 2003).

Eriksson and Lindström (2005, 2007), on the basis of their systematic review of the literature, reported that the SOC-29 was associated with quality of life and well-being in expected directions (with high levels associated with high sense of coherence), supporting its validity, and with changes in respondents' environments, and predicted a positive outcome over time, supporting its predictive validity, although studies were not all consistent. Overall, they concluded, from their review, that the SOC is a valid and cross-culturally applicable measure of how people manage life stress and maintain their health, although its structure remains unclear.

In a study of 189 US veterans, factor analysis of the scale revealed that all 29 items loaded on one true factor at 0.40 or above (eigenvalue given: 12.45) (see Antonovsky 1993). Gana and Garnier (2001) evaluated the French version of the 13-item scale in over 600 adults and reported a three-correlated factor model which included manageability, meaningfulness and comprehensibility. Eriksson and Lindström (2005) reported that the factorial structure of the full SOC appeared to be multidimensional, rather than unidimensional.

Reliability

The 29-item version of the scale was tested for reliability in 26 studies reported by Antonovsky (1993). The Cronbach alpha measure of internal consistency was 0.82–0.95. The 13-item version was used in 16 studies, and the Cronbach's alpha was 0.74–0.91. Some of the studies reported the test-retest correlations, which were stable at 0.54 over two years (Antonovsky 1993). Langius *et al.* (1994) and Langius (1995), in studies of patients with oral or pharyngeal cancer, reported the Cronbach's alpha to be 0.88–0.89. Eriksson and Lindström (2005) reported that in 12 studies using the SOC-29, the Cronbach's alpha of internal consistency ranged from 0.70 to 0.95; test-retest correlations ranged from 0.69 to 0.78 (at one year), 0.64 (at three years), 0.42 to 0.45 (four years), 0.59 to 0.67 (five years), and 0.54 (10 years) indicating good stability at one year, but which reduced, although not consistently, over time. The authors commented that at 10 years the SOC appeared comparatively stable, although not as stable as the developer argued. Söderhamn *et al.* (2015) reported a high level of homogeneity for the Norwegian version of the SOC-29 item version with a Cronbach's alpha coefficient of 0.91 and statistically significant item-to-total correlations, the SOC-29 was found to be homogeneous.

Overall the SOC-29 is a valid, reliable and cross culturally applicable measure, and the 13-item version also appears to have good psychometric properties (Eriksson and Lindström 2005; Eriksson *et al.* 2007). It should be noted that at least 15 different versions of the SOC have been used in at least 33 languages in 32 countries (Eriksson and Lindström 2005). For example, different three-item versions of the SOC have been developed in Sweden (Lundberg and Nystrom 1995), Germany (Schumann *et al.* 2003), Japan (Togari *et al.* 2007), and, as stated above, the 29-item SOC has been tested with good results in Norway (Söderhamn *et al.* 2015).

WARWICK-EDINBURGH MENTAL WELL-BEING SCALE (WEMWBS)

A more recently developed measure is the WEMWBS. The scale was funded by the Scottish Executive National Programme for improving mental health and well-being, commissioned by NHS Health Scotland, developed by the University of Warwick and the University of Edinburgh, and the copyright is jointly owned by NHS Health Scotland, the University of Warwick and the University of Edinburgh. It was developed to measure population well-being and for use in evaluations of mental health promotion initiatives (Tennant *et al.* 2007), and is now included in the annual Scottish Health Survey.

The measure was developed by an expert panel drawing on academic literature, qualitative research with focus groups and psychometric testing of an existing measure (Tennant *et al.* 2007). In contrast to negatively worded measures of mental distress, the developers deliberately included only positively worded items relating to different aspects of positive mental health. They regarded 'good mental well-being' as more than avoiding mental health problems. However, psychological well-being is not at the exact opposite end of the continuum to psychological 'ill-being', or distress, indicating that research participants need to be asked about both (Winefield *et al.* 2012).

Content

The WEMWBS is a 14-item, positively worded measure with five-point response scales, for assessing a population's mental well-being. It covers both hedonic and eudaimonic perspectives: optimism, feeling useful, relaxed, interested in others, energy, dealing with problems, thinking clearly, feeling good about self, feeling close to others, confident, able to make own mind up, feeling loved, interested in new things, cheerful. A seven-item version has also been developed.

Examples of items are shown in Box 7.9.

Box 7.9 Examples from the WEMWBS

Below are some statements about feelings and thoughts.

Please tick the box that best describes your experience of each over the last 2 weeks.

I've been feeling optimistic about the future
I've been feeling interested in other people
I've been dealing with problems well
I've been feeling close to other people
I've been interested in new things

None of the time/Rarely/Some of the time/Often/All of the time

Scoring

Each item carries a score from none of the time (1), rarely (2), some of the time (3), often (4), to all of the time (5). All items are scored positively, and when summed give a minimum score of 14 and a maximum score of 70. No weighting is used. A higher score indicates a higher level of mental well-being.

The WEMWBS does not provide any cut-off points to indicate levels of mental well-being, on the grounds that current knowledge and understanding of mental well-being is insufficient to enable this.

Reliability

The WEMWBS was initially tested in a student population (98 per cent completed the well-being items) and Scottish population surveys, and in two national Scottish surveys (but a high proportion, 16 per cent, failed to complete the well-being items). Otherwise it performed equally well in each group. Cronbach's alpha was 0.89 in the student sample, and 0.91 in the population sample. The authors concluded this suggested some item redundancy. Test-retest correlation at one week was high at 0.83. No ceiling effects were found, and the distribution of scores was normal (Tennant *et al.* 2007). It has been reported to be responsive to change (Maheswaran *et al.* 2012).

The internal construct validity of the WEMWBS was tested further with Rasch techniques. This indicated that a seven-item Short Warwick-Edinburgh Mental Well-being Scale (SWEMWBS) provided a better fit to the Rasch model (Stewart-Brown *et al.* 2009).

Confirmatory factor analysis supported the hypothesized single-factor structure (Tennant *et al.* 2007). Given that the measure is composed of several distinct concepts, the single structure reported is questionable. Further robust psychometric studies are required.

Validity

Again, the WEMWBS was initially validated in a student population and in two national Scottish surveys, performing equally well in each. Good content validity was reported. It discriminated between population groups as hypothesized, and the scale correlated highly with other mental health and well-being scales (Tennant *et al.* 2007), supporting its construct validity. Deary *et al.* (2013) used data on 8,643 men and women from the

National Child Development Survey (1,958 birth cohort), and examined whether cognitive ability influenced responses to the WEMWBS at age 50. They split respondents into three groups according to cognitive ability and analysed the Mokken scaling properties of each group. They reported that only the medium and high cognitive ability groups had acceptable (≥0.3) invariant item ordering (HT statistic); the same pattern was found when the three groups were assessed within men and women separately. The authors concluded that more attention should be paid to the content validity of questionnaires to ensure they are applicable to people with different levels of mental ability.

Further research on the WEMWBS is ongoing.

SCALES OF SELF-ESTEEM

Among the most popular and commonly used measures of self-esteem are: the Self-Esteem Scale (Rosenberg 1965); the Tennessee Self-Concept Scale (Fitts 1965); and the Self-Esteem Inventory (Coopersmith 1967). Several other popular scales have been reviewed by Crandall (1973), Robinson and Shaver (1973), Wylie (1974) and George and Bearon (1980); the reader is referred to these authors for a more detailed review. Most scales appear to warrant further testing on a wider range of population types as the early studies were concentrated on studies of students, although they are now increasingly used in clinical studies.

THE SELF-ESTEEM SCALE

Rosenberg (1965) described self-esteem as self-acceptance or a basic feeling of self-worth, and developed the Self-esteem Scale, based on Guttman scaling, for a study of 5,024 students in public schools in New York. Little information exists about the development of the scale. Self-esteem scores were correlated with characteristics such as participation and leadership in school activities. The measure was intended to be brief, global and unidimensional. It has been widely used in varying settings. Evidence suggests that it is suitable for use with older people. A study of around 5,000 retired teachers and telephone company employees by Atchley (1976) reported that men had higher self-esteem than women. Kaplan and Porkorny (1969), in a study of 500 adults in Harris County, Texas, reported that age is unrelated to self-esteem. Ward (1977), on the basis of a study of 323 residents of Madison, Wisconsin, reported that predictors for women's self-esteem were current activities, age-related deprivations and health. Among the elderly (aged 60–92), attitudes towards old age are predictive of self-esteem, and, for men, income and education are predictive (Ward 1977).

Content

The scale consists of 10 items of which five items are positively worded and five are negatively worded, with responses reported along a four-point continuum from 'strongly agree' to 'strongly disagree'. Examples of items are shown in Box 7.10.

Box 7.10 Examples from the Self-esteem Scale

I feel that I'm a person of worth, at least on an equal plane with others.
I feel that I have a number of good qualities.
All in all, I am inclined to feel that I am a failure.
I feel I do not have much to be proud of.
At times I think I am no good at all.
On the whole, I am satisfied with myself.
I take a positive attitude toward myself.

Strongly agree (1)/agree (2)/disagree (3)/strongly disagree (4)

Rosenberg, M. (1965) *Society and the Adolescent Self-Image*. Revised edition. Middletown, CT: Wesleyan University Press. With permission of University of Maryland. Not copyrighted. Free to use, but permission to use request is required via weblink which returns consent by reply. Request to use form can be accessed at: www.socy.umd.edu, http://socy.umd.edu/about-us/rosenberg-self-esteem-scale. Developer: Professor Morris Rosenberg. Information: www.bsos.umd.edu/socy/grad/rosenberg.doc, http://socy.umd.edu/about-us/rosenberg-self-esteem-scale, accessed 19 September 2015.

Scoring

The measure was designed as a 10-item Guttman scale. The category responses were originally designed to be scored from 0 to 6 (strongly agree to strongly disagree). However, there is no agreement over the method of scoring, and some users score responses dichotomously as 'agree' or 'disagree', and other researchers use a simple summing scale.

Validity

Rosenberg (1965) explicitly chose items for the scale which he felt had face validity. Rosenberg, in assessing its construct validity, also reported that positive self-esteem was predictive of several social and psychological characteristics, such as reduced shyness, depression and more assertiveness and social activities. He reported that the scale had acceptable predictive validity in relation to depression levels among volunteers assessed by nurses. Robinson and Shaver (1973) reported that the scale correlated 0.59–0.60 with Coopersmith's Self-Esteem Inventory, depending on the scoring method. It has also been reported to be significantly associated with depression (Schmitz *et al.* 2003), and to perform better than the Coopersmith Self-Esteem Inventory in predicting dieting disorder psychopathology (Griffiths *et al.* 1999).

Kaplan and Porkorny (1969) reported two uncorrelated factors which accounted for 45 per cent of the total variance. The items forming the first factor they called 'self-derogation', and they stated that the second factor reflected 'defense of individual worth'. Kohn (1969) reported similar results. A two-factor model was supported in factor analyses by Greenberger *et al.* (2003) in a study of over 700 ethnically diverse undergraduate students, who reported that it had high validity among different ethnic groups.

Reliability

Reliability (internal consistency and test-retest) has been shown to be good by Rosenberg (1965, 1986) who reported reproducibility coefficients of 0.85–0.92 and a scalability coefficient of 0.72; Ward (1977) reported a coefficient alpha of 0.74 for internal consistency; Silber and Tippett (1965) reported a test-retest reliability coefficient of 0.85 from administrations of the scale to 28 students with a two-week interval, and item correlations of 0.56 and 0.83.

In sum, the scale is attractive due to its brevity and simplicity but still requires further testing on wider populations for validity, reliability and sensitivity to change. Wylie (1974), in her extensive but early review of the scale, concluded that it is worthy of further research and development. Also, its method of scoring remains unresolved. It was highly recommended by George and Bearon (1980).

THE TENNESSEE SELF-CONCEPT SCALE (TSCS)

The TSCS is probably the most popular and most often used scale. It was developed for use in mental health rehabilitation in 1956 and revised in 1965 (Fitts 1965). Fitts (1965, 1972; Fitts and Warren 1996) based the scale on Maslow's theory that individuals who are more self-actualizing are more able to realize their true potentialities and to function in a more creative and effective manner. Fitts saw self-concept related to performance: the person who has a clear, consistent, positive and realistic self-concept will behave in a healthy, confident, constructive and effective way. This is dependent on other things being equal, and this, of course, is not always the case.

The scale was developed from other scales and open-ended items, and from self-descriptions from samples of psychiatric patients and non-patients. These were placed on an internal–external scale. Ninety remaining statements were independently classified by seven clinical psychologists into 15 categories. There was perfect agreement on their negative and positive content. The scale was initially tested on 626 people, aged 12–68.

Administration takes approximately 20 minutes, and is based on self-completion.

Content

The scale consists of a series of self-descriptive items covering physical self, moral-ethical self, personal self, family self and social self. These labels are divided into statements about internal self-concept: self-identity, self-acceptance and behaviour. The scale is intended to summarize an individual's feeling of self-worth, and the degree to which the image is realistic or deviant. Items tap both an internal and external dimension of self-concept. Version 2 of the TSCS (adult version) contains 82 items with five-point response categories ranging from 'Always false' to 'Always true'.

Details of the original scale are available in Fitts (1965), Roid and Fitts (1988) and Fitts and Warren (1996). Box 7.11 includes four items from version 2 of the scale (adult version).

Box 7.11 Examples from the Tennessee Self-Concept Scale (TSCS-2)

21. I have a healthy body.
 8. I am satisfied with my moral behaviour.
 3. I am a member of a happy family.
45. I am as sociable as I want to be.

Completely false (1)/mostly false (2)/partly false and partly true (3)/mostly true (4)/ completely true (5)

Scoring

The total score is a positive self-esteem score. Fitts (1965) reported a mean score, on the basis of his original sample of 628 adults, of 345.57 (potential range 90–450). A computerized scoring service is available from the publisher.

Validity

Correlations demonstrating convergent, discriminant and predictive validity were reported by Fitts (1965), Thompson (1972) and Roid and Fitts (1988). However, much of the evidence to support the scale comes from relatively early or unpublished studies. Correlations with an anxiety scale of −0.70 support the discriminant ability of the scale (Fitts 1965), and are confirmed by Thompson (1972). Fitts also reports a correlation of 0.68 with a scale of positive affect. Discriminant validity is partly suggested by a correlation of −0.21 with the F scale measure of authoritarianism; and predictive validity is suggested by its ability to distinguish between mental health and psychopathology (Fitts 1965). However, Wylie (1974) questioned the discriminant validity on the scale on the grounds of lack of sufficient information reported by Fitts (1965). While there are many relevant variables that correlate significantly with the scale, there are also many that do not (Reed *et al.* 1980).

The scale has been widely used on samples of juveniles and psychiatric patients, as well as normal adults. Self-esteem has been found to be higher among older people than among adults generally (Grant 1966). Goodrick *et al.* (1999) reported that the scale was able to predict improvement in severity of binge-eating.

Vincent (1968) undertook a factor analysis of the scale. Self-acceptance and personal-self loaded with several similar measures. Vacchiano and Strauss (1968) reported that their factor analysis of the scale revealed 20 factors. The factor structure remains unresolved (see McGuire and Tinsley 1981 and Roid and Fitts 1988). Applications of the scale do not show a consistent pattern of results to be able to support the definition of self-concept as defined by Fitts (Walsh 1984).

Reliability

Test-retest reliability tests show high correlations of 0.92 for the positive self-esteem score and 0.75 for the self-criticism scale over a two-week period in a study of 60 students (Fitts 1965). Wylie (1974) again criticized Fitts for lack of sufficient information to make independent judgements about the reliability of the scale. This has been rectified in a subsequent manual by Roid and Fitts (1988). Estimates of internal consistency (alpha coefficients) for the scale range between 0.66 and 0.94 for the total scale score and subsets of the scale, with most being between 0.70 and 0.87 (Stanwyck and Garrison 1982; Tzeng *et al.* 1985; Roid and Fitts 1988). However, inter-item correlations appear to be relatively low for the various subsets of items (from 0.14 to 0.35) (Tzeng *et al.* 1985), although this is within the range expected for such scales (Roid and Fitts 1988).

In sum, the scale appears usable with older people, although the low self-criticism scores obtained by the elderly should make the user cautious (George and Bearon 1980). It is a popular scale but potentially lengthy to administer.

COOPERSMITH SELF-ESTEEM INVENTORY (CSEI)

The Coopersmith Inventories were well researched (Coopersmith 1975, 1981a, 1981b), and are widely used in social science and by clinicians. Self-esteem is portrayed as a trait that is not evenly distributed in the population, but highly desirable to have. The manual of the scale offers several sources of population norms (Coopersmith 1981a). Coopersmith (1967) defined self-esteem as self-judgements of personal worth, a definition compatible with earlier definitions. The CSEI measures attitudes towards the self, encompassing several domains: social, academic, family and personal experiences. The scale was devised by five psychologists for use with children who classified items according to high or low esteem to derive a 50-item scale. Items were reduced to 25, after an item analysis based on the responses of 121 children. The correlation of the longer with the shorter version was 0.95. The scale is self-administered and takes approximately 10 minutes.

Content

The items consist of short statements which the subject rates as either 'like me' or 'unlike me'. It is multidimensional, covering leadership-popularity, self-derogation, family-parents, and assertiveness-anxiety. Examples are shown in Box 7.12.

Box 7.12 Examples from the CSEI (adults)

I can make up my mind without too much trouble.
I'm a lot of fun to be with.
I'm popular with people my own age.
It's pretty tough to be me.
Things are all mixed up in my life.

Reproduction by special permission of the publisher, Mind Garden, Inc., www.mindgarden.com, from the Coopersmith Self-Esteem Inventory Adult Form by Stanley Coopersmith Copyright © 1975, 2002 by Stanley Coopersmith. Further reproduction is prohibited without the publisher's written consent. The instrument can be obtained from the publisher; licence and manual fees are charged. Contact information: Mind Garden, 855 Oak Grove Avenue, Suite 215, Menlo Park, CA 94025, USA; website: http://mindgarden.com, accessed 16 October 2015; http://www.mindgarden.com/85-coopersmith-self-esteem-inventory, accessed 5 November 2015.

The 50-item scale has an additional eight lie-scale items (Coopersmith 1967). A similar 25-item version also exists, and this can be used with adults (aged 16+). The version for adults has been published by Robinson and Shaver (1973).

Scoring

The scoring format remains untested. The item responses 'like me' or 'unlike me' are allocated a value and simply summed. A score is derived by multiplying X, the raw score, by 2 on the short scale and 4 on the long scale. A totally positive score is 100 and a totally negative score is 0.

Validity

Convergent validity correlations between the scale and other self-esteem scales, based again on students, vary widely between 0.02 and 0.60 (Taylor and Reitz 1968; Ziller et al. 1969; Crandall 1973). More consistent correlations with the Rosenberg Self-Esteem Scale were reported by Robinson and Shaver (1973), again using students (total: 300) from 0.59 to 0.60. Hoffmeister (1976) compared two subscales of the Self-Esteem Questionnaire which he developed with the CSEI and reported correlations of 0.40 and 0.61. Correlations range between 0.44 and 0.75 when tested against a social desirability scale (Taylor and Reitz 1968), indicating that there is possible confounding with social desirability.

Correlations have been reported with scales measuring other concepts, which would be expected on theoretical grounds: Campbell (1967) reported a correlation of 0.31 with an achievement test; Boshier (1968) reported a correlation of 0.80 with the scale and liking one's first name; Wiest (1965) reported a correlation of 0.22 between the scale and the reporting of mutual liking between others and self. Other studies have reported correlations in the expected direction, for example, with psychiatric disorder in adolescents (Guillon *et al.* 2003), and binge-eating in obese hospital outpatients (Jirik-Babb and Geliebter 2003). Not all correlations are in the direction expected. For example, Trowbridge (1970) reported a higher mean on the scale for children who were socioeconomically disadvantaged. A gender bias on six of the scale items (25-item version) has been reported (Chapman and Mullis 2002), requiring caution in its use.

Wylie (1974) questioned Coopersmith's claims of validity for the scale, on the grounds of the large number of significance tests undertaken in its development and the non-reporting of the actual number of such tests. The number reaching statistical significance at the 0.5 level was unreported, thus making it impossible to estimate the number that could have occurred by chance alone.

Robinson and Shaver (1973), on the basis of two samples of students (total: 500), carried out two factor analyses of the scale which indicated its multidimensional nature. Four factors emerged: self-derogation, leadership-popularity, family-parents and assertiveness-anxiety. The family-parents factor was reported to be the most stable and least ambiguous. Kokenes (1974) estimated the validity of the subscales by factor analysis of the responses of 7,600 school children and reported that the four bipolar dimensions obtained were highly congruent with the test's subscales.

Reliability

The scale was originally administered to 87 school children. Early testing for test-retest reliability reported high coefficients at 0.88 over five weeks and 0.70 over three years, based on the samples of pre-adolescent school children (Coopersmith 1967). Thus it is a stable measure over time and is not suitable for longitudinal use where changes require measurement (Coopersmith 1967). Split-half reliability tests also show high correlations: 0.90 (Taylor and Reitz 1968). Spatz and Johnson (1973) administered the 50-item child version to 600 students and reported internal-consistency coefficients in excess of 0.80. However, internal consistency was reported to be low in another study of 453 college students (Crandall 1973), a probable consequence of its multi-dimensionality.

In sum, the scale appears to have been initially well researched and is widely used. A major methodological limitation has been its restricted use with samples of students for the testing of the reliability and validity of the adult version (Adair 1984).

EXAMPLE

An example of the use of measures of subjective well-being is shown in Box 7.13.

Box 7.13 Example of descriptive study using subjective well-being outcome measures

Brajković *et al.* (2011) aimed to investigate self-reported life satisfaction in elderly retirees in the community and in a retirement home, and associations with gender, type of residence, living arrangement, self-rated health status, loneliness and sense of humour.

Their sample comprised 300 elderly retirees from Zagreb, Croatia. Their inclusion criteria were that people were able to perform everyday activities independently (e.g. dressing, bathing, walking, eating), and to have been retired for at least five years. Those with physical disabilities or serious physical illness not associated with the normal ageing processes were excluded.

Their measures included some of those reviewed in this book, namely the UCLA Loneliness Scale, the Life Satisfaction Index, and the SF-36 Health Survey questionnaire.

They reported that people who lived in a retirement home had higher life satisfaction compared with those who lived in their own households. Those who had children also had higher life satisfaction. Those who had poorer self-rated health and who reported feelings of loneliness had worse life satisfaction. Sociodemographic variables, self-rated health status, self-rated loneliness and a sense of humour explained 52.8 per cent of variance in life satisfaction. No differences in life satisfaction were found with respect to gender, marital status or living arrangement.

Their conclusion recommended preventative activities.

CHAPTER 8

MEASURING BROADER QUALITY OF LIFE

CHAPTER COVERAGE

QUALITY OF LIFE

Measurement of quality of life (QoL) is relevant to the evaluation of outcomes of health and social care interventions, and of conditions which can affect a person's whole life.

In addition, the worldwide emphasis on health promotion, and enhancement of population well-being, has led to the need to use broader health and social care outcome measures, including QoL. Strategies for mental health promotion in particular are related to improving QoL and the potential for health rather than focusing on amelioration of symptoms and deficits (Bowling 2014c – see also https://www.gov.uk/government/publications/chief-medical-officer-cmo-annual-report-public-mental-health, accessed 4 January 2016).

This chapter, then, focuses on broader, generic measures of QoL. These are theoretically distinct from measures of broader health status and health-related QoL which have often dominated the QoL field. Health is valued highly by people, but good health is just one of the areas nominated by the public as giving their life quality (Bowling 1995, 2005b; Bowling *et al.* 2003).

Regardless of conceptual distinctions, many investigators have used measures of broader health status to measure health-related QoL or even broader QoL. This has been justified on the basis of the untested assumption that broader measures of health status (e.g. the SF-36) include the main areas in which health can affect one's life (Ware *et al.* 1993; Bowling 1995), and which are relevant for health services. However, it does lead to conceptual confusion. In addition, a plethora of disease-specific QoL measures has been developed, with little standardization of measurement approaches between studies (Garratt *et al.* 2002). A pragmatic approach has prevailed in the literature on QoL, which has meant that the definition of terms has been neglected, and the selection of measurement scales often appears to be ad hoc.

An increasing number of investigators are unhappy with the traditional use of measures, or proxy measures, of QoL which focus on functioning rather than addressing the complexity of people's views and expectations, and which are theoretical. For example, Staniszewska (1999) compared cardiac patients' expectations of their health care with the domains of the SF-36 and reported that patients adopted a broader approach than that contained within the eight domains of the SF-36 questionnaire, and mentioned expectations of the manageability of their condition and of reassurance, and emphasized the future (knowing what will happen to their condition, increasing their chances of living). This has also led to the development of more individualized measures, which are presented, with standardized approaches, in this chapter.

QoL spans a broad range of topics and disciplines (see Chapter 1). It is made up of both positive and negative experiences and affect. It is a dynamic concept, which poses further challenges for measurement. When measuring changes in QoL, several variables need to be taken into account, including actual changes in circumstances of interest (e.g. health) and regression to the mean. Other factors which require consideration include stable personality characteristics. For example, optimism bias might help people to cope with, and adjust to, deteriorating circumstances, leading to an optimistic evaluation of their QoL as higher (Pearlin and Schooler 1978; Scheier and Carver 1985; Diener *et al.* 1991; Sprangers and Schwartz 1999; Brissette *et al.* 2002).

Relevant cognitive or affective processes in changing circumstances also include making comparisons of one's situation with others who are better or worse off, cognitive dissonance reduction (defensive preference for the circumstances experienced), reordering of goals and values and response shift. Consciously or unconsciously, people may adjust to deteriorating circumstances because they want to feel as good as possible about themselves. The roots of this process are in control theory, with goals of homeostasis. Response shift refers to the process whereby internal standards and values are changed – and hence the perception of QoL (Sprangers and Schwartz 1999). Albrecht and Devlieger (1999) focused on the issue of why so many people with serious and persistent disabilities report their QoL to be good or excellent, when their lives would be viewed as undesirable by external observers. Their in-depth interviews with people indicate that consideration of QoL was dependent upon finding a balance between body, mind and the self (spirit), and on establishing and maintaining harmonious relationships, supporting the theory of homeostasis.

Some investigators of QoL use the 'then-test' technique to test for changes in internal standards. With this method, respondents are asked about their perceptions of their situation at baseline (Tn), and then again at follow-up (Tn + 1), along with retrospective questions at follow-up about how they perceive themselves to have been at baseline (then-test for Tn). Analysis and comparison of the scores indicates the response shift and the change in QoL (Sprangers et al. 1999; Joore et al. 2002). The reliability and validity of this method has yet to be fully tested.

Psychological outlook is also likely to be an influencing factor. Bowling et al. (2007) reported, from their national survey of people aged 65+ in Britain, that about a fifth of respondents reported fairly to very severe levels of functional difficulty, and almost two-thirds of this group rated their QoL positively – compared to those with similar levels of poor functioning who rated their QoL negatively. The former group were more likely to feel in control of their lives, adopting a 'can do', positive approach, using coping strategies of acceptance and compensation (Baltes and Baltes 1990).

The subjectivity and complexity of QoL presents a challenge not only to the design of QoL measurement scales, and their composition (content validity), but also to their scoring and/or weighting. If measurement scales give equal weighting to the various sub-domains of QoL it is unlikely that the domains will have equal significance to different social groups and individuals within these. Even where scales are weighted it is unlikely that the weightings will be equally applicable to different social groups and individuals. Moreover, the literature comparing standardized weighted and unweighted cardinal (i.e. summed) scales – whether of life events, life satisfaction or health status – consistently reports no benefit of more complex weighted methods over simple summing of scores in relation to the proportion of explained variance or sensitivity to change over time (Andrews and Crandall 1976; Jenkinson et al. 1991). And little experimental work has been carried out testing the different values which can be attached to weights – such as relative importance, satisfaction or goal achievement and gap ('social comparisons' and 'expectancy') ratings of individuals.

This chapter examines broader scales of QoL that have largely been developed outside disease-specific contexts. The exceptions are the LASA and Spitzer scales, which were developed for use with cancer patients. These are presented here because researchers across disciplines often adapt their format (unacknowledged) (i.e. the use of the LASA response scale and the global QoL Spitzer Uniscale). Broad scales of QoL have also been developed in mental health; as they are disease-specific and limited to research in mental health they are not included here (these have been reviewed in *Measuring Disease* (Bowling 2001)).

Broader, multi-dimensional lay-based models and measures have also been developed for use at population level. The most recently developed and well-tested in both adult and older population samples are: the CASP-19 (control, autonomy, satisfaction, pleasure); the World Health Organization's WHOQOL and WHOQOL-OLD; and the Older People's Quality of Life questionnaire (OPQOL). A more recent development is the measurement of QoL in social care (ASCOT). These measures are reviewed here.

THE WORLD HEALTH ORGANIZATION'S MEASURES

The Constitution of the WHO (1948a, 1948b) defined health as 'a state of complete physical, mental and social well-being not merely the absence of disease . . .' Thus it followed that a measure of health outcomes should include not just assessment of clinical changes but also of broader well-being and health-related QoL.

The WHO, in collaboration with 15 centres worldwide, developed two instruments for measuring QoL – the WHOQOL-100 and the WHOQOL-BREF – which were intended for use in a wide range of cultural settings, enabling different populations to be compared (WHOQOL Group 1994, 1996). While developed for use in clinical practice, clinical and policy research on outcomes, and audit, the WHOQOL instruments were designed broadly to reflect the WHOQOL Group's (1993) definition of QoL as based on individual's perceptions of their position in the context of their culture and value systems, and in relation to their goals, expectations, standards and concerns. They regarded QoL as not confined to domains of health but as broad ranging and affected by a person's physical health, psychological state, personal beliefs, social relationships and relationship to their environment.

The WHOQOL was developed from statements collected from patients with a range of conditions, professionals, and healthy people, and was initially piloted by expert review and qualitative fieldwork. It was subsequently tested for validity and reliability on 250 patients and 50 healthy respondents in the 15 participating centres. The original instrument contained 300 items, and this was reduced to 100, which form the current instrument – WHOQOL-100. The WHOQOL-BREF, a 26-item version of the WHOQOL-100, was developed using data from the field trials of the parent instrument (WHOQOL Group 1998b).

The core WHOQOL instruments assess QoL across situations. Modules were also developed which collect more detailed information from specific groups (e.g. elderly people, refugees, people with specific diseases such as cancer, HIV/Aids). The WHOQOL-100 is administered by an interviewer, although the WHOQOL-BREF can be self-administered. The full instrument takes 10–20 minutes administration time. It is available in over 20 different languages, and each translation was tested for cultural equivalence. A methodology is available for further translations. A manual is also available from the developers.

WHOQOL-100

WHOQOL-100 initially contained six broad domains of QoL, 24 facets of QoL (four items per facet), and four general items covering subjective overall QoL and overall health. These produced 100 items in total. The six specific domains were overall QoL and general health: (1) physical health (energy and fatigue; pain and discomfort; sleep and rest); (2) psychological (bodily image and appearance; negative feelings; positive feelings; self-esteem; thinking, learning, memory and concentration); (3) level of independence (mobility; activities of daily living; dependence on medicinal substances and medical aids; work capacity); (4) social relations (personal relationships; social support; sexual activity); (5) environment (financial resources; freedom, physical safety and security; health and social care: accessibility and quality; home environment; opportunities for acquiring new information and skills; participation in, and opportunities for, recreation/leisure; physical environment (pollution/noise/traffic/climate); transport); (6) spirituality/religion/personal beliefs (single facet: spirituality/religion/personal beliefs). Hagerty *et al.* (2001) criticized the WHOQOL Group's apparent prior decision to include six domains, without providing any justification, and for the absence of respondents' importance ratings in the scoring of QoL (despite the definition underpinning the WHOQOL implying individual-level evaluation).

Analyses of the factor structure of the WHOQOL-100 indicated that domains 1 and 3 and domains 2 and 6 could be merged, thereby creating four domains of QoL instead of six: physical, psychological, social relationships and environment. These reflect the current grouping and scoring and were supported in cross-cultural studies (WHOQOL Group 1998b; Power *et al.* 1999). All items are rated on a five-point scale. The time reference for the questions is 'in the last two weeks'.

Content

The WHOQOL-100 now contains four broad domains of QoL, 24 facets of QoL (four items per facet), and four general items covering subjective overall QoL and overall health). These produce 100 items in total. The four domains are: physical, psychological, social relationships and environment.

All items are rated on a five-point scale. As noted, the time reference for the questions is 'in the last two weeks'. Examples from the WHOQOL-100 are shown in Box 8.1.

Box 8.1 Examples from the WHOQOL-100

The following questions ask you to say how satisfied, happy or good you have felt about various aspects of your life over the past two weeks. For example, about your family life or the energy that you have. Decide how satisfied or dissatisfied you are with each aspect of your life and circle the number that best fits how you feel about this. Questions refer to the past two weeks.

How satisfied are you with the quality of your life?
In general, how satisfied are you with your life?
How satisfied are you with your health?
How satisfied are you with the energy you have?

Very dissatisfied/dissatisfied/neither satisfied nor dissatisfied/satisfied/very satisfied.

The following questions ask about **how much** you have experienced certain things in the last two weeks, for example, positive feelings such as happiness or contentment. If you have experienced these things an extreme amount circle the number next to 'An extreme amount'. If you have not experienced these things at all, circle the number next to 'Not at all'. You should circle one of the numbers in between if you wish to indicate your answer lies somewhere between 'Not at all' and 'Extremely'. Questions refer to the last two weeks.

How safe do you feel in your daily life?
Not at all/Slightly/Moderately/Very/Extremely

Do you feel you are living in a safe and secure environment?
Not at all/Slightly/Moderately/Very much/Extremely

How much do you worry about your safety and security?
Not at all/A little/A moderate amount/Very much/An extreme amount

How comfortable is the place where you live?
Not at all/Slightly/Moderately/Very/Extremely

How much do you like it where you live?
Not at all/A little/A moderate amount/Very much/An extreme amount

© World Health Organization. Reproduced with permission, www.who.int/msa/qol.

Written permission obtained to cite these items was obtained from: The WHOQOL Group, Department of Mental Health, WHO, CH-1211, Geneva 27, Switzerland.

The WHOQOL instruments are available in more than 20 languages. The appropriate language version, and permission for using it, can be obtained from the appropriate national centre. (See www.who.int/mental_health/publications/whoqol/en/. A user agreement form is available online WHOQOL@who.int. Permission to use the UK instrument must be obtained from Professor Suzanne Skevington, WHO Centre for the Study of Quality of Life, University of Bath, Bath, BA2 7AY, UK; s.m.skevington@bath.ac.uk.)

Full length (Power *et al.* 1999) and shorter (WHOQOL Group 1998b) versions have been developed and tested, as well as a version for older people (WHOQOL-OLD) (Skevington 1999; Power *et al.* 1999, 2005). The WHOQOL has been used with different cultural groups across the world (http://www.euro.who.int/ageing/quality).

Scoring

The WHOQOL-100 produces scores relating to specific (positive feelings, social support, financial resources) and main domains (physical, psychological, social relationships) of QoL, a score for overall QoL and a score for general health. Scores are produced for: physical, psychological, social relationships and environment. Details on scoring are reported in manuals available from the WHOQOL Group (Programme on Mental Health, World Health Organization, CH-1211 Geneva 27, Switzerland). Syntax files for checking and cleaning data, and computing facet and domain scores are available from the WHOQOL Group.

Validity

The WHOQOL instruments have been reported to have good discriminant and content validity, although work on their validity and reliability is continuing (WHOQOL Group 1998a, 1998b). They appear to be well accepted by respondents.

There are many studies of the psychometric performance of the instrument. The difficulty with reviewing the overall psychometric properties is that the studies all relate to different language versions, and different disease or population groups. For example, Pibernik-Okanovic (2001) tested the discriminant validity of the WHOQOL-100 with a small sample of diabetic patients in Croatia and reported that, at two months follow-up, it was sensitive to improvement in condition in patients whose treatment had been changed, in comparison with controls. The WHOQOL-100 was reported to have good concurrent validity, greater comprehensiveness and good responsiveness to clinical change, in comparison with the SF-36, in a study of over 100 outpatients with chronic pain in the UK (Skevington *et al.* 2001).

Although results are not all consistent, investigators in various countries have reported that the WHOQOL-100 can successfully discriminate between patient groups across a wide range of conditions, and has generally good psychometric properties (e.g. Struttmann *et al.* 1999; Skevington *et al.* 2001).

It was reported earlier that factor analysis of the WHOQOL-100 supported four domains of quality of life instead of six: physical, psychological, social relationships and environment.

Reliability

The WHOQOL Group (1998a) reported on the initial psychometric properties of the WHOQOL-100; both published and unpublished data show that the instrument was shown to have good test-retest and face reliability, and high internal consistency (Power *et al.* 1999; Skevington 1999). Szabo (1996) reported that all except one of the domains of the WHOQOL-100 achieved Cronbach's alphas over the threshold of acceptability of between 0.82–0.95.

Pibernik-Okanovic's (2001) study of diabetic patients in Croatia found that the WHOQOL-100 produced Cronbach's alphas of 0.76 to 0.95 for the four domains.

While the WHOQOL-100 is lengthy, the advantage is its breadth of scope and applicability in different cultures. A short version is available, also with good psychometric properties, but short forms are always weaker than full versions. The manual, appropriate language version of the instrument, scoring instructions and syntax files for their computation, permission for use and other details of the instruments can be obtained from the relevant national centre (see WHO website: http://www.who.int) or from the WHOQOL Group at the WHO in Geneva.

WHOQOL-BREF

Content

The WHOQOL-BREF contains two items for overall QoL and general health and one item from each of the 24 facets in the WHOQOL-100, and can be self-administered.

Scoring

The WHOQOL-BREF produces domain but not facet scores. Details on scoring are reported in manuals available from the WHOQOL Group, Programme on Mental Health, World Health Organization, CH-1211 Geneva 27, Switzerland. Syntax files for checking and cleaning data, and computing facet and domain scores are also available from the WHOQOL Group.

Validity and reliability

The WHOQOL-BREF was tested by de Girolamo *et al.* (2000) in over 300 people who were in contact with health services in Italy. They reported that only the physical and psychological domains were able to discriminate between healthy and unhealthy respondents. Domain scores produced by the WHOQOL-BREF have been reported to correlate highly (0.89) with the four domains of the WHOQOL-100 domains scores; and this shorter instrument was reported to have good discriminant and content validity, internal consistency and test-retest reliability in cross-sectional surveys of adults carried out in 23 countries (WHOQOL Group 1998b; Skevington *et al.* 2004). The WHOQOL-BREF can successfully discriminate between patient groups across a wide range of conditions, and has generally good psychometric properties (Fleck *et al.* 2000; Leplege *et al.* 2000).

Test-retest reliability of the WHOQOL-BREF was tested by de Girolamo *et al.*'s (2000) study in Italy, and they reported correlations of between 0.76 and 0.93 for the domains. They also reported internal consistency with alphas ranging from 0.65 to 0.80. Leplege *et al.* (2000), on the basis of their study of over 2,000 patients in different types of clinic in France, reported that the homogeneity of the short version was lower than the full instrument, but was still acceptable: item scale correlations were greater than 0.40 for two-thirds of the items; and the Cronbach's alpha for all domains on the WHOQOL-BREF were over 0.65. Assessments of the discriminant ability of the WHOQOL-BREF, using item response theory, with a sample of students in Iran, reported that the reverse coded items had poorer discriminatory power than un-recoded items (Vahedi 2010). It is possible that the items were less discriminatory in a healthy population, or it supports the view that the use of both positively and negatively worded items in the same scale adversely affects measurement consistency. However, a general rule in questionnaire design is to vary the direction of scale item wording, or responses, to order to avoid 'response sets' (i.e. people's tendencies to endorse responses positioned on the far right or far left of a questionnaire – see Bowling 2014b). Examples of items are in Box 8.2.

Box 8.2 Examples from the WHOQOL-BREF

The following questions ask about how much you have experienced certain things in the last two weeks.

How much do you feel that pain prevents you from doing what you need to do?

How much do you enjoy life?

Not at all/ A little/ A moderate amount/ Very much/ An extreme amount

The following questions ask you to say how good or satisfied you have felt about various aspects of your life over the last two weeks.

How satisfied are you with your sleep?

How satisfied are you with your personal relationships?

Very dissatisfied/ Dissatisfied/ Neither satisfied nor dissatisfied/ Satisfied/ Very satisfied

The following question refers to how often you have felt or experienced certain things in the last two weeks.

How often do you have negative feelings, such as blue mood, despair, anxiety, depression?

Never/ Seldom/ Quite often/ Very often/ Always

© World Health Organization. Reproduced with permission, www.who.int/msa/qol and www.who.int/mental_health/media/en/76.pdf, accessed 6 October 2015. Written permission to cite these items was obtained from the WHOQOL Group, Department of Mental Health, WHO, CH-1211, Geneva 27, Switzerland.

The WHOQOL instruments are available in more than 20 languages. The appropriate language version, and permission for using it, can be obtained from the appropriate national centre (see www.who.int/mental_health/publications/whoqol/en/). A user agreement form is available online (see WHOQOL@who.int). Permission to use the UK instrument (cited here) must be obtained from Professor Suzanne Skevington, WHO Centre for the Study of Quality of Life, University of Bath, Bath, BA2 7AY, UK (s.m.skevington@bath.ac.uk).

WHOQOL-OLD

The WHOQOL-OLD was developed from the parent instrument: the World Health Organization's WHOQOL Group's WHOQOL-100, and cross-cultural studies (see Power et al. 1999). It was tested on convenience samples of older people across cultures (Power et al. 2005). The WHOQOL-OLD has been used with different cultural groups across the world (see http://www.euro.who.int/ageing/quality).

Content

It is a multi-faceted measure of QoL and comprises seven subscales (24 items): sensory abilities, autonomy, past present and future activities, social participation, death and dying, and intimacy (four items per subscale). Response scales are five-point and vary in their wording ('Not at all' to 'An extreme amount'/'Completely'/'Extremely'; 'Very poor' to' Very good'; 'Very dissatisfied' to 'Very satisfied'; 'Very unhappy' to 'Very happy').

Scoring

The WHOQOL-OLD produces domain but not scores for the individual facets. Details on scoring are reported in manuals available from the WHOQOL Group, Programme on Mental Health, World Health Organisation, CH-1211 Geneva 27, Switzerland. Syntax files for checking and cleaning data, and computing facet and domain scores are available from the WHOQOL Group.

Examples of some of the items are shown in Box 8.3.

Box 8.3 Examples from the WHOQOL-OLD

How much freedom do you have to make your own decisions?

Not at all   A little   A moderate amount   Very much   An extreme amount

To what extent do you feel in control of your future?

Not at all   A little   A moderate amount   Very much   An extreme amount

How much do you feel that the people around you are respectful of your freedom?

Not at all   A little   A moderate amount   Very much   An extreme amount

© World Health Organization. Reproduced with permission, www.who.int/msa/qol and http://www.who.int/substance_abuse/research_tools/whoqolbref/en/, accessed 6 October 2015. Written permission obtained to cite these items was obtained from the WHOQOL Group, Department of Mental Health, WHO, CH-1211, Geneva 27, Switzerland.

The WHOQOL instruments are available in more than 20 languages. The appropriate language version, and permission for using it, can be obtained from the appropriate national centre (see www.who.int/mental_health/publications/whoqol/en/). A user agreement form is available online (see WHOQOL@who.int). Permission to use the UK instrument (cited here) must be obtained from Professor Suzanne Skevington, WHO Centre for the Study of Quality of Life, University of Bath, Bath, BA2 7AY, UK (s.m.skevington@bath.ac.uk).

Validity and reliability

The WHOQOL-OLD was tested by Bowling (2009b) and Bowling and Stenner (2011) along with their Older People's Quality of Life (OPQOL) questionnaire and the CASP-19 in national population surveys of people aged 65+ living at home in Britain, including an ethically diverse sample. The construct validity of the three QoL measures was tested by correlating them with independent self-rated QoL and self-ratings on several of its domains. Before the three QoL scales were administered, respondents were asked to rate their QoL overall, and in relation to their health, social relationships, independence, control and freedom, home and neighbourhood, psychological/emotional well-being, financial circumstances and leisure, and social activities. The WHOQOL-OLD correlated weakly to moderately well between −0.128 and −0.466 (both p <0.01) in the samples (minus sign reflects direction of coding), with those with better WHOQOL-OLD scores reporting higher global QoL (Bowling 2009b). The WHOQOL-OLD also correlated with most of the QoL domain self-ratings in the British population sample, but often failed to correlate significantly with the QoL domain self-ratings in the ethnically diverse sample (Bowling 2009b).

In Bowling's population survey analyses, the WHOQOL-OLD satisfied the 0.70<0.90 threshold for internal consistency reliability with Cronbach's alpha in the British population sample aged 65+ (alpha 0.849), but not in the ethnically diverse sample (alpha 0.415). The subscales to total correlation ranges, across samples, for the WHOQOL-OLD were highly significant (Spearman's rho 0.291–0.761; all p <0 .01) (Bowling 2009b; Bowling and Stenner 2011). The reliability criterion for item-total correlations (the correlation of the item with the scale total with that item omitted) is that the item should correlate with the total scale by at least 0.20. Fourteen of the 24 WHOQOL-OLD items failed this criterion in the ethnically diverse sample only. As expected, all items correlated more highly with similar, than dissimilar, items in the scales. All subscale to total score Spearman's rho correlations, within each sample, were highly significant at p <.01 (WHOQOL-OLD rho 0.291–0.761).

LEIPAD QUESTIONNAIRE

The LEIPAD was developed under the auspices of the European Office of the World Health Organization to assess multidimensional QoL in older people, which reflects various aspects of daily functioning (e.g. physical, mental, social and occupational) (de Leo et al. 1998a, 1998b). The name of the instrument derives from the institutions of its main developers in LEIden and PADua. Field testing of the instrument, on over 500 patients attending GPs, was conducted in Italy, The Netherlands and Finland.

The developers recognized that QoL assessment had become narrow in focus because of the interest in QoL as a clinical outcome indicator. This narrow focus was not regarded as useful for older people, and a wider measure which incorporated a person's material, physical, social, emotional and spiritual well-being was said to be preferable. These areas were said to become more closely interrelated with age due to the increased changes in experiencing various adverse events simultaneously. The aim of the developers of LEIPAD was to develop an instrument that was sensitive to change and which assessed QoL subjectively from the older person's perspective, as well as containing some more objective items. Thus the core of the LEIPAD is a self-report questionnaire requesting self-evaluations of existing state and effects on daily life. De Leo et al. (1998a) argued that existing multidimensional instruments developed for use with older people were too long (although these are assessment instruments, not health-related QoL questionnaires), and broader health status scales omitted relevant dimensions (e.g. cognitive status).

The original LEIPAD contained 37 items, which were taken from existing questionnaires or created 'ad hoc' by the developers, especially those with expertise in psychogeriatric medicine. Thus it was not developed with older people, but was based on 'expert' views of the important items and dimensions to include. These items initially covered 10 areas: self-perceived physical health, mental health, emotional health, self-esteem, expectations for the future, activities and instrumental activities of daily living (ADL, IADL), interpersonal and social functioning, recreational activities, financial situation and religiousness/spirituality. This early version had a single scoring system for all items (the response categories were: Not at all/A little/Somewhat/Much/Very much, with a corresponding five-point scale ranging from 0 (high level of well-being) to 4 (low level of well-being). Objective data were included in order to collect background information: sociodemographic characteristics, personality characteristics, the Mini-Mental State (Folstein et al. 1975), current illnesses and medications, indicators of religiousness/life sense. The authors argued that personality characteristics and mental status could be used to distinguish between valid and invalid self-reports.

The instrument was revised and two items were added to make 39 items: sleeping and sexual functioning. The scoring was simplified (a four-point scale from 0 to 3 was used). Following testing with over 200 people, further revisions were undertaken and the number of items was increased to 51. Questions were included on tiredness/energy, concentration, irritability, temper, tendency to argue, resentment, negative self-concept, satisfaction with relationships, trust in others, sexual interest, finances and satisfaction with health care – the latter question was later removed along with an earlier question on incontinence. This led to the current 49-item version, which was tested with almost 600 people aged 65 and over in Italy, The Netherlands and Finland.

Content

The current version of the questionnaire comprises 49 self-assessment items, 31 of which form seven core subscales: physical function (five items), self-care (six items), depression and anxiety (four items), cognitive functioning (five items), social functioning (three items), sexual functioning (two items) and life satisfaction (six items). The remaining 18 items act as the moderators for assessing the influence of social desirability bias and personality on respondents' scores: self-perceived personality disorders (five questions from Hyler and Rieder's (1987) Personality Diagnostic Questionnaire – Revised); anger, resentment, irritability (four items); social desirability (three items from the Crowne and Marlowe (1964) questionnaire); religious faith (two items); self-esteem (three items). Administration of the total scale takes about 15–20 minutes. Some examples are given below in Box 8.4.

Box 8.4 Examples from the LEIPAD

Social Functioning Scale
How satisfied are you with your social ties or relationships?
Do you feel emotionally satisfied in your relationships with other people?
Is there someone to talk with about personal affairs when you want to?

Self-esteem Scale
Taking everything into consideration, do you feel inferior to other people?
How often do you avoid things (refrain from doing things) because you feel inferior?
'I tend to have a negative opinion of myself.'

Reprinted with permission from the author and Taylor & Francis LLC (http://wwwt&fonline.com).
Source: de Leo, D., Diekstra, R.F.W., Lonnqvist, L. *et al.* (1998) LEIPAD, an internationally applicable instrument to assess quality of life in the elderly. *Behavioral Medicine*, 24: 17–27. Developer: Professor Diego De Leo, Australian Institute for Suicide Research and Prevention, Mt Gravatt Campus, Griffith University, 176 Messines Ridge Road, Mt Gravatt QLD 4122, Australia; d.deLeo@griffith.edu.au.

Availability: free to use without permission with acknowledgement of the source above.

Scoring

Each subjective item is scored from 0 to 3, with 0 = the best condition and 3 = the worst.

The item scores are summed to form the subscale scores; and the subscale scores are: physical function (score: 0–15), self-care (0–18), depression and anxiety (0–12), cognitive functioning (0–15), social functioning (0–9), sexual functioning (0–6) and life satisfaction (0–18). Again, 0 = best and the highest = worst.

The responses to the moderator scale items are dichotomous (yes/no) and scored as 0 or 1 (0 = no problem and highest = worst). The item scores are summed to form the subscale scores; the subscale scores are: self-perceived personality disorders (0–6), anger, resentment, irritability (0–4), social desirability (0–3), religious faith (0–2) and self-esteem (0–3). A global index of the scales can be computed with 0 = best and 93 = worst.

Validity

The field testing was with almost 600 people aged 65 and over in Italy, The Netherlands and Finland (de Leo *et al.* 1998a). The scale was tested against the Rotterdam Questionnaire which is widely used in Europe, and measures psychological stress, physical stress and daily activity. Significant, and high, correlations were obtained on the LEIPAD subscales and similar subscales on the Rotterdam Questionnaire, in support of the validity of the LEIPAD.

Rouhani and Zoleikani (2013) used the LEIPAD (49 items) in a study of people aged over 60 in Iran. In support of its validity, they reported that several expected variables were correlated with the LEIPAD, including age, marital status, income and literacy. A French version was tested by Jalenques *et al.* (2013) with a general population sample of 195 elderly people, and it was reported that concurrent validity was supported by expected correlations with the RAND Medical Outcomes Study SF-36.

The factor structure was tested by the developers on their entire sample aged 65 and over, and then in the subsamples from each of the three countries (de Leo *et al.* 1998a). This showed that the stability of a three-factor solution was insufficient. A two-factor structure of the scale was supported, and accounted for more than half of the total variance: psychosocial functioning (life satisfaction, depression and anxiety, and cognitive functioning) and physical functioning (self-care and physical function). However, exploratory factor analysis by Jalenques *et al.* (2013) using the French version, extracted eight factors providing a multidimensionality structure with five misclassifications of items in the seven theoretical scales.

Reliability

The results of the field testing showed that the scale had fairly high internal consistency for the subscales (de Leo *et al.* 1998a). The subjective subscale internal consistency coefficients were: physical function (Cronbach's alpha: 0.74), self-care (Cronbach's alpha: 0.74), depression and anxiety (Cronbach's alpha: 0.78), cognitive functioning (Cronbach's alpha: 0.70), social functioning (Cronbach's alpha: 0.78), sexual functioning (two items: Pearson's r = 0.43) and life satisfaction (Cronbach's alpha: 0.61, the lower internal consistency reflects the diverse life domains asked about).

The moderator subscale coefficients were: self-perceived personality disorders (Cronbach's alpha: 0.63), anger, resentment, irritability (Cronbach's alpha: 0.62), social desirability (Cronbach's alpha: 0.60), religious faith (two items; correlation: 0.62) and self-esteem (Cronbach's alpha: 0.63). These coefficients were lower than for the subjective subscales, but the developers considered them to be adequate. The study of the French version by Jalenques *et al.* (2013) reported good acceptability, with response rates superior to 93 per cent, good internal consistency (Cronbach's alphas 0.73 to 0.86) and strong test-retest reliability (ICCs higher than 0.80 for six scales and 0.70 for one).

The attraction of the instrument is that it is simple to understand. It is also intended to be multidimensional and relevant for older people. A QoL questionnaire for older people, which is not disease focused, is a positive development.

CASP-19 (CONTROL, AUTONOMY, SELF-REALIZATION AND PLEASURE)

The CASP-19 was designed by Higgs and his colleagues (Higgs *et al.* 2003; Hyde *et al.* 2003) to measure QoL in early old age. The name of the instrument reflects its content: **C**ontrol, **A**utonomy, **S**elf-realization and **P**leasure. The authors used the following definitions of their concepts: control as the ability to actively intervene in one's environment; autonomy as the right of an individual to be free from the unwanted interference of others; self-realization and pleasure as capturing the active and reflexive process of being human.

They developed their measure theoretically, based on Maslow's human needs satisfaction model. Maslow (1954) proposed a hierarchy of shared human needs necessary for maintenance and existence (physiological, safety and security, social and belonging, ego, status and self-esteem, and self-actualization). Maslow (1962) argued that once their basic needs are satisfied, human beings pursue higher needs such as self-actualization and esteem. Hence Hörnquist (1982) argued that as human needs are the foundations for QoL, QoL can be defined in terms of human needs and the satisfactory fulfilment of those needs. Some investigators of QoL in mental health have also incorporated a needs-based satisfaction model (Bowling 1995).

There were three phases of scale development. The first involved consultation with a panel of experts in gerontology and methodology to assess the face validity of the theoretically relevant items which had been selected by the authors for inclusion. These items were then piloted with focus groups of older people as a check on content validity, structure and duration of completion (Hyde *et al.* 2003). Finally, the 22-item scale was completed by post by almost 300 people aged 65–75 (Hyde *et al.* 2003). After analysis, the scale was reduced to 19 items, concentrating on four theoretically derived domains (19 items): control (four items), autonomy (five items), pleasure (five items), self-realization (five items), with four-point Likert response scales 'Often' to 'Never'. Thus it was developed for use with an older population sample, but has also been used successfully in several population surveys, including the English Longitudinal Survey of Ageing (ELSA) (Blane *et al.* 2008). The measure has been used in over 20 countries, including large-scale surveys and two randomized controlled trials (RCTs) (see Hyde *et al.* 2015). A number of other foreign language versions are being tested (personal communication from author).

Content

The CASP-19 was developed as a four-dimensional measure, and is self-administered. As noted above, it concentrates on four domains: control (four items), autonomy (five items), pleasure (five items) and self-realization (five items), with four-point Likert response scales for each item: 0 (never), 1 (not very often), 2 (sometimes) 3 (often).

Some of the items are shown in Box 8.5.

Box 8.5 CASP-19

Control
My age prevents me from doing the things I would like to.
I feel that what happens to me is out of my control.
I feel left out of things.
I feel I can do the things that I want to.

Autonomy
Family responsibilities prevent me from doing what I want to.
I feel that I can please myself what I can do.
My health stops me from doing the things I want to do.
Shortage of money stops me from doing the things that I want to.

Reprinted with permission of the developer. The CASP is in the public domain and is free to use. The developer can be contacted: Dr Martin Hyde, Department of Sociology, Room 3.047, Arthur Lewis Building, University of Manchester, M13 9PL; Twitter: @HydeM1976.

Scoring

Each scale item carries a score of 0–3. Both negatively and positively worded items are included; negatively worded items are reverse coded so that all item responses are in the same direction for summing. The 19 items are summed, to make a score range of 0–57. The range of the scale is defined at the extremes as 0 = 'complete absence of QoL' and 57 (defined in different descriptive terms) = 'total satisfaction of all four domains'. Scores for the 19 items were well distributed along the range of scores, although there was a slight negative skew.

Validity

Validity and reliability were assessed using the postal survey data (Hyde *et al.* 2003). Concurrent validity was partly tested with correlations of the scale with the eight-item Index of Life Satisfaction, which tapped some of the same topics, and a strong, positive association between the two scales was found (r = 0.67).

Several surveys have supported the construct validity of the CASP-19, including reported associations between the CASP-19 and health and functioning (see Hyde *et al.* 2015). The CASP-19 was tested by Bowling (2009b) and Bowling and Stenner (2011) along with the OPQOL and WHOQOL-OLD in national population surveys of people aged 65+ living at home in Britain, including an ethnically diverse sample. The OPQOL, CASP-19, and WHOQOL-OLD total scores all correlated moderately to highly with each other (rho: 0.380–0.732; all p <.01) (Bowling 2009b), in support of their construct validity. The construct validity of the three QoL measures was also tested by correlating them with independent self-rated QoL and self-ratings on several of its domains. Before the three QoL scales were administered, respondents were asked to rate their QoL overall, and in relation to their health, social relationships, independence, control and freedom, home and neighbourhood, psychological/emotional well-being, financial circumstances and leisure, and social activities. The CASP-19 correlated with the overall QoL ratings between –0.273 and –0.577 (both p <0.01) in the samples (minus sign reflects direction of coding), with those with better CASP scores reporting higher global QoL, supporting its construct validity. The CASP-19 also correlated with most of the QoL domain self-ratings in the British population sample, although with fewer of the domain self-ratings in the ethnically diverse sample (Bowling 2009b).

Kim *et al.*'s (2015) study, of older people in Central and Eastern Europe, while reporting high ceiling effects, supported the construct validity of the CASP-19 and three versions of CASP-12. All correlations between CASP-19 and physical health, physical functioning and depression were statistically significant, in expected directions.

Exploratory factor analysis of the original 22-item instrument confirmed the pattern of item loadings across the four conceptual domains (Higgs *et al.* 2003). Hyde *et al.* (2003)

reported that separate factor analysis of the four summed scores for the four domains revealed strong loadings supporting a single underlying QoL factor. However, Kim *et al.*'s (2015) analyses of survey population data in Central and Eastern Europe reported that a two-factor structure for the CASP-19 provided a substantially better fit to the data than the four-factor model (and see later, CASP-12).

Reliability

The postal survey indicated that the scale had moderate to high internal consistency. Once two of the original items had been removed from the control subscale ('Other people take my opinions seriously' and 'I feel that I am a respected person') the homogeneity of the scale improved from Cronbach's alpha 0.29 to 0.59. Similarly, once one item ('At times I think I am no good at all') had been removed from the self-realization subscale the homogeneity improved from 0.59 to 0.77. The coefficients of the remaining two subscales were unchanged by the removal of items (coefficients not given, but the range of the Cronbach's alphas for all four subscales was given as between 0.6 and 0.8). Thus the scale was reduced from 22 to 19 items across the four subscales. The inter-correlations between the subscales ranged from 0.35 to 0.67.

In the studies by Bowling (2009b), comparing the OPQOL, WHOQOL-OLD and CASP-19, the subscales to total correlation ranges, across samples, for the CASP-19 were: rho 0.549 to 0.834. All subscale to total score Spearman's rho correlations, within each sample, were highly significant at p <0.01 (Bowling and Stenner 2011).

All but one of the CASP items met the criteria for acceptability with item-total correlations (the correlation of the item with the scale total with that item omitted; the item should correlate with the total scale by at least 0.20) in the British population survey, although five of the 19 CASP items failed to meet this in the ethnically diverse sample. The CASP-19 also satisfied the 0.70<0.90 threshold for internal consistency reliability with Cronbach's alpha in the British population sample aged 65+ sample (alpha 0.866), but not in the ethnically diverse sample (alpha 0.553).

Kim *et al.*'s (2015) analyses also supported the reliability of the CASP-19 and three versions of CASP-12, in their population samples of older people in Central and Eastern Europe. They reported the Cronbach's alphas for the CASP-19 subscales met the 0.70 criteria for acceptability in each country (ranging from 0.83 to 0.86). Each subscale, except autonomy (which had low Cronbach's alpha reliability coefficients), had acceptable to high reliability. When they combined the control and autonomy domains to form a 12-item scale, the alpha coefficients increased to between 0.56 to 0.68 in each country (Czech Republic, Russia, Poland) for version 1 of the CASP-12, and to between 0.58 and 0.69 for version 2 of the CASP-12, and to between 0.76 and 0.80 for version 3 of the CASP-12.

The attraction of the CASP-19 is its strong conceptual base in a theory of human need. It is a useful instrument as it measures the domains of control, autonomy, self-realization and pleasure in older people, domains also suggested as important for 'successful ageing' (Baltes and Baltes 1990). Few other measures cover control and autonomy adequately in a practical instrument.

CASP-12

A short version of the CASP has been developed (Wiggins *et al.* 2008), containing 12 items in the four CASP domains – control (three items), autonomy (three items), pleasure (three items), and self-realization (93 items). The items are summed, with a high score representing good QoL. There have been three suggested revisions of the CASP-12 (Borsch-Supan *et al.* 2005; Wiggins *et al.* 2008; Sexton *et al.* 2013).

While the CASP was developed as a four-dimensional scale, Sexton *et al.* (2015) reported that, using the CASP-12 in the Irish Longitudinal Study of Ageing, these four dimensions formed either a single factor model, or two distinct dimensions: control/autonomy and self-realization/pleasure. They argued that the four dimensions were not sufficiently conceptually or empirically distinctive.

Hamrén *et al.* (2015) used the CASP-12 (version 2) in a survey of people aged 55+ in Ethiopia. They added a fifth response item ('Always'), in order to reduce the skewed distributions, as recommended by Sexton *et al.* (2013). They reported that confirmatory factor analysis of the CASP-12 provided reasonable support for an 11-item four-factor model when the item on 'shortage of money' was removed which was responsible for the model obtaining an initially poor fit. They then summed the remaining 11 CASP items to form a CASP-11 for further analysis.

LINEAR ANALOGUE SELF-ASSESSMENT (LASA)

LASAs, or Visual Analogue Scales (VAS) as they are also called, have been adapted and used in several different ways to assess people's QoL, including that of cancer patients. For example, an early application of LASA was by Priestman and Baum (1976) in their study of the subjective effects of endocrine therapy in 13 women with advanced breast cancer.

Singh *et al.* (2014) summarized single-item numerical linear analogue self-assessment scales in relation to their advantages (e.g. brevity, reduced patient burden, patient-based quantification, in effect, rather than using predetermined metric formula) and disadvantages (dependent on patients' capabilities for completion, lack of detail, debate surrounding reliability of single items).

Content

LASA scales employ lines, the length of which are taken to denote the continuum of some emotional or physical experience, or to represent a global state, such as overall QoL. The lines are usually 10 cm long with stops at right angles to the line extremes (see description by Cella 1995). The use of 10 cm lines permits measurement of a wider spread than shorter lines (e.g. 5 cm), as some people tend to place their mark in the middle ranges. Anchoring descriptors are placed at each end of the line (representing the extremes of the experience) and respondents mark their current state on that experience somewhere on that line. The score is the measured number of millimeters from the zero end of the scale to the patient's indication of where they fall. Some investigators ask respondents to circle a number along the LASA (not all show the horizontal line as well as numbers). These are also known as numerical LASA scales or VAS. It is a technique that has been easily administered to 5-year-old children (Scott *et al.* 1977), although some people may find them difficult (Huskisson 1974). Examples of items from LASA scales are shown in Box 8.6.

Box 8.6 Examples of LASA items used to measure QoL

a) Based on two of Locke *et al.*'s (2007) five single-item LASAs
Respondents are asked to circle the number (0–10) best reflecting their response to LASA items to describe their feelings during the past week, including today.

Item 2. Emotional well-being (including depression, anxiety, stress etc.)

Item 5. Overall well-being over the past week.

The horizontal LASA is anchored at each end by 0 (As good as can be) and 10 (As bad as can be), with the digits 0, 1, 2, 3, 4, 5, 6, 7, 8, 9, 10 displayed and equally spaced along the line.

The original LASAs are reprinted in full in: Locke, D.E.C., Decker, P.A., Sloan, J.A. *et al.* (2007) Validation of single-item linear analog scale assessment of quality of life in neuro-oncology Patients. *Journal of Pain and Symptom Management*, 34: 628–38, Appendix A.

With permission of the first author: Dr D.E.C. Locke.

b) Spitzer QoL Index Uniscale
The respondent is asked to place an X on the line to rate quality of life:

_____

lowest quality of life   highest quality of life

With permission of co-author: Dr Renaldo Battista (and see Spitzer QL Index, next).

See information on performance in: Spitzer, W.O., Dobson, A.J., Hall, J. *et al.* (1981) Measuring the quality of life of cancer patients. *Journal of Chronic Disease*, 34, 585–97.

Scoring

The respondent is generally instructed to mark a point (e.g. with a cross) along the LASA line that corresponds to their response. The distance from the lowest point anchor mark (usually coded as 0) to their mark provides a numeric score for the item. The items are summed. Or, if numbers are displayed on the LASA, respondents are asked to circle a number (e.g. as with Locke *et al.*'s 2007 LASA in Box 8.6). LASAs in which the numbers are displayed along the line are also known as a 0 to 10 numerical VAS.

Validity

LASAs have been been shown to be able to detect treatment response in cancer patients (Coates *et al.* 1987; Butow *et al.* 1991; Demetri *et al.* 2002). In a drug trial in palliative care, a LASA showed parallel changes to a longer, psychometrically sound cancer-specific QoL (the EORTC QLC-C30) (Hedley *et al.* 2002). Slevin *et al.* (1988) in their testing of the scale, however, reported that the LASA scale correlated poorly with the Hospital Anxiety and Depression (HAD) scale. Slevin *et al.* suggested that this was due to the HAD items being less applicable to cancer patients. Gough *et al.* (1983) assessed 100 patients with advanced cancer in Australia, using a single LASA item 'How would you rate your general feeling of well-being today?', a 21-item LASA, and a self- and interviewer-administered five-item QL Index (Spitzer's) (which covered activity, daily living, health, support and outlook). Each patient was evaluated four times at four-weekly intervals for 12 weeks. The correlation coefficients for the four methods ranged from 0.38 to 0.86. The single-item LASA question correlated moderately to well with all three questionnaires (0.38 to 0.67). The LASA-21 correlated from 0.46 to −0.65 with the other items. However, shorter scales are inevitably less stable (Bernhard *et al.* 2001).

Locke *et al.* (2007) investigated the psychometric properties of single-item LASAs with 205 patients with newly diagnosed high-grade gliomas, who had enrolled in the three clinical trials. They found that LASA items correlated strongly with similar scales on other, well-validated, multi-item scales that are frequently used in cancer patients, thereby supporting the concurrent validity and construct validity of the LASA. Singh *et al.* (2014) analysed baseline data from over 900 people participating in 36 clinical trials and six observational studies with various populations, including healthy volunteers, cancer trial patients (patients with advanced incurable cancer or patients receiving treatment with curative intent), hospice patients and their caregivers. The overall QoL LASA used was rated 0 (as bad as it can be) to 10 (as good as it can be). They reported that overall QoL was weakly but highly significantly correlated with performance status; it was significantly associated with tumor response. They concluded that their study indicated that the single-item measure of overall QoL had acceptable content and construct validity as an indicator of well-being.

There are many references in the early literature relating to the validity of the VAS techniques in general (Melzack 1983). The wide range of such measures available for assessing QoL in relation to cancer was reviewed by Hauser and Walsh (2008). They concluded that their use as single-item measures of QoL in cancer patients is reliable, and responsive to change, and that these scales may best represent an individual's global QoL without the constraints of predetermined domains. Their main criticisms were that they are more difficult to complete than are other rating scales and have the potential for measurement error.

Reliability

Slevin *et al.* (1988) tested LASA scales against the HAD scale, the Karnofsky Index and the Spitzer Quality of Life Index, with 108 cancer patients in London, and reported that the LASAs showed similar concordance coefficients when taken as a whole, compared with being divided into four equal parts, i.e. the continuous scale is no more sensitive than the four-point scale. Two different groups of 25 patients also filled in the same forms on a single day, and daily for five consecutive days, during a period when their clinical state was expected to remain stable. Professionals completed the scales in relation to the same patients. The LASA was found to be easily reproducible, and had greater reproducibility than the other scales.

Although the scale is simple and has been reported to be reproducible and able to discriminate between groups, patients may sometimes need time to accustom themselves to representing their feelings along a continuum.

Investigators have used a range of different LASAs (Pandey *et al.* 2000) in both clinical and non-clinical studies. Locke *et al.* (2007), in their study of over 200 patients with newly diagnosed high-grade gliomas, investigated the psychometric properties of single-item linear analogue scale assessments (LASAs) for QoL. They included Priestman and Baum (1976) LASAs on physical ability and mood, along with others: QoL overall, physical, emotional, spiritual, intellectual. They reported that the LASA QoL scales were strongly, and highly significantly, associated in expected directions with established scales measuring mood, mental status, symptom distress and functioning. The data suggest that single-item LASA scales are valid for assessing QoL of cancer patients and are an appropriate alternative if shorter instruments are needed.

In another adaptation, Bernhard *et al.* (2001) investigated compared QoL LASAs for physical well-being, mood and coping in their study of 84 patients in Sweden with early breast cancer, with follow-up after chemotherapy at three or six months. They compared single-item QoL LASAs with the Sickness Impact Profile, the HAD, and measures of mood. Discriminant validity was investigated by multitrait-multimethod correlation, responsiveness by standardized response mean. They reported that discriminant validity of each of these indicators, including the QoL LASAs, was supported at baseline, but for each measure it was weaker after treatment. The QoL LASA indicators were confirmed to be responsive to cytotoxic side-effects, mental distress and psychosocial dysfunction in patients with early breast cancer.

Overall, LASAs have been reported to provide reliable and valid measurements, although single-item LASAs are inevitably less reliable than the use of a full scale (Bowling 2005c).

SPITZER'S QUALITY OF LIFE INDEX (QL INDEX)

Another scale which involves using a VAS, in addition to simple category scales, is Spitzer's QL Index (Spitzer *et al.* 1981). It covers comparable dimensions to most broader health-status scales: activity, performance of ADL, perception of health, support from family and friends and outlook on life. A uniscale for rating overall QoL during the previous week is also included, and this is often used separately. Although the developers specified that it was to be used to rate the QoL of cancer patients, the index and uniscale are presented here because they have been widely used in other clinical and non-clinical contexts. In particular, the uniscale has frequently been used or adapted to rate QoL.

Spitzer *et al.* (1981) identified components of health-related QoL empirically by questioning lay people as well as health professionals. They formed three advisory panels each with 43 members from Sydney, Australia. These consisted of cancer patients and their relatives, patients with chronic diseases and their relatives, healthy people aged between 20 and 59, and 60+, physicians, nurses, social workers and other health professionals and members of the clergy. One panel received an open-ended questionnaire designed to elicit spontaneous beliefs about factors that could enhance or decrease the QoL. The second panel received a more structured questionnaire seeking views on various aspects of defined QoL. The third panel assessed the results from the first two and the relative importance of the main factors. The factors that were rated as the most important formed the first drafts of the QL Index which were tested on 339 people from outpatients clinics. This resulted in the following dimensions of QoL being incorporated within the definitive QL Index: activity; performance of ADL; perception of health; support from family and friends; and outlook on life.

Its authors caution that it is not suitable for measuring or classifying the QoL of ostensibly healthy people (Spitzer *et al.* 1981), although the uniscale is often used with this group. The index is short and easily administered. The average completion time is one minute. There are numerous applications of this scale in clinical settings.

Content

The QL Index consists of five items. Each item represents a different domain of life functioning: activity, performance of ADL, perception of health, support from family and friends and outlook on life. Respondents are requested to tick the statements which apply to them. Respondents only have the option of one tick per statement to indicate that it applies to them. There are problems with interpretation if respondents can do some tasks but not others. A version exists for clinicians to complete on behalf of patients. Completion takes about a minute.

The scale also comprises a visual analogue rating uniscale in which the respondent places a cross on a horizontal line to indicate their QoL during the past week (anchored at each end from lowest quality to highest quality). This is repeated by the clinician to provide a proxy rating of the respondent's QoL. Standardized descriptions of the anchor terms are provided. Examples of the items are presented in Box 8.7.

Box 8.7 Examples from Spitzer QL index and uniscale

Activity
I do not work in any capacity nor do I study nor do I manage my own household.

Daily living
I am able to eat, wash, go to the toilet and dress without assistance. I drive a car or use public transport without assistance.

Health
I lack energy or only feel 'up to par' some of the time.

Support
I have good relationships with others and receive strong support from at least one family member and/or friend.

Outlook on life
I generally look forward to things and am able to make my own decisions about my life and surroundings.

These statements are also adapted for the clinician to make proxy ratings of the patient's status.

Spitzer QoL Uniscale: *the respondent is asked to place an X on the line to rate quality of life:*

_____

lowest quality of life   highest quality of life

With permission of co-author, Dr Renaldo Battista. See: Spitzer, W.O., Dobson, A.J., Hall, J. *et al.* (1981) Measuring the quality of life of cancer patients. *Journal of Chronic Disease*, 34: 585–97.

Scoring

The scoring of the Spitzer QL Index is simple. The scale consists of five items, with three options for replies. The item responses comprise scores 0–2, giving an overall score of 0 to 10. The scale can be summed into a single score or each item can be presented separately.

Validity

Spitzer *et al.* (1981) asked 68 lay people and professionals (e.g. physicians) to assess the scope and format of the instrument; most judged it to be satisfactory and the authors judged the scale to have content validity. They also tested the scale for validity by inviting 150 physicians to rate 879 patients. Less than two-thirds of the physicians (59 per cent) reported that they were 'very confident' of the accuracy of their scores. However, the analysis of physicians' scores showed that the close clustering of high scores among healthy subjects, the spread of scores among those who were definitely ill, and the low scores of those who were seriously ill, made clinical sense and provided evidence of its discriminative ability. Convergent validity was judged to be adequate by Spitzer *et al.* (1981) by comparing physicians' and patients' ratings. When the physicians' ratings were compared to patients' self-ratings, the correlation was moderately high (0.61). The authors reported that the scale was able to discriminate between healthy people and patients with varying conditions. The authors did not intend it to be appropriate for measuring global QoL in healthy populations, and they reported that it does not discriminate adequately among well people (Spitzer *et al.* 1981).

Gough *et al.* (1983) reported that the uniscale correlated over r = 0.60 with the Karnofsky Performance Index. The scale and the uniscale are also correlated moderately to highly on other global-functioning and disease-specific QoL (Spitzer *et al.* 1981; Mor *et al.* 1984; Morris *et al.* 1986; Mor 1987; Sloan *et al.* 1998). Mor (1987), on the basis of three samples of newly diagnosed cancer patients (total: 2,046), reported a correlation between the QL Index and the Karnofsky Performance Index of 0.63; the correlation was moderate probably because of the multidimensional nature of the QL Index. The item correlations of the scale with the Karnofsky scale ranged from 0.13 to 0.57. The correlation coefficients were not high enough in these studies to be confident that these scales cover the same dimensions. The QoL Index has also been reported to be able to predict mortality among cancer patients (Mor *et al.* 1984, Morris *et al.* 1986), although Mor (1987) concluded that it was not sufficiently sensitive for use as an outcome indicator of care. It has been used in an Australian study of outcome of breast cancer patients and was shown to be capable of discriminating between patients on intermittent therapy and those receiving continuous therapy (Coates *et al.* 1987). However, Levine *et al.* (1988) reported that it did not sufficiently discriminate between patients with breast cancer who had completed or had not yet completed their treatment.

Morris and Sherwood (1987) in the USA administered the QL Index to different samples of cancer patients at different stages of the disease. Over 2,000 patients were included in the study. A strong correlation was reported between the Karnofsky performance-status rating and the QL Index, in support of construct validity and discriminative ability. The QL Index was also able to successfully distinguish between cancer patients who were newly diagnosed, those under active treatment, and those nearing the terminal stages of the disease. However, the authors did not feel it was sufficiently sensitive for use as an outcome variable in studies evaluating the effect of a treatment or intervention on patients' lives. This was mainly because of the insensitivity of the social functioning index of the scale. Wood-Dauphinee and Williams (1991) reviewed the literature on the QoL Index and the uniscale and cited several studies that supported its convergent validity and discriminative ability on the basis of correlations with other scales, and its ability to discriminate between healthy and sick people, and sensitivity to the stages of the disease progress. Lim and Morad (1998) reported that significant gradients in the Spitzer QL Index scores were observed by age, serum albumin, comorbid disorders, previous hospitalization, capacity for self-care and rehabilitation status, supporting its construct validity. Bonnetain *et al.* (2006), in a study of 259 patients included in a randomized multicenter phase III trial for oesophageal cancer, reported that the QL Index did not discriminate between surviving patients at two years, who had initially received different treatments (surgical or non-surgical).

Reliability

Spitzer *et al.* (1981), on the basis of 150 physicians' ratings of 879 patients, reported that assessment of internal consistency demonstrated a high coefficient (0.77), and the correlation for inter-rater reliability was high (0.81). The scale has been shown to have reasonable inter-item reliability (Mor *et al.* 1984; Morris *et al.* 1986; Mor 1987). The stability of the scale is more questionable. Slevin *et al.* (1988) administered the index along with the Linear Analogue Self-Assessment (LASA) quality-of-life VAS, the Karnofsky Performance Index and the HAD. The scales were completed by 108 patients and their doctors at the same time. Two different groups of 25 patients filled in the same questionnaires on a single day, and daily for five consecutive days. Reproducibility was not as good as the Karnofsky Performance Index. The Karnofsky, which correlated with the Spitzer Index (patients' rating of quality of life: 0.49), demonstrated greater reproducibility than any of the other scales. The variability in their results from repeated testing questions the reliability of the Spitzer QL Index. Large discrepancies between patients' and doctors' ratings of the patients' QoL have been reported by Slevin *et al.* (1988), questioning the validity of proxy ratings. Sloan *et al.* (1998) reported, on the basis of patients with advanced cancer participating in a clinical trial of treatment, that doctors' ratings on the uniscale were lower than the patients' own ratings. This indicates that patients with advanced cancer rate their lives more highly than the doctors who rated them. Moinpour *et al.* (2000) also reported poor agreement between patients' and families' ratings of the patients' QoL using the QL Index. They concluded that proxies are a poor substitute for capturing patients' perspective on their QoL. This view has been supported in studies of proxy ratings using other scales. For example, in a study of patients' and friends'/relatives' (proxies) ratings of the patient using the EuroQol, Dorman *et al.* (1997b) reported that while moderate agreement between ratings was found for directly observable domains, agreement was less good for the more subjective domains. Lim and Morad (1998) reported Spitzer's QL Index had acceptable measurement properties in their study of 59 dialysis patients. Inter-rater agreement for the total score was good with a mean intra-class correlation coefficient 0.66 (range 0.47–0.81), although agreement for dimension scores was less good. Intra-rater agreement was generally better than inter-rater agreement.

Slevin *et al.* (1988) argued that the QoL Index contained inappropriate questions for measuring the QoL of cancer patients, and that the continued popularity of the Spitzer scale, despite poor reliability and validity of the scales, stems from researchers' tendency to rely on significance values when assessing their scales, rather than on the size of the correlation value. The QL's reliance on just five items means that it does not adequately account for the different dimensions of health-related QoL. It has been criticized for excluding spiritual and financial domains (McMillan 1996). The scale's reproducibility requires further investigation and a major disadvantage is the confusion of several dimensions within one item. However, the scale has been popular despite limitations (Addington-Hall *et al.* 1990).

INDIVIDUALIZED MEASURES OF QUALITY OF LIFE

The conceptual and methodological difficulties inherent in QoL research, and the reliance on psychometric testing for scale development at the expense of the relevance of scale items to the individual (Hunt 1999), supports the case for capturing individuals' own values and experiences. More qualitative or semi-structured methods to explore QoL have long existed (e.g. the use of diaries; in-depth interviews with critical incident and life history approaches; repertory grid techniques). Given the need for meaningful quantitative measures in research on health outcomes, some investigators have also attempted to reconcile qualitative and quantitative approaches (Guyatt *et al.* 1987; O'Boyle *et al.* 1992; Browne 1999; Ruta *et al.* 1999). These individualized measures ask people themselves about the most important things in their lives, or about the most important effects of their condition on their lives, and ask them to prioritize or weight the areas mentioned (Joyce *et al.* 1999).

Individualized measures require the use of methods of scoring and weighting which are complex. The individualized weighting procedures also require interviewer administration for valid results and optimum response rates. While individualized measures are a welcome development on a complex topic, Fitzpatrick (1999) argued that the hypothesis that they provide more reliable and valid measures of QoL than standardized measures has yet to be confirmed. Tugwell *et al.* (1990) also argued that any superiority of more individualized approaches over standardized approaches can be explained by the fact that standardized instruments contain more 'noise' from items that are less relevant or irrelevant to patients.

SCHEDULE FOR THE EVALUATION OF INDIVIDUAL QUALITY OF LIFE (SEIQoL)

The SEIQol is a generic, individualized QoL scale (O'Boyle *et al.* 1993; Browne *et al.* 1997). It is based on the rationale that it works within the value system of the individual being assessed, rather than the value systems of others. It derived its cognitive aspects from theoretical studies of perception and their extension to social judgement theory (Joyce *et al.* 2003). While the SEIQoL is a generic measure of QoL, and is not a health-related or disease-specific measure, it has been used with many groups of patients in studies of clinical outcome, as well as with older people and carers (e.g. McGee *et al.* 1991; O'Boyle *et al.* 1992; Coen *et al.* 1993, 1999; Browne *et al.* 1994; Hickey *et al.* 1996, 1997; O'Boyle 1996, 1997a, 1997b; Waldron *et al.* 1999; Scholzel-Dorenbos 2000; Tovbin *et al.* 2003; Wettergren *et al.* 2003). It also influenced the development of the Audit of Diabetes Dependent Quality of Life (ADDQoL) which measures individual's perceptions of the impact of their diabetes on their QoL (Bradley *et al.* 1999). The SEIQoL was reported to be acceptable to people, although administration by an interviewer is required which, due to expense, often limits studies to relatively small numbers.

Content and scoring

The SEIQoL enables individuals to nominate the areas of life they consider to be the most important to their QoL, based on their own values. Respondents are asked to nominate five areas of QoL that are important to them, then they are asked to rate their current status in each area, as well as their global QoL, against vertical VAS, which are then tabulated into bar charts by the interviewer using a laptop computer (see Box 8.8).

In the direct weighting (SEIQoL-DW) method, the respondents weight the relative importance of each area using a hand-held disc which can be scored and which provides the relative weights for each area. This is known as the direct weighting procedure (O'Boyle *et al.* 1993). The disc consists of five stacked, centrally mounted, interlocking laminated discs. Each disc is a different colour and is labelled by the interviewer with one of the five areas of life selected by the respondent. The coloured discs can be rotated over each other to produce a dynamic pie chart where the relative size of each coloured 'area of life' represents the weight the respondent attaches to that area. There is a

100-point scale on the circumference of the disc, and the proportion that each coloured area represents can be scored from this to produce the individual weighting of the importance the individual attaches to each area of life.

Box 8.8 Examples from the SEIQoL-DW

What are the *five most important areas* of your life at present – the things which make your life a relatively happy or sad one at the moment . . . The things that you feel determine the quality of your life?

Now that you have named the five most important areas in your life, I am going to ask you to *rate* how each of these are for you at the moment. First I will show you an example of how the rating is done . . .

I would like you to show me how important the five areas of life you have mentioned are *in relation to each other*, by using this disc (indicate SEIQoL-DW). People often value some areas of life as more important than others. This disc allows you to show me how important each area in your life is by giving the more important areas a larger area of the disc and the less important areas a smaller area of the disc.

© Department of Psychology, Royal College of Surgeons in Ireland, 1993. Reproduced with permission of the developer. The administration manual (O'Boyle *et al.* 1993) is free and downloadable at e-publications@RCSI: http://epubs.rcsi.ie/psycholrep/39, accessed 13 October 2015. Contact: Carole Carolan, Department of Psychology, Royal College of Surgeons in Ireland, St Stephen's Green, Dublin 2, Ireland; email ccarolan@rcsi.ie.

Weighting

QoL weights for the importance of domains may be derived alternatively, using human judgement analysis techniques (based on vignettes of conditions) during the interview, although the shorter direct weighting procedure described above is generally preferred in order to reduce researcher and respondent burden. It is interviewer administered, and takes up to 30 minutes to explain and administer (O'Boyle *et al.* 1993; Browne *et al.* 1997).

Validity

Validity has been partly assessed. O'Boyle *et al.* (1992) indicated that the SEIQoL was sensitive to individuals' QoL. Participants in a study of 56 healthy people aged 65 and over were able to understand and complete the SEIQoL correctly. However, health status was not correlated with the perceived importance of health on the SEIQoL at baseline, and the correlation was low at 12-month follow-up interview. The weight placed on the importance of health did not increase over the 12-month study period, despite a significant decline in health status (Browne *et al.* 1994). In research on hip replacement, health was unexpectedly nominated more frequently by controls than patients (O'Boyle *et al.* 1992). Among a healthy population, relationships, health, family and finances were the most frequently nominated (by over 50 per cent), and among gastro-intestinal clinic attenders, family, work, social and leisure activities, and health, were the most frequently nominated domains (McGee *et al.* 1991). These differences in values appear to justify the use of an individualized scale.

The scale was applied by O'Boyle *et al.* (1992) in a prospective intervention study of 20 patients undergoing unilateral total hip replacement surgery, with a six-month follow-up. Comparisons were made with matched, non-patient controls. The scale showed improvements in scores after surgery. However, the SEIQoL can present difficulties when measuring change. QoL is a dynamic concept and patients may rate different areas as important at different stages in their condition. Therefore, in order to assess change in prospective studies, the recommended practice in the user's manual is that new cues are elicited at each assessment. Cues nominated at baseline should then be given to the respondent and the SEIQoL procedure repeated. This is necessary in order to enable direct comparison between assessments (O'Boyle *et al.* 1993).

Lintern *et al.* (2001) compared the results of the PGI, the SEIQol and the SF-36 in patients with multiple sclerosis. They reported that the SEIQoL scores related more closely to SF-36 dimensions of health and vitality and the PGI scores related closely to the SF-36 dimension of physical functioning. They suggested that these differences may reflect the conceptual bases of the instruments. Neudert *et al.* (2001) asked patients with amyotrophic lateral sclerosis to rate their perceptions of the validity of the SEIQoL, the Sickness Impact Profile and the SF-36, using VAS ratings. The validity of the SEIQoL was rated as higher than both the Sickness Impact Profile and the SF-36, indicating that patients felt that the SEIQoL was more likely to measure their QoL. A study by Smith *et al.* (2000), however, reported that the SEIQoL, the SF-36 and two disease-specific instruments all lacked sensitivity to changes in clinical condition over time in a study of cardiac patients.

Reliability

Test-retest of both the direct weighting procedure and the human judgement analysis weightings was carried out using 40 healthy volunteers at baseline, at 7–10 days and 14–20 days later. The weights produced by the two different methods differed, on average, by 7.2 to 7.8 points over time. The direct weights varied over time by 4.5 points and the human judgement analysis weights varied by 8.4 points (Browne *et al.* 1997). The authors of the scale pointed out that the results suggested stability among some respondents. The results indicated that most people were consistent but individuals varied. One problem with reliability testing in the case of the SEIQoL is that both weighting methods lead to a total of 100. On repeat testing, if the weight provided for a particular area of life changes, then so must the weight for one or more of the other domains.

The open-ended questions in the SEIQoL have inspired the design of other semi-structured questionnaires for exploring the QoL. For example, Bowling (1995) asked a national sample of adults to list the five most important areas of life, and to prioritize them. Because it was uncertain whether the important things in life to people equated with QoL, Bowling *et al.* (2003) subsequently asked a national sample of people aged 65

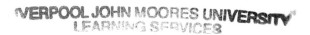

and over a series of open-ended questions directly on QoL, and confirmed that the domains closely overlapped. The questions they used were:

1 Thinking about your life as a whole, what is it that makes your life good – that is, the things that give your life quality? You may mention as many things as you like.
2 What is it that makes your life bad – that is the things that reduce the quality in your life? You may mention as many things as you like.
3 Thinking of all these good and bad things you have just mentioned, which one is the most important to you?
4 What single thing would improve the quality of your life?
5 What single thing would improve the overall quality of life for people of your age?

A strong case could be made for the use of the SEIQoL as the core component of disease-specific measures, although more work is required in view of its potential complexity. A manual and computerized version of the instrument is available (O'Boyle et al. 1993). It has been translated for use in other countries, including Sweden and Denmark (Scholzel-Dorenbos 2000; Ventegodt et al. 2003; Wettergren et al. 2003).

PATIENT GENERATED INDEX (PGI)

The other main individualized measure, the PGI, was developed by Ruta and his colleagues who aimed to 'develop an instrument that could be used to quantify the difference between an individual's hopes and expectations and reality in a way that has meaning and relevance in their daily lives' (Ruta 1992; Ruta et al. 1994b, 1999; Garratt and Ruta 1999). It rests on the recognition that assessment of QoL is subjective, and the measure is based on 'gap' or 'comparisons' theory (Calman 1984). Within this model, QoL is expressed as the extent to which hopes and ambitions are matched by experience, and the aim of an intervention is to narrow the gap between expectations and reality. It was based partly on Guyatt et al.'s (1987) disease-specific scale in which patients are asked about the five most important activities that are affected by their condition, and on the priority evaluation methods used by town planners to assess community preferences, in which people allocate points between a set of characteristics – from shopping facilities to garden size (Ruta et al. 1999).

Content and scoring

The PGI is completed in three steps. In step 1, respondents are asked to specify the five most important areas of their life ('affected by their condition' if disease or disease-specific versions are used). Step 2 asks them to rate how bad (badly affected) they are in each chosen area on a scale of 0–100 (0 represents the worst they can imagine for themselves and 100 represents exactly as they would like to be). A sixth box enables them to rate all other areas of life. In step 3, respondents are asked to imagine that they can improve some or all of their selected areas. They are then given 'points' (the number varies with the version – generic, health related or disease specific – of the scale used) to spend across one or more areas that they would most like to improve. The points, then, represent the relative importance of potential improvements in that area, and represent the individualized weighting. The PGI is less suitable for self- or postal administration because of its complexity; as many people self-complete it incorrectly (Macduff and Russell 1998), interviewer administration is required.

Box 8.9 Examples from the PGI (health)

Step 1: Identifying areas
We would like you to think of the most important areas of your life (that are affected by your HEALTH).* Please write up to FIVE areas in the boxes below.

(*Note: Health is referred to in the health-related quality of life version, but not in the generic version; in the disease-specific versions the specific condition is referred to.)

Step 2: Scoring each area
In this part we would like you to score the areas you mentioned in Step 1. This score should show how badly affected you were over the past MONTH. Please score each area out of 10 (10 = Exactly as you would like to be . . . 1 = The worst you could imagine).

Step 3: Spending points
We want you to imagine that any or all the areas of your life could be improved. You have 12 imaginary points to spend to show which areas you would like to see improve. Spend more points on areas you would like to see improve and less on areas that are not so important.

You don't have to spend points in every area. You can't spend more than 12 points in total.

Background source: Ruta, D.A., Garratt, A.M., Leng, M. *et al.* (1994) A new approach to the measurement of quality of life: the patient-generated index. *Medical Care*, 32: 1109–26.
The PGI can be used without permission. For information see https://eprovide.mapi-trust.org, accessed 22 October 2015.

To generate an index, the self-ratings for each area are multiplied by the proportion of points awarded to that area and summed to give a score between 0 and 100. The score aims to represent the extent to which reality matches expectations in the areas in which respondents most value improvement. This, then, represents the authors' construct of QoL (Ruta *et al.* 1999). Self-administered and interviewer-administered versions are available, as well as generic, health- and disease-specific versions.

Validity

The PGI was initially tested with 20 patients, and a checklist version of areas of life was generated for a postal questionnaire version. This was further tested in a postal survey of 20 more patients, who were subsequently interviewed, and the questionnaire later modified. A further postal survey of 74 people identified by GPs as suffering from low back pain resulted in 47 per cent being returned completed; 27 per cent were returned partly completed and 31 per cent were returned blank, indicating that the exercise is too complex or burdensome for self-completion (Ruta et al. 1999). The response rates for self-completion, as opposed to interviewer administration, of the PGI have been reported to be almost two-thirds that of Ware et al.'s (1993) SF-36 Health Survey. There is some evidence that non-responders to the postal versions of the PGI are less well educated, in lower socioeconomic groups (measured by housing tenure) and are more likely to be retired than responders (Ruta et al. 1999). There is evidence that respondents with perceived health problems who complete the PGI correctly are younger and spent longer in education than those with health problems who do not complete it correctly (Macduff and Russell 1998).

The index correlated well with the RAND SF-36 scales measuring pain, social functioning and role limitations attributable to physical problems, and with the clinical questionnaire used. The scores reflected GPs' assessments of severity. The PGI was also applied and tested by the developers with patients with low back pain, menorrhagia, suspected peptic ulcers and varicose veins (Ruta et al. 1999). In these main validation studies, the correlations between the PGI scores and the domains of Ware et al.'s (1993) SF-36 scores were weak to moderate, although still highly significant in most cases ($r = 0.06$ to 0.39). The PGI was reported to detect small to moderate changes in three of the four conditions studied over a 12-month period. It was more responsive to change than the SF-36. Ruta et al. (1999) thus claimed that the PGI is as sensitive to individuals' QoL as standardized measures. Further tests by the developers for construct validity showed small or non-significant results. It was unknown whether this reflected the weakness of their hypotheses, the smaller sample sizes, or the weakness of the PGI (Ruta et al. 1999).

Tully and Cantrill (2000) also tested the validity of the PGI with over 1,000 people aged 65 and over with arthritis, using a postal survey and follow-up interviews with a sub-sample. Their response rates were high at 78 per cent and 83 per cent respectively. They reported that the PGI met four and failed to meet six of their criteria for validity. While their hypotheses were confirmed for associations between the PGI and the Arthritis Impact Measurement Scales, severity of arthritis, and those who had sought medical care and those who had not, the PGI failed to detect changes in health status or distinguish between respondents taking analgesia or not. Follow-up interviews with a sub-sample of respondents also revealed that there were problems with respondents' interpretation of instructions.

In contrast, Haywood et al. (2003), in a postal survey application of the PGI to patients with ankylosing spondylitis, reported that the instrument had acceptable completion rates, data quality was adequate, the PGI correlated significantly with other QoL questionnaires, and it achieved moderate levels of responsiveness to changes in health. Camilleri-Brennan et al. (2002) administered the PGI, pre- and three months post-operatively, to 33 patients with rectal cancer. The PGI correlated significantly with several domains of other QoL questionnaires, it was responsive to improvement in condition after surgery, and was more responsive to change than the SF-36.

It was stated earlier (see SEIQoL) that Lintern et al. (2001), in their comparison of scales, found that the PGI scores related closely to the SF-36 dimension of physical functioning, whereas the SEIQoL scores related more closely to SF-36 dimensions of health and vitality. They suggested that these differences may reflect the conceptual bases of the instruments.

Witham *et al.* (2008) used the PGI in a longitudinal study of 75 day hospital patients aged 65+, with no cognitive impairment, in Scotland. To assess its construct validity, they hypothesized that QoL would worsen with self-reported function and worsening function (measured using the Barthel Index, Functional Limitations Profile and HADS). The PGI correlated moderately and highly significantly with the Functional Limitations Profile at each wave ($r = -0.44$ to -0.51, $p < 0.001$), but weakly with the Barthel score at each wave ($r = 0.09$ to 0.18, not statistically significant). The PGI correlation with the HADS anxiety score at baseline was weak and not significant ($r = 0.039$), but it correlated moderately and significantly with the HADS depression score ($r = 0.37$, $p = 0.002$). It did not correlate significantly with number of co-morbid conditions or medications. However, the correlations with the other measurement scales in expected directions supported the construct validity of the PGI. Tavernier *et al.* (2011) examined the PGI with 86 adults with cancer in the USA, receiving their first course of radiation therapy in hospital outpatients. Overall, the PGI was moderately and significantly associated with cancer distress and QoL measures, in the expected directions, supporting the construct validity of the PGI. Martin *et al.*'s (2007) structured review of the PGI concluded that it appeared valid.

Reliability

Test-retest results at two weeks (post return of a 12-month follow-up questionnaire) with patients with low back pain, menorrhagia, suspected peptic ulcers and varicose veins were reported to be adequate by the developers (Ruta *et al.* 1999). Haywood *et al.* (2003), in their postal survey of patients with ankylosing spondylitis, reported that the test-retest reliability coefficients of the PGI were high (0.80). Tully and Cantrill (2000), in their postal survey of over 1,000 patients aged over 65 years with arthritis, reported the test-retest reliability coefficient to be lower at 0.55, increasing to 0.67 when respondents who had misinterpreted the instructions were excluded (detected at the follow-up interviews). They concluded that the instrument elicited patient concerns about their condition that other, more structured, questionnaires may not identify.

Witham *et al.* (2008), in their longitudinal study of 75 day hospital patients aged 65+, without cognitive impairment, in Scotland, tested the PGI for reliability. It was administered by a trained nurse at baseline, at one week, and at final attendance. Completion rate was high at 99 per cent at baseline, and then 100 per cent of those who were still eligible/remaining in the day hospital at follow-ups. Mean completion times ranged between 4.2 to 5.0 minutes at each wave. They reported that the PGI had moderate reliability. Test-retest scores in patients who reported no change in their QoL at week one was $r = 0.72$ when new PGI domains could be selected, and lower at $r = 0.61$ when baseline domains were presented for reassessment. Thus re-presenting the domains of QoL selected at baseline for re-scoring did not improve reliability. Responsiveness coefficients suggested low responsiveness. Responsiveness to change as measured by effect size was also low for the PGI. In Tavernier *et al.*'s (2011) study with cancer patients receiving radiotherapy, the PGI was responsive to those reporting high or low distress. A small-to-moderate effect size was found in those who had an increase (effect size = 0.51) or decrease (effect size = 0.38) in the PGI over time. A structured review of the validity, reliability and responsiveness of the PGI by Martin *et al.* (2007) concluded that reliability was adequate for group comparisons, but the evidence was unclear for its responsiveness.

A systematic review by Tang *et al.* (2014) of cancer studies using individualized questions identified four papers that used the PGI, out of 2,167 initially identified. The authors reported that a theme across these studies was of concerns of patients mentioned in response to the PGI, but not identified by standardized QoL measures. However, despite such advantages, individualized measures can present difficulties when measuring change, as QoL is dynamic, and patients may rate different areas as important at different stages in their condition. As Sprangers and Schwartz (1999) stated, patients confronted with a life-threatening or chronic condition need to accommodate to their illness, and a mediator in this process is response shift. This involves changing internal standards, values and conceptualizations of QoL. Also, as with the SEIQoL, on repeat testing, if the score (weight) provided for a particular area of life changes, then so must the weight for one or more of the other domains.

OLDER PEOPLE'S QUALITY OF LIFE QUESTIONNAIRE (OPQOL)

The OPQOL questionnaire is unique in being developed bottom-up from the views of a national random sample of 999 people aged 65+, living at home in Britain, and qualitative follow-up interviews with 80 people. The QoL survey questionnaire started with open-ended questions to elicit people's perceptions of QoL: about what gave their lives quality, what took quality away from their lives, and their relative importance. Their thematically coded responses were then compared with psychosocial theory (Bowling *et al.* 2003). The responses to these open-ended questions, and themes raised during the in-depth follow-up interviews, were then assessed against theoretical concepts of QoL (Bowling *et al.* 2003; Bowling and Gabriel 2004; Bowling 2005b). All responses were thematically coded in detail ('root and branch' themes and sub-themes). These open-ended questions, which are of value when examining people's own views of their QoL, are shown in Box 8.10, along with the seven-point QoL uniscale used.

Box 8.10 Open-ended questions and QoL uniscale item, to elicit views of QoL

'Thinking about your life as a whole, what is it that makes your life good – that is, the things that give your life quality? You may mention as many things as you like.'

'What is it that makes your life bad – that is the things that reduce the quality in your life? You may mention as many things as you like.'

'Thinking about all these good and bad things you have just mentioned which one is the most important to you?'

Again, thinking about the good and bad things you have mentioned that make up your quality of life, which of the answers on this card best describes the quality of your life as a whole?

(1) So good, it could not be better
(2) Very good
(3) Good
(4) Alright
(5) Bad
(6) Very bad
(7) So bad, it could not be worse

And what single thing would improve the quality of your life?

'And what single thing, in your opinion, would improve the overall quality of life for people of your age?'

Source: Bowling *et al.* 2003; Bowling 2005b and see www.ilcuk.org.uk/files/pdf_pdf_159.pdf, accessed 5 August 2015. © Ann Bowling.

Items are free to use without permission, with acknowledgement of source and referencing of original publications: Bowling, A., Gabriel, Z., Dykes, J. *et al.* (2003) Let's ask them: definitions of quality of life and its enhancement among people aged 65 and over. *International Journal of Aging and Human Development*, 56: 269–306.

The main things mentioned by people, and included in the OPQOL, were categorized into main and sub-themes by two researchers, independently, with cross-checking. The main themes were: social relationships, social roles and activities, activities/hobbies enjoyed alone, health, psychological outlook and well-being, home and neighbourhood, financial circumstances and independence (Bowling *et al.* 2003). Smaller numbers of people mentioned a wide range of other things. The responses were consistent with older people's views to the reverse question about what took quality away from life.

Detailed sub-themes were also categorized to reflect the context – i.e. why the theme was raised. The themes and sub-themes are detailed in Bowling (2005b). The domains and items included in the OPQOL reflect this common core of main constituents of QoL.

Apart from published studies in Britain, China and Italy (see below), the OPQOL is currently being used in surveys across the world, including Australia, the USA (California), Finland and Sweden.

Content

The full OPQOL is a 32- to 35-item QoL measure, with the longer 35-item version reflecting additional items on children, religion and culture which were prioritized by ethically diverse older people. The 32 or 35 items represent: 1) life overall (four items), 2) health (four items), 3) social relationships and participation (seven in 32-item version, eight in 35-item version – additional item on children), 4) independence, control over life, freedom (five items), 5) area: home and neighbourhood (four items), 6) psychological and emotional well-being (four items), 7) perceived financial circumstances (four items), 8) religion/culture (two items, 35-item version – additional items on religion/culture) (Bowling 2009b; Bowling and Stenner 2011). A short, 13-item version – the OPQOL-Brief – has also been developed and tested (Bowling *et al.* 2013).

The shorter OPQOL-Brief includes 13 of the OPQOL items (see Box 8.11), prioritized by older people as the most important and which were among the most psychometrically robust items (Bowling *et al.* 2013).

Box 8.11 OPQOL-Brief and OPQOL

The OPQOL-Brief consists of these 13 items from the full OPQOL (which were rated as most important by older people); five-point response scales are used. Each item in the full OPQOL and the OPQOL-Brief is in the form of a statement, and respondents are asked to do the following.

Please indicate the extent to which you agree or disagree with each of the following statements.

Against the items is a five-point Likert response scale: Strongly agree (coded 1), Agree (coded 2), Neither agree nor disagree (coded 3), Disagree (coded 4), Strongly disagree (coded 5).

I enjoy my life overall
I look forward to things
I am healthy enough to get out and about
My family, friends or neighbours would help me if needed
I have social or leisure activities/hobbies that I enjoy doing
I try to stay involved with things
I am healthy enough to have my independence
I can please myself what I do
I feel safe where I live
I get pleasure from my home
I take life as it comes and make the best of things
I feel lucky compared to most people
I have enough money to pay for household bills

OPQOL and OPQOL-Brief: Copyrighted © A. Bowling. Access: the OPQOL questionnaires are free to download and use from the International Longevity Centre UK website, and no permissions are needed, just with acknowledgement of source and original publications. Full OPQOL: Bowling, A. (2009) Psychometric properties of the Older People's Quality of Life Questionnaire validity. *Current Gerontology and Geriatrics Research*, open access Volume 2009, Article ID 298950, 12 pages, doi:10.1155/2009/298950, www.hindawi.com/journals/cggr/2009/298950.abs.htm. Bowling A. and Stenner, P. (2011) Which measure of quality of life performs best in older age? A comparison of the OPQOL, CASP-19 and WHOQOL-OLD. *Journal of Epidemiology and Community Health*, 65: 273–80, open access, doi:10.1136/jech. 2009.087668. OPQOL-Brief: Bowling, A., Hankins, M., Windle, G., Bilotta, C. and Grant, R. (2013) A short measure of quality of life in older age: the performance of the brief Older People's Quality of Life questionnaire (OPQOL-brief). *Archives of Geriatrics and Gerontology*, 56(1): 181–7, http://dx.doi.org/10.1016/j.archger, accessed

8 December 2012. Contact details: Professor Ann Bowling, Faculty of Health Sciences, University of Southampton, S017 1BJ. Access: links to selected OPQOL documents, questionnaire, scoring and UK population norms can be accessed, and materials downloaded at no cost at the Archive of International Longevity Centre UK (ILC-UK) website. Weblinks are cited with permission of ILC-UK. The full OPQOL questionnaire, scoring details, the OPQOL-Brief, and other information about the research, can be found and downloaded via: http://www.ilcuk.org.uk/index.php/ publications/publication_details/good_neighbours_measuring_quality_of_life_in_old_age. Direct link to the report: www.ilcuk.org.uk/images/uploads/publication-pdfs/pdf_pdf_159.pdf. Direct link to the full OPQOL questionnaire: http://www.ilcuk.org.uk/files/pdf_pdf_161.pdf. All accessed 19 December 2015. Also see: https://eprovide.mapi-trust.org/ accessed 21 July 2016.

Scoring

The items in each 1–5 point response scale are summed to create a total OPQOL or OPQOL-Brief score. As questions were worded either positively or negatively, then before summing reverse coding of positively worded items is required (in order to reverse their 5–1 codes to 1–5). Higher scores represent higher QoL. Subscale items can also be summed for subscale scores. The questionnaire, norms and scoring are freely available for use, and can be found on the web Archive of the International Longevity Centre UK (see Box 8.11).

Validity

Three British population surveys of older people, including an ethnically diverse sample, were used to test the acceptability, reliability, validity and factor structure of the full and short versions of the OPQOL (Bowling 2009b; Bowling and Stenner 2011; Bowling et al. 2013). Two of these surveys were based on face-to-face interviews and the other was administered by post.

In terms of acceptability to respondents, an open-ended postal questionnaire item asked respondents how easy or difficult they found the OPQOL to complete, and almost all indicated that they found the questionnaire very easy to complete. Item completion was at acceptable levels – item non-response for all three QoL scales was between 1–3 per cent in both interview surveys, although, as expected, slightly higher in the self-administered postal survey (5–11 per cent) (Bowling 2009b).

The distributions of grouped scale scores on each instrument showed a tendency to span middle values, although, as expected, these were more distributed towards middle-poor QoL for the ethnically diverse sample, and towards middle-good QoL for the British population sample. Few OPQOL scores were distributed at the extreme ends, as would be expected (people dislike perceiving themselves as extremes). The item distributions also show that responses to most items spanned the full range, although more of the ethnically diverse respondents opted for middle categories, thus 'sitting on the fence', compared with other respondents, whose responses were more likely to be at the positive end of the scale (Bowling 2009b).

Each version of the OPQOL has been tested for reliability and validity in three national population samples of people aged 65+, including an ethnically diverse population sample. Two of these surveys used face-to-face interview methods, and one used postal administration; these surveys also provided population norms for the OPQOL in Britain (Bowling 2009b; Bowling *et al.* 2010, 2013; Bowling and Stenner 2011). The OPQOL has also been used in an intervention trial of exercise in the UK (Iliffe *et al.* 2014), and with geriatric outpatients in Italy, and was able to predict their outcomes at follow-up (Bilotta *et al.* 2010, 2011, 2012). The OPQOL has also been used and tested in China with older people living alone (Chen *et al.* 2014).

The OPQOL has good psychometric properties overall, and performed better among ethnically diverse groups than two other measures of QoL administered (CASP-19 and WHOQOL-OLD) (Bowling and Stenner 2011).

Construct validity (also known as concurrent validity) was tested by correlating the OPQOL with variables QoL was expected to be associated with, based on the literature. As hypothesized, the total scores for three QoL scales administered to a population sample of people aged 65+ in Britain, and an ethnically diverse population sample aged 65+ in Britain (the OPQOL, CASP-19 and WHOQOL-OLD) all correlated moderately to highly with each other (rho 0.380–0.732; all p <0 .01).

The OPQOL was further tested for construct validity by Bowling (2009b) and Bowling and Stenner (2011) along with the CASP-19 and WHOQOL-OLD in national population surveys of people aged 65+ living at home in Britain, including an ethnically diverse sample. The construct validity of the three QoL measures was tested by correlating them with independent self-rated QoL and self-ratings on several of its domains. Before the three QoL scales were administered, respondents were asked to rate their QoL overall, and then in relation to their health, social relationships, independence, control and freedom, home and neighbourhood, psychological/emotional well-being, financial circumstances and leisure, and social activities. Each rating was on a five-point response scale ranging from 'Very good' to 'Very bad'). The OPQOL was highly significantly associated with the global and domain ratings. The correlations were between –0.389 and –0.659 (both p <0.01) in the three samples (minus sign reflects direction of coding), with those with better OPQOL scores reporting higher global QoL.

In each of the three national population samples, the OPQOL was significantly associated, in expected directions, with several hypothesized variables (Bowling 2005b); for example, respondents with higher OPQOL scores reported better health and functional status, help and support, and were more likely to be married and in higher socioeconomic groups. Older age was inversely associated with QoL on each measure across samples, with younger people scoring a better QoL. There were no associations with sex, again as expected, supporting discriminant validity (see Bowling 2009b for detailed statistics). These results support the construct validity (convergent and discriminant) of the OPQOL.

A further test of construct validity was scale-scale and subscale-subscale correlations (using Spearman's rho) between the OPQOL, CASP-19, and WHOQOL-OLD to assess construct validity further. It was expected that the scales and subscales, where a comparable domain of QoL was assessed, would correlate significantly with each other. Higher correlations would not necessarily be expected as the content of each measure differed. The OPQOL, CASP-19, and WHOQOL-OLD total scores all correlated moderately to highly with each other in expected directions (rho 0.380 to 0.732; all p <0.01). The subscales to scale total correlation ranged, across samples, for the OPQOL from rho

0.235 to 0.786 (all p < 0.01). Subscales within the OPQOL correlated significantly with each other, using Spearman's rho, when expected theoretically. For example, the OPQOL 'psychological well-being and outlook' subscale correlated significantly with the OPQOL 'life overall' subscale in each of the three samples (Spearman's rho: 0.232, 0.554, 0.380 in each sample; all p < 0.01). Similarly, given that poor health and frailty can limit one's independence, the OPQOL 'health and functioning' subscale correlated significantly with the OPQOL 'control, independence, and freedom' subscale: Spearman's rho: 0.138, 0.489, 0.460 (all p < 0.01) in the samples (Bowling and Stenner 2011). Multiple regression models further supported the validity and underlying constructs of the OPQOL (Bowling and Stenner 2011).

Milte *et al.* (2014), in a mixed methods study of 21 older adults from a day rehabilitation facility in Southern Adelaide, Australia, reported that their qualitative analysis of focus group transcripts supported the value of health and psychological well-being, and social (independence, safety) domains to participants' QoL. They found a fairly strong, positive association between EQ-5D scores and the OPQOL-Brief (Spearman's rho: 0.730; p < 0.01). Kaambwa *et al.* (2015), in a study of 87 older adults living in five care homes in Australia, reported moderate convergent validity for a number of instrument dimensions in relation to the OPQOL-Brief, ASCOT and EQ-5D-3L. The strongest relationship (r = 0.57) was between 'enjoy life' (OPQOL-Brief) and 'social contact' (ASCOT). The overall intraclass correlation coefficient (ICC) was 0.54 and Bland-Altman scatter plots showed that 3–6 per cent of normalized Z-scores were outside the 95 per cent limits of agreement – this indicated moderate agreement between all three instruments (agreement highest between the OPQOL-Brief and the ASCOT). Chen *et al.* (2014), in their study in China, reported that the convergent validity of the OPQOL was supported by moderate correlations with functional ability, social support and loneliness, with Spearman's rho of –0.50, 0.49 and –0.53, respectively. The discriminant validity was confirmed by differentiating QoL scores between the depressed and non-depressed groups.

Principal components analysis (PCA) revealed the presence of nine, rather than the expected eight, components of the OPQOL where the eigenvalues exceeded 1, explaining cumulatively 60.583 per cent of the total variance in QoL between respondents. Confirmatory factor analysis is still required (see detailed PCA statistics in Bowling and Stenner 2011). Chen *et al.* (2014), in China, reported that exploratory factor analysis indicated that the OPQOL formed the expected eight factors accounting for 63.77 per cent of the variance.

Reliability

The OPQOL satisfied the 0.70<0.90 threshold for internal consistency reliability with Cronbach's alpha in all three population samples at 0.748, 0.876 and 0.901 (Bowling and Stenner 2011). The test-retest reliability of the OPQOL was assessed by mailing a second copy of the questionnaire, plus items about any recent life changes, to a sub-sample of 50 consenting QoL longitudinal survey respondents four weeks after they had returned the first questionnaire; 31 respondents returned the questionnaire within the required time period. The four-week test-retest correlations, assessed among QoL follow-up survey respondents, ranged from moderate to high (r = 0.403 to 0.782). Lower correlations were explained by reported life changes in the intervening month, demonstrating the difficulties of test-retest exercises in older populations (Bowling 2009b).

The reliability criterion for item-total correlations (the correlation of the item with the scale total with that item omitted) is that the item should correlate with the total scale by at least 0.20. With three exceptions, the OPQOL items met this criterion for all three samples; as Cronbach's alpha was not improved by the removal of these three items, and they performed well otherwise (in validity tests), they were retained. As expected, all items correlated more highly with similar, than dissimilar, items in the scales (Bowling and Stenner 2011). The subscales to scale total correlation ranges, across samples, for the OPQOL were rho 0.235 to 0.786 (all p <.01) (acceptability criteria for reliability = r >0.20) (Bowling 2009b).

Chen *et al.* (2014), in their study in China (of over 500 older people living alone), reported that the Cronbach's alpha coefficient of the OPQOL was 0.90 for the total scale and over 0.70 for most of its dimensions. The two-week test-retest reliability ranged from 0.53 to 0.87.

OLDER PEOPLE'S QUALITY OF LIFE QUESTIONNAIRE – BRIEF (OPQOL-BRIEF)

The OPQOL-Brief was developed and tested by Bowling *et al.* (2013). The shorter OPQOL-Brief includes 13 of the OPQOL items (see Box 8.11 earlier), which were prioritized by older people as the most important and which were among the most psychometrically robust. It was tested in a national British population survey of people aged 65+.

Validity

Comparisons were made with the OPQOL-Brief and other measures of QoL in older age: the CASP-19 and WHOQOL-OLD. The Spearman's rank correlations for the OPQOL-Brief with the CASP-19 was rho 0.661 (p <0.001) and with the WHOQOL-OLD it was rho 0.642 (p <0.001) (the respective correlation between the OPQOL-35 and the WHOQOL-OLD was rho 0.699 (p <0.001), and rho 0.739 (p <0.001) with the CASP-19). These correlations support the validity of the OPQOL-Brief.

In further support of the validity of the OPQOL-Brief, it was moderately and highly significantly associated, in expected directions, with variables hypothesized to influence QoL, using Spearman's rank-order correlation coefficients. These included self-rated active ageing (rho –0.503, p <0.001), self-rated health status (rho –0.517, p <0.001), physical functioning (degree of ability walking 400 yards, performing heavy housework, shopping/carrying heavy bags, going up/down steps/stairs summed) (rho –0.432, p <0.001), self-rated global QoL (rho –0.560, p <0.001), numbers of helpers and supporters (rho 0.342, p <0.001), numbers of social activities (rho 0.439, p <0.001), socioeconomic status and age (rho: –120, p <0.001), and age (rho –0.125, p <0.001). Thus, in support of the scale's convergent validity, those with optimal health status, physical functioning, global QoL ratings, more helpers and supporters, and more social activities, and to a lesser extent, those in higher socioeconomic groups and who were younger, had higher OPQOL-Brief scores, indicating better QoL. There was no significant correlation with sex (rho –0.03), again supporting discriminant validity.

The reliability and validity of the 13 items included in the OPQOL-Brief were compared with the remaining 22 (i.e. excluded from the OPQOL-Brief) items from the full OPQOL. The Cronbach's alpha of the 13-item OPQOL-brief was 0.856, compared with a lower alpha of 0.757 for the 22 discarded items, supporting the stronger internal consistency of the OPQOL-Brief (despite having fewer items than the 22 comparison variable – Cronbach's alpha is inflated by larger numbers of items). The Spearman's correlation between the OPQOL-Brief and global self-rated QoL was rho 0.753, and between the remaining 22 items summed and global self-rated QoL, it was rho 0.564, supporting the stronger validity of the former. The number of missing cases in the OPQOL-13 was just six out of 589 responders, compared with 27 in the summed 22-item discarded items. When the OPQOL-Brief was plotted against the discarded 22 items summed (i.e. in effect, an 'OPQOL-22'), it showed several outliers. An improved pattern was found between the OPQOL-Brief (13 items) against the full OPQOL-35, supporting the internal consistency of the OPQOL-Brief, and the decision to exclude the 22 items (see details in Bowling *et al.* 2013).

Analysis of the structure and scaling of the OPQOL-Brief was undertaken using PCA and Mokken scaling. The PCA on the correlation matrix of OPQOL-13 questions yielded two components with eigenvalues over 1 (4.9 and 1.3); together they explained 48 per cent of variance. As factor analysis methods (PCA) do not test whether the items form a scale, the extent to which the 13 items formed a homogenous scale was further examined using the Mokken scaling procedure (Sijtsma and Molenaar 2002). The Mokken scaling confirmed that the items formed a monotone homogenous scale with a homogeneity coefficient of $H = 0.36$, exceeding the minimum practical threshold of $H = 0.3$.

Reliability

The reliability of the OPQOL-Brief was tested in a British population sample aged 65+ (Bowling *et al.* 2013), and was also shown to be highly reliable. Cronbach's alpha measure of internal consistency exceeded the 0.70 threshold at 0.856 for the 13 items (n = 583 cases included in analysis). Item-item reliability correlations for the OPQOL-Brief ranged between r 0.174 and 0.598, with similar variables achieving highest correlations (e.g. 'I enjoy my life overall' with 'I look forward to things': r 0.598) and dissimilar variables achieving lower correlations (e.g. 'I am healthy enough to get out and about' with 'My family, friends, neighbours would help me if needed': r 0.174), as would be expected. Items were not over-correlating, suggesting that there was no item redundancy. The item-total reliability correlations for the 13 items all exceeded the threshold for acceptability (range: r 0.36 for 'I have enough money to pay for household bills' to r 0.67 for 'I enjoy life overall'). Cronbach's alpha for the OPQOL-Brief of 0.856 was not improved if any of the items were deleted, and all were retained.

The measure is copyrighted, and is free to download and use without permission, just acknowledgement of source and referencing of original publications (see Boxes 8.11 and 8.12).

Box 8.12 OPQOL and OPQOL-Brief access

OPQOL-brief: copyrighted @ A. Bowling.

The OPQOL and OPQOL-Brief questionnaires are free to download and use and no permissions are needed.

For the OPQOL and OPQOL-Brief, the developer's request is that the sources are credited.

The full OPQOL questionnaire, scoring details, the OPQOL-Brief and other information about the research can be found and downloaded via:

http://www.ilcuk.org.uk/index.php/publications/publication_details/good_neighbours_measuring_quality_of_life_in_old_age

The link for actual PDF of the OPQOL-Brief is above and can also be accessed here: http://www.ilcuk.org.uk/images/uploads/publication pdfs/OPQOL_brief_questionnaire_and_responses.pdf

Weblinks cited with permission of ILC-UK.

See also:

https://eprovide.mapi-trust.org/ accessed 21 July 2016. A Welsh translation of the full OPQOL has also been developed, see: http://micym.org/llais/measure/index accessed 21 July 2016.

ADULT SOCIAL CARE OUTCOMES TOOLKIT FOR ASSESSING SOCIAL CARE-RELATED QoL (ASCOT)

ASCOT was developed specifically for use in social care (Netten 2011), and to fill an acknowledged gap in measurement tools, given the absence of dedicated social care outcome measures. It was developed within an economic framework following the extra-welfarist approach (Brouwer *et al.* 2008), and with the aim of developing a utility scale for use in measuring cost-effectiveness of interventions. This approach was intended to ensure that measures are sensitive to the impact of care, and suitable for measuring the value of outcomes. The developers argued that studies in social care tend to use health outcome measures, such as the EQ-5D, to assess cost-effectiveness, but these focus on people's functional abilities, rather than on the impact of support on their QoL. ASCOT was therefore developed as a measure of social care-related QoL (SCRQoL) to measure the full range of social care outcomes; it was envisaged to be more sensitive than the EQ-5D (Netten *et al.* 2012). SCRQoL refers to those aspects of people's QoL that are relevant to and the focus of social care interventions (Netten *et al.* 2011). ASCOT was reviewed in brief by Bowling (2014a, 2014b).

The design of ASCOT was based on expert review with social care stakeholders to identify the relevant attributes to include (Netten 2011). This was to ensure ASCOT's sensitivity to outcomes of interest to policy-makers and relevance to the evaluation of social care interventions. Its development included a literature review of service users' understanding of social care outcomes, and finally cognitive interviews were conducted in order to check social care service users' understanding of terms in ASCOT, and clarify items where needed (Netten *et al.* 2012). Netten *et al.* (2012) and Malley *et al.* (2012) proposed that in order to measure the value of social care services a measure should reflect the compensatory activity of social care, be sensitive to client choice and capture SCRQoL, and reflect those aspects of QoL that are the focus of social care support.

Content

ASCOT is a multi-attribute preference-weighted measure of SCRQoL. It includes eight distinct attributes, or domains: personal cleanliness and comfort, food and drink, control over daily life, personal safety, accommodation cleanliness and comfort, social participation and involvement, occupation and dignity. It also includes a preference-weighted measure of SCRQoL for use in economic evaluations. There is one item per attribute. Each attribute has four response options, reflecting four outcomes, which distinguish between Sen's (1985) functioning needs and capabilities. The top two reflect states where outcomes are fully realized but differ in the extent to which respondents have choice over how the outcome is realized, or not. The scoring for the measure is based on population preference weights in order to reflect the relative importance of different aspects of SCRQoL reflected in the domains.

The importance of the relative domains for scoring was established with preference studies of the domains with 500 members of the public, and 450 people who had received services (equipment). In support of hypotheses, SCRQoL was higher in the general population sample. Preferences were not associated with age or service use. It was designed to be preference-weighted to reflect the relative importance of the SCRQoL states in order to be capable of generating a single score for use in cost-effectiveness analyses (Netten *et al.* 2012). Some examples of items and responses are shown in Box 8.13.

Box 8.13 Examples from the ASCOT

Control over daily life
I have as much control over my daily life as I want – I have no control over my daily life

Personal cleanliness and comfort
I feel clean and am able to present myself the way I like – I don't feel at all clean or presentable

Social participation
I have as much social contact as I want with people I like – I have little social contact with people and feel socially isolated

Dignity
The way I'm helped and treated makes me think and feel better about myself – the way I'm helped and treated completely undermines the way I think or feel about myself.

Sources: Netten, A., Beadle-Brown, J., Caiels, J., Forder, J., Malley, J., Smith, N., Trukeschitz, B., Towers, A., Welch, E. and Windle, K. (2011) *Adult Social Care Outcomes Toolkit v2.1: Main guidance*, PSSRU Discussion Paper 2716/3. Canterbury: Personal Social Services Research Unit, University of Kent. Netten, A., Burge, P., Malley, J., Potoglou, D., Towers, A., Brazier, J., Flynn, T., Forder, J. and Wall, B. (2012) Outcomes of social care for adults: developing a preference-weighted measure. *Health Technology Assessment*, 16: 1–165, http://dx.doi.org/10.3310/hta16160. Note on registration and copyright: only users who register on the ASCOT website may download the ASCOT tools. Registration is free, as is the use of ASCOT for non-commercial purposes. See www.pssru.ac.uk/ascot/

Contact: Personal Social Services Research Unit, University of Kent at Canterbury, UK; ascot@kent.ac.uk, accessed 22 October 2015.

Validity and reliability

A survey of older people receiving publicly-funded home care services was conducted by face-to-face interview in several sites across England to assess the validity of ASCOT; 301 people in 10 areas of England were interviewed (10 per cent by proxy) (Malley *et al*. 2012). Hypothesis testing was used to test construct validity for each ASCOT attribute. Some evidence for construct validity was reported. A strong relationship between QoL and general well-being in each of the domains was found. The survey also demonstrated the feasibility of its use among older people, although the need for some proxy respondents indicated a need for a proxy version.

While service and policy relevance is essential, the deliberate top-down development of this measure has the consequence that broader user relevance is less certain, although its validity is supported in relation to different service user groups (Malley and Netten 2009; Milte *et al*. 2014).

Versions appropriate for different care settings are available, as well as a carer version – the ASCOT-Carer. Initial testing with 387 unpaid carers, who completed a face-to-face or telephone interview, supported the construct validity by statistically significant relationships between ASCOT-Carer and scores on instruments of related constructs, as well as with characteristics of the carer and care recipient. The Cronbach's alpha of 0.87 (seven items) indicates that the internal reliability of the instrument is satisfactory.

A toolkit for ASCOT is available that also includes data entry tools that can be used to enter data collected with these instruments and generate sample and individual ASCOT scores for current, expected and gain in SCRQoL, and for capacity to benefit (see www.pssru.ac.uk/ascot/). Assessment of reliability is ongoing/planned.

EXAMPLE

Box 8.14 Example of trial using multiple secondary outcome measures, including QoL and health-related QoL

Iliffe *et al*. (2014) conducted a pragmatic, three-arm parallel design, cluster-controlled trial, with allocation at the level of consenting general practices in three areas of the UK.

Consenting patients aged ≥ 65 years were eligible to be included in the trial if they were independently mobile and able physically to take part in a group exercise. Several exclusion criteria applied (see Iliffe *et al.* 2014 for details at http://www.journalslibrary. nihr.ac.uk/hta/volume-18/issue-49#abstract, accessed 17 September 2015). Blinding of participants was not possible due to the type of intervention.

The primary objective was to evaluate the effect of home-based and community-based exercise programmes for older people, compared with usual care, on attainment of recommended physical activity levels at 12 months after the intervention ended.

The primary outcome was the proportion of participants reaching/exceeding the national recommended target of ≥ 150 minutes of moderate to vigorous physical activity per week at 12 months after the intervention ended.

The secondary outcomes included direct health benefits (i.e. functional status, psychological status, falls – rates, number and nature, fear of falling), self-efficacy and assessments of importance of physical activity, health-related QoL and costs. Among the measures used, and included in this book, were the Older People's Quality of Life questionnaire (OPQOL) and the EQ-5D; social networks were measured using the brief Lubben Social Network Scale (LSNS).

Apart from differences between groups in their attitudes towards exercise, the results of the secondary outcome measures were consistent in that there were no statistically significant differences between intervention arms and the usual-care arm in self-efficacy, mental and physical well-being, QoL, balance confidence, social networks, falls risk or functional abilities.

References

Aaronson, N.K. (1993) The EORTC QLQ-C30, A quality of life instrument for use in international clinical trials in oncology (abstract). *Quality of Life Research*, 2: 51.

Aaronson, N.K., Acquadro, C., Alonson, J. *et al.* (1992) International quality of life assessment (IQOLA) project. *Quality of Life Research*, 1: 349–51.

Abbey, A. and Andrews, F.M. (1986) Modelling the psychological determinants of life quality, in F.M. Andrews (ed.) *Research on the Quality of Life*. Ann Arbor, MA: Survey Research Center, Institute for Social Research, University of Michigan.

Abbott, R.A., Ploubidis, G.B., Huppert, F.A. *et al.* (2006) Psychometric evaluation and predictive validity of Ryff's psychological well-being items in a UK birth cohort sample of women. *Health and Quality of Life Outcomes*, 4: 76.

Abernethy, A.P., Shelby-James, T., Fazekas, B.S. *et al.* (2005) The Australian-modified Karnofsky Performance Status (AKPS) scale: a revised scale for contemporary palliative care clinical practice. *BMC Palliative Care*, 4: 7.

Ada, L., Dean, C.M., Hall, J.M. *et al.* (2003) A tread-mill and overground walking programme improves walking in persons residing in the community after stroke: a placebo-controlled randomised trial. *Archives of Physical Medical Rehabilitation*, 84: 1486–91.

Adair, F.L. (1984) Coopersmith Self-Esteem Inventories, in D.J. Keyser and R.C. Sweetland (eds) *Test Critiques*, Vol. I. Kansas City, MI: Test Corporation of America.

Adams, B.L. (1969) Analysis of a life satisfaction index. *Journal of Gerontology*, 24: 470–4.

Adams, B.N. (1967) Interaction theory and the social network. *Sociometry*, 30: 64–78.

Adams, K.B., Matto, H.C. and Sanders, S. (2004) Confirmatory factor analysis of the Geriatric Depression Scale. *The Gerontologist*, 44: 818–26.

Addington-Hall, J. and Kalra, L. (2001) Measuring quality of life. Who should measure quality of life? *British Medical Journal,* 322: 1417–20.

Addington-Hall, J.M., MacDonald, L.D. and Anderson, H.R. (1990) Can the Spitzer Quality of Life Index help to reduce prognostic uncertainty in terminal cancer? *British Journal of Cancer*, 62: 695–9.

Affleck, J.W., Aitken, R.C.B., Hunter, J. *et al.* (1988) Rehabilitation status: a measure of medico-social dysfunction. *Lancet*, i: 230–3.

Agrell, B. and Dehlin, O. (1989) Comparison of six depression rating scales in geriatric stroke patients. *Stroke*, 20: 1190–4.

Albrecht, G.L. and Devlieger, P.J. (1999) The disability paradox: high quality of life against all odds. *Social Science and Medicine*, 48: 977–88.

Alden, D., Austin, C. and Sturgeon, R. (1989) A correlation between the Geriatric Depression Scale long and short forms. *Journal of Gerontology*, 44: 124–5.

Alonso, J., Anto, J.M., Gonzalez, M. *et al.* (1992) Measurement of a general health status of non-oxygen-dependent chronic obstructive pulmonary disease patients. *Medical Care*, 30: 125–35 (suppl. 5).

American Psychiatric Association (2013) *Diagnostic and Statistical Manual of Mental Disorders* (5th edn). Arlington, VA: American Psychiatric Publishing.

American Psychological Association (1974) *Standards for Educational and Psychological Tests*. Washington, DC: APA.

Anderson, R. (1988) The quality of life of stroke patients and their carers, in R. Anderson and M. Bury (eds) *Living with Chronic Illness: The Experience of Patients and Their Families*. London: Unwin Hyman.

Anderson, J., Sullivan, F. and Usherwood, T.P. (1990) The Medical Outcomes Study Instruments (MOSI) – use of a new health status measure in Britain. *Family Practice*, 7: 205–18.

Anderson, J.P., Kaplan, R.M., Coons, S.J. and Schneiderman, L.J. (1998) Comparison of the quality of wellbeing scale and the SF-36 results among two samples of ill adults: AIDS and other illnesses. *Journal of Clinical Epidemiology*, 51: 755–62.

Anderson, R.T., Aaronson, N.K. and Wilkin, D. (1993) Critical review of the international assessments of health-related quality of life. *Quality of Life Research*, 2: 369–95.

Andersson, E. (1993) The Hospital Anxiety and Depression Scale: homogeneity of the subscales. *Journal of Social Behavior and Personality*, 21: 197–204.

Andrews, F.M. (1974) Social indicators of perceived life quality. *Social Indicators Research*, 1: 279–99.

Andrews, F.M. (ed.) (1986) *Research on the Quality of Life*. University of Michigan: Institute for Social Research, Michigan.

Andrews, F.M. and Crandall, R. (1976) The validity of measures of self-reported well-being. *Social Indicators Research*, 3: 1–19.

Andrews, F.M. and McKennel, A.C. (1980) Measures of self-reported well-being: their affective, cognitive and other components. *Social Indicators Research*, 18: 127–55.

Andrews, F.M. and Robinson, J.P. (1991) Measures of subjective well-being, in J.P. Robinson, P.R. Shaver and L.S. Wrightsman (eds) *Measures of Personality and Social Psychological Attitudes*. London: Academic Press, Inc.

Andrews, F.M. and Withey, S.B. (1974) Developing measures of perceived life quality: results from several national surveys. *Social Indicators Research*, 1: 1–26.

Andrews, F.M. and Withey, S.B. (1976) *Social Indicators of Well-being: Americans' Perceptions of Life Quality*. New York: Plenum Press.

Andrews, G., Peters, L. and Teeson, M. (1994) *The Measurement of Consumer Outcome in Mental Health: A Report to the National Health Information Strategy Committee*. Sydney: Clinical Research Centre for Anxiety Disorders.

Anke, A.G. and Fugl-Meyer, A.R. (2003) Life satisfaction several years after severe multiple trauma – a retrospective investigation. *Clinical Rehabilitation*, 17: 431–42.

Antonovsky, A. (1987) *Unravelling the Mystery of Health: How People Manage Stress and Stay Well*. San Francisco: Jossey-Bass Publishers.

Antonovsky, A. (1990) A somewhat personal odyssey in studying the stress process. *Stress Medicine*, 6: 71–80.

Antonovsky, A. (1993) The structure and properties of the Sense of Coherence Scale. *Social Science and Medicine*, 36: 725–33.

Antonucci, T.C. (1986) Hierarchical mapping technique. *Generations: Journal of the American Society on Aging*, 10: 10–12.

Arfwidsson, L., Elia, G., D'Laurell, B. *et al.* (1974) Can self-rating replace doctors' rating in evaluating antidepressive treatment? *Acta Psychiatrica Scandinavica*, 50: 16–22.

Argyle, M., Martin, M. and Crossland, J. (1989) Happiness as a function of personality and social encounters, in J.P. Forgas and J.M. Innes (eds) *Recent Advances in Social Psychology: An International Perspective*. North Holland: Elsevier Science Publishers.

Arnau, R.C., Meagher, M.W., Norris, M.P. and Bramson, R. (2001) Psychomatic evaluation of the Beck Depression Inventory-II with primary care medical patients. *Health Psychology*, 20: 112–19.

Aspray, T.J.I., Stevenson, P., Abdy, S.E. *et al.* (2006) Low bone mineral density measurements in care home residents – a treatable cause of fractures. *Age and Ageing*, 35: 37–41.

Atchley, R.C. (1976) Selected social and psychological differences between men and women in later life. *Journal of Gerontology*, 31: 204–11.

Aure, O.F., Nilsen, J.H. and Vasseljen, O. (2003) Manual therapy and exercise therapy in patients with chronic low back pain: a randomised, controlled trial with 1-year follow-up. *Spine*, 28: 525–31.

Aydemir, G., Tezer, M.S., Borman, P. *et al.* (2006) Treatment of tinnitus with transcutaneous electrical nerve stimulation improves patients' quality of life. *Journal of Laryngology and Otology*, 120: 442–5.

Ayis, S., Gooberman-Hill, R. and Ebrahim, S. (2003) Long-standing and limiting long-standing illness in older people: associations with chronic diseases, psychosocial and environmental factors. *Age and Ageing*, 32: 265–72.

Aylard, P.R., Gooding, J.H., McKenna, P.J. and Snaith, R.P. (1987) A validation study of three anxiety and depression self assessment scales. *Psychosomatic Research*, 31: 261–8.

Bagby, R.M., Rydner, A.G., Schuller, D.R. and Marshall, M.B. (2004) The Hamilton Depression Rating Scale: has the gold standard become a lead weight? *American Journal of Psychiatry*, 161: 2163–77.

Baker, F. and Intagliata, J. (1982) Quality of life in the evaluation of community support systems. *Evaluation and Program Planning*, 5: 69–79.

Balaswamy, S. and Richardson, V.E. (2001) The cumulative effects of life events, personal and social resources on subjective well-being of elderly widowers. *International Journal of Aging and Human Development*, 53: 311–27.

Ball, R. and Steer, R.A. (2003) Mean Beck Depression Inventory-II scores of out-patients with dysthymic or recurrent-episode major depressive disorders. *Psychological Reports*, 93: 507–12.

Baltes, P. and Baltes, M. (1990) Psychological perspectives on successful aging: the model of selective optimisation with compensation, in P. Baltes and M. Baltes, *Successful Aging: Perspectives from the Behavioral Sciences*. New York: Cambridge University Press.

Banks, M.H. (1983) Validation of the General Health Questionnaire in a young community sample. *Psychological Medicine*, 13: 349–53.

Bardelli, D. and Saracci, R. (1978) Measuring the quality of life in cancer clinical trials: a sample survey of published trials, in P. Armitage and D. Bardelli (eds) *Methods and Impact of Controlled Therapeutic Trials in Cancer*. Geneva: Unione Internationale Contre le Cancer. Technical Report Series, No. 36.

Barrera, M. (1980) A method for the assessment of social support networks in community survey research. *Connections*, 3: 8–13.

Barrera, M. (1981) Social support in the adjustment of pregnant adolescents: assessment issues, in B.H. Gottlieb (ed.) *Social Networks and Social Support*. Beverly Hills, CA: Sage Publications.

Barrera, M. and Ainlay, S. (1983) The structure of social support: a conceptual and empirical analysis. *Journal of Community Psychology*, 11: 133–43.

Barrera, M. and Baca, L.M. (1990). Recipient reactions to social support: contributions of enacted support, conflicted support and network orientation. *Journal of Social and Personal Relationships,* 7: 541–51.

Barrera, M., Baca, L., Christiansen, J. *et al.* (1985) Informant corroboration of social support network data. *Connections*, 8: 9–13.

Barrera, M., Sandler, I.M. and Ramsay, T.B. (1981) Preliminary development of a scale of social support: Studies on college students. *American Journal of Community Psychology*, 9: 435–46.

Barry, M.M. (1997) Well-being and life satisfaction as components of quality of life in mental disorders, in H. Katschnig, H. Freeman and N. Sartorius (eds) *Quality of Life in Mental Disorders*. John Wiley & Sons, Chichester.

Bech, P. (1981) Rating scales for affective disorder: their validity and consistency. *Acta Psychiatrica Scandinavica*, suppl. 295: 1–101.

Bech, P., Gram, L.F., Dein, E. *et al.* (1975) Quantitative rating of depressive states. *Acta Psychiatrica Scandinavica*, 51: 161–70.

Bech, P., Kastrup, M. and Rafaelsen, O.J. (1986) Mini-compendium of rating scales for states of anxiety, depression, mania, schizophrenia and corresponding DSM-III syndromes. *Acta Psychiatrica Scandinavica*, 73 (suppl.): 1–37.

Beck, A.T. (1970) *Depression: Causes and Treatment*. Philadelphia, PA: University of Pennsylvania Press.

Beck, A.T. and Beck, R.W. (1972) Screening depressed patients in family practice: a rapid technique. *Postgraduate Medicine*, 52: 81–5.

Beck, A.T., Mendelson, M., Mock, J. *et al.* (1961) Inventory for measuring depression. *Archives of General Psychiatry*, 4: 561–71.

Beck, A.T., Rial, W.Y. and Rickels, K. (1974) Short form of depression inventory: cross validation. *Psychological Reports*, 34: 1184–6.

Beck, A.T., Steer, R.A. and Garbin, M.G. (1988) Psychometric properties of The Beck Depression Inventory: twenty-five years of evaluation. *Clinical Psychology Review*, 8: 77–100.

Beck, A.T., Steer, R.A. and Brown, G.K. (1996a) *Manual for the Beck Depression Inventory-II*. San Antonio, Texas: Psychological Corporation.

Beck, A.T., Steer, R.A., Ball, R. and Ranieri, W. (1996b) Comparison of Beck Depression Inventories-IA and -II in psychiatric out-patients. *Journal of Personality Assessment*, 67: 588–97.

Becker, M. (1974) The health belief model and personal health behaviour. *Health Education Monographs*, 2: 32–73.

Beckie, T.M. and Hayduk, L.A. (1997) Measuring quality of life. *Social Indicators Research*, 42: 21–39.

Bedford, A. and Deary, I.J. (1997) The personal disturbance scale (DSSI/SAD): development, use and structure. *Journal of Personality and Individual Differences*, 22: 493–510.

Bedford, A., Foulds, G.A. and Shefield, B.F. (1976) A new personal disturbance scale (DSSI/SAD). *British Journal of Social and Clinical Psychology*, 15: 387–94.

Benjamin, S., Decalmer, P. and Haran, D. (1982) Community screening for mental illness: a validity study of the General Health Questionnaire. *British Journal of Psychiatry*, 140: 174–80.

Benner, P. (1985) Quality of life: a phenomenological perspective on explanation, prediction, and understanding in nursing science. *Advances in Nursing Science, Special Issue: Quality of Life*, 8: 1–14.

Bentham, J. ([1834] 1983) *Deonotology*. Oxford: Clarendon Press.

Berg, R.L., Hallauer, D.S. and Berk, S.N. (1976) Neglected aspects of the quality of life. *Health Services Research*, 11: 391–5.

Berglund, G., Liden, A., Hansson, M.G. *et al.* (2003) Quality of life in patients with multiple endocrine neoplasia type 1 (MEN 1). *Family Cancer*, 2: 27–33.

Bergner, M. (1988) Development, testing and use of the Sickness Impact Profile, in S.R. Walker and R.M. Rosser (eds) *Quality of Life Assessment and Application*. Lancaster: MIT Press.

Bergner, M. (1993) Development, testing and use of the Sickness Impact Profile, in S.R. Walker and R.M. Rosser (eds) *Quality of Life Assessment: Key Issues in the 1990s* (2nd edn). Dordrecht: Kluwer Academic.

Bergner, M., Bobbitt, R.A., Kressel, S. *et al.* (1976a) The Sickness Impact Profile: conceptual formulation and methodology for the development of a health status measure. *International Journal of Health Services*, 6: 393–415.

Bergner, M., Bobbitt, R.A., Pollard, W.E. *et al.* (1976b) The Sickness Impact Profile: validation of a health status measure. *Medical Care*, 14: 57–67.

Bergner, M., Bobbitt, R.A., Carter, W.B. *et al.* (1981) The Sickness Impact Profile: development and final revision of a health status measure. *Medical Care*, 19: 787–805.

Berkanovic, E., Hurwicz, M.L. and Landsverk, J. (1988) Psychological distress and the decision to seek medical care. *Social Science and Medicine*, 27: 1215–21.

Berkman, L.F. and Glass, T. (2000) Social integration, social networks, social support and health, in L.F. Berkman and I. Kawachi (eds) *Social Epidemiology*. New York: Oxford University Press.

Berkman, L.F. and Syme, S.L. (1979) Social networks, host resistance and mortality: a nine-year follow-up study of Alameda County residents. *American Journal of Epidemiology*, 109: 186–204.

Berkman, P.L. (1971) Life stress and psychological well-being: a replication of Langner's analysis in the Midtown Manhattan study. *Journal of Health and Social Behaviour*, 12: 35–45.

Bernhard, J., Sullivan, M., Hurny, C. *et al.* (2001) Clinical relevance of single item quality of life indicators in cancer clinical trials. *British Journal of Cancer*, 84: 1156–65.

Berrios, G.E. and Bulbena-Villarasa, A. (1990) The Hamilton Depression Scale and the numerical description of the symptoms of depression, in P. Bech and A. Coppen (eds) *The Hamilton Scales*. New York: Springer-Verlag.

Berwick, D.M., Budman, S., Damico-White, J. *et al.* (1987) Assessment of psychological morbidity in primary care: explorations with the General Health Questionnaire. *Journal of Chronic Diseases*, 40: 71S–9S.

Berwick, D.M., Murphy, J.M., Goldman, P.A. *et al.* (1991) Performance of five-item mental health screening test. *Medical Care*, 29: 169–76.

Bigelow, D.A., McFarland, B.H. and Olson, M.M. (1991) Quality of life of community mental health program clients: validating a measure. *Community Mental Health Journal*, 27: 43–55.

Biggs, J.T., Wylie, L.T. and Ziegler, V.E. (1978) Validity of the Zung self-rating depression scale. *British Journal of Psychiatry*, 132: 381–5.

Bild, B.K. and Havighurst, R.J. (1976) Life satisfaction. *Gerontologist*, 16: 70–5.

Bilotta, C., Bowling, A., Casè, A. *et al.* (2010) Dimensions and correlates of quality of life according to frailty status: a crosssectional study on community-dwelling older adults referred to an outpatient geriatric service in Italy. *Health & Quality of Life Outcomes*, 8: 56.

Bilotta, C., Bowling, A., Nicolina, P. *et al.* (2011) Older People's Quality of Life (OPQOL) scores and adverse health outcomes at a one-year follow-up. A prospective cohort study on older outpatients living in the community in Italy. *Health and Quality of Life Outcomes*, 9: 72.

Bilotta, C., Bowling, A., Nicolina, P., Case, A. and Vergani, C. (2012) Quality of life in older outpatients living alone in the community in Italy. *Health and Social Care in the Community*, 20: 32–41.

Bjelland, I., Dahl, A.A., Haug, T.T., Neckelmann, D. *et al.* (2002) The validity of the Hospital Anxiety and Depression Scale: an updated literature review. *Journal of Psychosomatic Research*, 52: 69–77.

Björvell, H., Aly, A., Langius, A. and Nordstrom, G. (1994) Indicators of changes in weight and eating behaviour in severely obese patients treated in a nursing behavioural program. *International Journal of Obesity*, 18: 521–5.

Black, S.E., Blessed, J.A., Edwardson, J.A. *et al.* (1990) Prevalence rates of dementia in an ageing population: are low rates due to the use of insensitive instruments? *Age and Ageing*, 19: 84–90.

Blanchflower, D.G. and Oswald, A.J. (2001) *Wellbeing over time in Britain and the USA*. Warwick: University of Warwick, Research Paper No. 616, Department of Economics.

Blanchflower, D.G. and Oswald, A.J. (2004) Well-being over time in Britain and the USA. *Journal of Public Economics*, 88: 1359–86.

Blane, D., Gopalakrishnan, N. and Montgomery, S.M. (2008) Quality of life, health and physiological status and change at older ages. *Social Science and Medicine*, 66, 1579–87.

Blay, S.L., Ramos, L.R. and Mari-Jde, J. (1988) Validity of a Brazilian version of the Older Americans Resources and Services (OARS) mental health screening questionnaire. *Journal of the American Geriatrics Society*, 36: 687–92.

Blazer, D.G. (1982) Social support and mortality in an elderly community population. *American Journal of Epidemiology*, 115: 684–94.

Blumenthal, M.D. (1975) Measuring depressive symptomatology in a general population. *Archives of General Psychiatry*, 32: 971–8.

Blunch, N.J. (2013). Introduction to structural equation modeling using IBM SPSS statistics and AMOS. 2nd ed. California, Thousand Oaks: Sage.

Bombardier, C., Ware, J., Russell, J. *et al.* (1986) Auranofin therapy and quality of life in patients with rheumatoid arthritis. *American Journal of Medicine*, 81: 565–78.

Bond, J. and Carstairs, V. (1982) *Services for the Elderly*. Scottish Health Service Studies no. 42. Edinburgh: Scottish Home and Health Department.

Bond, M., Bowling, A., McKee, D. *et al.* (2003) Is age a predictor of access to cardiac services? *Journal of Health Services Research and Policy*, 8: 40–7.

Bonnetain, F., Bouché, O., Michel, P. *et al.* (2006) A comparative longitudinal quality of life study using the Spitzer quality of life index in a randomized multicenter phase III trial (FFCD 9102): chemoradiation followed by surgery compared with chemoradiation alone in locally advanced squamous resectable thoracic esophageal cancer. *Annals of Oncology*, 17: 827–34.

Borgatta, E.F. and Montgomery, R.J.V. (1987) *Critical Issues in Ageing Policy: Linking Research and Values*. Beverly Hills, CA: Sage Publications.

Borsch-Supan, A. Brugiavini, A., Jurges, H. *et al.* (2005) *Health, Ageing and Retirement in Europe: First Results from the Survey of Health, Ageing and Retirement in Europe*. Mannheim: Mannheim Research Institute of the Economics of Aging.

Boshier, R. (1968) Self esteem and first names in children. *Psychological Reports*, 22: 762.

Boury, J., Larkin, K. and Krummel, D. (2004) Factors related to postpartum depressive symptoms in low-income women. *Women and Health*, 39: 19–34.

Bowling, A. (1990) The prevalence of psychiatric morbidity among people aged 85 and over living at home. *Social Psychiatry and Psychiatric Epidemiology*, 25: 132–40.

Bowling, A. (1991) Social support and social networks: their relationship to the successful and unsuccessful survival of elderly people in the community. An analysis of concepts and a review of the evidence. *Family Practice*, 8: 68–83.

Bowling, A. (1994) Social networks and social support among older people and implications for emotional well-being and psychiatric morbidity. *International Review of Psychiatry*, 6: 41–58.

Bowling, A. (1995) What things are important in people's lives? A survey of the public's judgements to inform scales of health-related quality of life. *Social Science and Medicine*, Special Issue 'Quality of Life', 10: 1447–62.

Bowling, A. (2001) *Measuring Disease: A Review of Disease-specific Quality of Life Measurement Scales* (2nd edn). Buckingham: Open University Press.

Bowling, A. (2005a) Mode of questionnaire administration can have serious effects on data quality, *Journal of Public Health Medicine*, 27: 281–91.

Bowling, A. (2005b) *Ageing well. Quality of life in old age*. Maidenhead: Open University Press.

Bowling, A. (2005c). Just one question: if one question works why ask several? Editorial. *Journal of Epidemiology and Community Health*, 59: 342–5.

Bowling, A. (2006) Successful ageing from older people's perspectives. Results from a British survey of ageing. *European Journal of Ageing*, 3: 123–36.

Bowling, A. (2008) Enhancing later life: how older people perceive active ageing. *Ageing and Mental Health*, 12: 293–301.

Bowling A. (2009a) Perceptions of active ageing in Britain: divergences between minority ethnic and whole population samples. *Age and Ageing*, 38: 703–10.

Bowling, A. (2009b) Psychometric properties of the Older People's Quality of Life Questionnaire: validity. *Current Gerontology and Geriatrics Research*, www.hindawi.com/journals/cggr/2009/298950.abs.html (accessed on 8 August 2016).

Bowling, A. (2011) Do older and younger people differ in their reported well-being? A national survey of adults in Britain. *Family Practice*, 28: 145–55.

Bowling, A. (2014a) *Quality of life: Measures and Meanings in Social Care Research.* Methods Review 16. National Institute for Health Research: School for Social Care Research, London, http://www.sscr.nihr.ac.uk/PDF/MR/MR16.pdf (accessed on 8 August 2016).

Bowling, A. (2014b) *Research Methods in Health. Investigating Health and Health Services* (4th edn). Maidenhead: Open University Press.

Bowling, A. (2014c) Appendix 1: The definition and measurement of wellbeing and quality of life in mental health promotion and outcomes, in *Annual Report of the Chief Medical Officer, 2013*, Professor Dame Sally Davies, Public mental health priorities. Making mental health services more effective and accessible. London: Department of Health, https://www.gov.uk/government/publications/chief-medical-officer-cmo-annual-report-public-mental-health (accessed on 8 August 2016).

Bowling, A. and Browne, P. (1991) Social support and emotional well-being among the oldest old living in London. *Journal of Gerontology*, 46: S20–32.

Bowling, A. and Cartwright, A. (1982) *Life after a Death: A Study of the Elderly Widowed*. London: Tavistock Press.

Bowling, A. and Charlton, J. (1987) Risk factors for mortality after bereavement: a logistic regression analysis. *Journal of the Royal College of General Practitioners*, 37: 551–4.

Bowling, A. and Dieppe, P. (2005) What is successful ageing and who should define it? *British Medical Journal,* 331: 1548–51.

Bowling, A. and Ebrahim, S. (eds) (2005) *Handbook of Health Research Methods: Investigation, Measurement and Analysis*. Maidenhead: Open University Press.

Bowling, A. and Farquhar, M. (1995) Changes in network composition among older people living in Inner London and Essex. *Journal of Health and Place*, 3: 149–66.

Bowling, A. and Gabriel, Z. (2004) An integrational model of quality of life in older age. A comparison of analytic and lay models of quality of life. *Social Indicators Research*, 69: 1–36.

Bowling, A. and Grundy, E. (1997) Activities of daily living: changes in functional activity in three samples of elderly and very elderly people. *Age and Ageing*, 26: 107–14.

Bowling, A. and Grundy, E. (1998) Longitudinal studies of social networks and mortality in later life. *Reviews in Clinical Gerontology*, 8: 353–61.

Bowling, A. and Stenner, P. (2011) Which measure of quality of life performs best in older age? A comparison of the OPQOL, CASP-19 and WHOQOL-OLD. *Journal of Epidemiology and Community Health*, 65: 273–80.

Bowling, A. and Windsor, J. (1997) The discriminative power of The Health Status Questionnaire-12 (HSQ-12) in relation to age, sex and longstanding illness: findings from a survey of households in Britain. *Journal of Epidemiology and Community Health*, 51: 564–73.

Bowling, A. and Windsor, J. (2001) Towards the good life. A population survey of dimensions of quality of life. *Journal of Happiness Studies*, 2: 55–81.

Bowling, A. and Windsor, J. (2008). The effects of question order and response-choice on self-rated health status in the English Longitudinal Study of Ageing (ELSA). *Journal of Epidemiology and Community Health*, 62: 81–5.

Bowling, A., Leaver, J. and Hoeckel, T. (1988) *The Needs and Circumstances of People Aged 85+ Living at Home in City and Hackney*. London: Department of Public Health, City and Hackney Health Authority.

Bowling, A., Farquhar, M., Grundy, E. and Formby, J. (1992) Psychiatric morbidity among people aged 85+ in 1987. A follow-up study at two and a half years: associations with changes in psychiatric morbidity. *International Journal of Geriatric Psychiatry*, 7: 307–21.

Bowling, A., Farquhar, M., Grundy, E. and Formby, J. (1993) Changes in life satisfaction over a two and a half year period among very elderly people living in London. *Social Science and Medicine*, 36: 641–55.

Bowling, A., Farquhar, M. and Grundy, E. (1994a) Associations with changes in level of functional ability. *Ageing and Society*, 14: 53–73.

Bowling, A., Farquhar, M. and Grundy, E. (1994b) Changes in the ability to get outdoors among a community sample of people aged 85+ in 1987: results from a follow-up study in 1990. *International Journal of Health Sciences*, 5: 13–23.

Bowling, A., Farquhar, M. and Grundy, E. (1996) Associations with changes in life satisfaction among three samples of elderly people living at home. *International Journal of Geriatric Psychiatry*, 11, 1077–87.

Bowling, A., Bond, M., Jenkinson, C. and Lamping, D. (1999) Short Form-36 (SF-36) Health Survey Questionnaire: Which normative data should be used? Comparisons between the norms provided by the Omnibus Survey in Britain, The Health Survey for England and the Oxford Health and Lifestyle Survey. *Journal of Public Health Medicine*, 21: 255–70.

Bowling, A., Bannister, D., Sutton, S., Evans, O. and Windsor, J. (2002) A multi-dimensional model of QoL in older age. *Ageing and Mental Health*, 6: 355–71.

Bowling, A., Gabriel, Z., Dykes, J. *et al.* (2003) Let's ask them: definitions of quality of life and its enhancement among people aged 65 and over. *International Journal of Aging and Human Development*, 56: 269–306.

Bowling, A, See-tai S, Morris, R. and Ebrahim S. (2007) Quality of life among older people with poor functioning. The influence of perceived control over life. *Age and Ageing*, 36: 310–15.

Bowling, A. Iliffe, S., Kessel, A., Higginson, I. (2010) Fear of dying in an ethnically diverse society: cross-sectional studies of people aged 65+ in Britain. *Postgraduate Medical Journal*, 86: 197–202, www.pmj.bmj.com/content/86/1014/197.full (accessed on 8 August 2016).

Bowling, A., Hankins, M., Windle, G. *et al.* (2013) A short measure of quality of life in older age: The performance of the brief Older People's Quality of Life questionnaire (OPQOL-brief). *Archives of Geriatrics and Gerontology*, 56(1): 181–7.

Bradburn, N.M. (1969) *The Structure of Psychological Wellbeing*. Chicago, IL: Aldine Publishing.

Bradburn, N.M. and Caplovitz, D. (1965) *Reports on Happiness: A Pilot Study of Behaviour Related to Mental Health*. Chicago, IL: Aldine Publishing.

Bradley, C., Tod, C., Gorton, T. *et al.* (1999) The development of an individualized questionnaire measure of perceived impact of diabetes on quality of life: the ADDQoL. *Quality of Life Research*, 8: 79–91.

Bradlyn, A.S., Harris, C.V., Warner, J.E. *et al.* (1993) An investigation of the validity of the Quality of Well-Being Scale with pediatric oncology patients. *Health Psychology*, 12: 246–50.

Bradwell, A.R., Carmal, M.H. and Whitehead, T.P. (1974) Explaining the unexpected: abnormal results of biochemical profile investigations. *Lancet*, ii: 1071–4.

Brajković, A., Gregurek, R., Kušević, Z. *et al.* (2011) Life satisfaction in persons of the third age after retirement. *Collegium Antropologicum,* 35: 665–71.

Brazier, J.E. and Roberts, J.R, (2004) The estimation of a preference-based index from the SF-12. *Medical Care*, 42: 851–9.

Brazier, J.E., Harper, R., Jones, N. *et al.* (1992) Validating the SF-36 health survey questionnaire: a new outcome measure for primary care. *British Medical Journal*, 305: 160–4.

Brazier, J., Harper, R., Waterhouse, J. *et al.* (1993a) Comparison of outcome measures for patients with chronic obstructive pulmonary disease. Paper presented to the Fifth European Health Services Research Conference, Maastricht, December.

Brazier, J.E., Jones, N. and Kind, P. (1993b) Testing the validity of the EuroQol and comparing it with the SF-36 health survey questionnaire. *Quality of Life Research*, 2: 169–80.

Brazier, J.E., Roberts, J. and Deverill, M. (2002) The estimation of a preference-based measure of health from the SF-36. *Journal of Health Economics*, 21: 271–92.

Brazier, J., Roberts, J., Tsuchiya, A. and Busschbach, J. (2004). A comparison of the EQ-5D and SF-6D across seven patient groups. *Health Economics*, 13: 873–84.

Bridgwood, A. (2000) *People aged 65 and Over*. Results of an independent study carried out on behalf of the Department of Health as part of the 1998 General Household Survey. London: Office for National Statistics.

Brink, T.L., Curran, P., Dorr, M.L. *et al.* (1983) Geriatric Depression Scale reliability: order, examiner and reminiscence effects. *Clinical Gerontology*, 2: 57–60.

Brissette, I., Cohen, S. and Seeman, T.E. (2000) Measuring social integration and social networks, in S. Cohen, L.G. Underwood and B.H. Gottlieb (eds) *Social Support Measurement and Intervention. A Guide for Health and Social Scientists*. Oxford: Oxford University Press.

Brissette, I., Scheier, M.F. and Carver, C.S. (2002) The role of optimism in social network development, coping, and psychological adjustment during a life transition. *Journal of Personality and Social Psychology*, 82: 102–11.

Brissette, I., Leventhal, H. and Leventhal, E.A. (2003) Observer ratings of health and sickness: can other people tell us anything about our health that we don't already know? *Health Psychology*, 22: 471–8.

Brodman, K., Erdmann, A.J., Jr and Wolff, H.G. (1949) *Cornell Medical Index Health Questionnaire*. New York: Cornell University Medical College.

Brodman, K., Erdmann, A.J., Jr, Wolff, H.G. and Miskovitz, P.F. (1986) *Cornell Medical Index Health Questionnaire*. 1986 Revision. New York: Cornell University Medical College.

Bronfort, G. and Bouter, L.M. (1999) Responsiveness of general health status in chronic low back pain: a comparison of the COOP charts and the SF-36. *Pain*, 83: 201–9.

Brook, R.H., Ware, J.E., Davies-Avery, A. *et al.* (1979a) Overview of adult health status measures fielded in RAND's health insurance study. *Medical Care*, 17 (supplement), 1–131.

Brook, R.H., Ware, J.E., Davies-Avery, A. *et al.* (1979b) *Conceptualization and Measurement of Health for Adults in the Health Insurance Study*, vol. VIII, Overview. Santa Monica, CA: RAND Corporation, R-1987/8-HEW.

Brookings, J.B. and Bolton, B. (1988) Confirmatory factor analysis of the Interpersonal Support Evaluation List. *American Journal of Community Psychology*, 16: 137–47.

Brooks, R. (1996) EuroQol: the current state of play. *Health Policy*, 37: 53–72.

Brorsson, B. and Asberg, K.H. (1984) Katz Index of Independence in ADL: reliability and validity in short-term care. *Scandinavian Journal of Rehabilitative Medicine*, 16: 125–32.

Brouwer, W.B., Culyer, A.J., van Exel, N.J. and Rutten, F.F. (2008) Welfarism vs. extra-welfarism. Journal of Health Economics, 27: 325–38.

Brown, B., Bhrolchain, M. and Harris, T. (1975) Social class and psychiatric disturbance among women in an urban population. *Sociology*, 9: 225–54.

Brown, G.L. and Zung, W.W.K. (1972) Depression scales: self or physician rating? A validation of certain clinically observable phenomena. *Comprehensive Psychiatry*, 13: 361–7.

Brown, J., Bowling, A. and Flyn, T. (2004) *Models of Quality of Life: A Taxonomy, Overview and Systematic Review of Quality of Life*. Sheffield: Department of Sociological Studies, European Forum on Population Aging Research.

Brown, J.H., Lewis, M.D., Kazis, E. *et al.* (1984) The dimensions of health outcomes: a cross validated examination of health status measurement. *American Journal of Public Health*, 74: 159–61.

Browne, J.P. (1999) Selected methods for assessing individual quality of life, in C.R.B. Joyce, H.M. McGee and C.A. O'Boyle (eds) *Individual Quality of Life. Approaches to Conceptualisation and Assessment*. The Netherlands: Harwood Academic Publishers.

Browne, J.P., O'Boyle, C.A., McGee, H.M. *et al.* (1994) Individual quality of life in the healthy elderly. *Quality of Life Research*, 3: 235–44.

Browne, J.P., O'Boyle, C.A., McGee, H.M. *et al.* (1997) Development of a direct weighing procedure for quality of life domains. *Quality of Life Research*, 6: 301–9.

Bruce, B. and Fries, J.F. (2003a) The Stanford Health Assessment Questionnaire (HAQ): a review of its history, issues, progress and documentation. *Journal of Rheumatology*, 30: 167–78.

Bruce, B. and Fries, J.F. (2003b) The Stanford Health Assessment Questionnaire: dimensions and practical applications. *Health and Quality of Life Outcomes* (BioMed Central Ltd), 1: 20.

Bucquet, D., Condom, S. and Ritchie, K. (1990) The French version of the Nottingham Health Profile: a comparison of item weights with those of the source version. *Social Science and Medicine*, 30: 829–35.

Bullinger, M. (1995) German translation and psychometric testing of the SF-36 Health Survey: preliminary results from the IQOLA project. *Social Science and Medicine* (Special Issue 'Quality of Life'), 10: 1359–66.

Burchhardt, C.S., Woods, S.L., Schultz, A.A. *et al.* (1989) Quality of life of adults with chronic illness: a psychometric study. *Research on Nursing and Health*, 12: 347–54.

Bureau-Chalot, F., Novella, J-L., Jolly, D. *et al.* (2002) Feasibility, acceptability and internal consistency reliability of the Nottingham Health Profile in dementia patients. *Gerontology*, 24: 220–5.

Burnam, M.A., Wells, K.B., Leake, B. and Landsverk, J. (1988) Development of a brief screening instrument for detecting depressive disorders. *Medical Care*, 26: 775–89.

Burström, K., Johannesson, M., Diderichsen, F. *et al.* (2001) Swedish population health-related quality of life results using the EQ-5D. *Quality of Life Research*, 10: 621–35.

Bush, J.W. (1984) General health policy model: Quality of well-being (QWB) scale, in N.K. Wenger, M.E. Mattson and C.D. Furbergetal (eds) *Assessment of Quality of Life in Clinical Trials of Cardiovascular Therapies*. New York: Le Jacq.

Butow, P., Coates, A., Dunn, S., Bernhard, J. and Hurny, C. (1991) On the receiving end IV: validation of quality of life indicators. *Annals of Oncology*, 2: 597–603.

Buxton, M. (1983) The economics of heart transplant programmes: measuring the benefits, in G. Teeling Smith (ed.) *Measuring the Social Benefits of Medicine*. London: Office of Health Economics.

Buxton, M., Acheson, R.M., Caine, N. et al. (1985) Costs and Benefits of the Heart Transplantation Programmes at Harefield and Papworth Hospitals. London: Her Majesty's Stationery Office.

Byrne, D.G. (1978) Cluster analysis applied to self reported depressive symptomatology. Acta Psychiatrica Scandinavica, 57: 1–10.

Caine, N., Sharples, L.D., English, T.A.H. and Wallwork, J. (1990) Prospective study comparing quality of life before and after heart transplantation. Transplantation Proceedings, 22: 1437–9.

Caine, N., Harrison, S.C.W., Sharpies, L.D. and Wallwork, J. (1991) Prospective study of quality of life before and after coronary artery bypass grafting. British Medical Journal, 302: 511–16.

Cairl, R.E., Pfeiffer, E., Keller, D.M. et al. (1983) An evaluation of the reliability and validity of the functional assessment inventory. Journal of the American Geriatric Society, 31: 607–12.

Caldwell, R.A. and Reinhart, M.A. (1988) The relationship of personality to individual differences in the use of type and source of social support. Journal of Social and Clinical Psychology, 6: 140–6.

Calman, K.C. (1984) Quality of life in cancer patients – a hypothesis. Journal of Medical Ethics, 10: 124–7.

Camilleri-Brennan, J., Ruta, D.A. and Steele, R.J. (2002) Patient generated index: new instrument for measuring quality of life in patients with rectal cancer. World Journal of Surgery, 26: 1354–9.

Campbell, A. (1976) Subjective measures of well-being. American Psychologist, 31: 117–24.

Campbell, A. (1981) The Sense of Well-being in America. New York: McGraw-Hill.

Campbell, A., Converse, P.E. and Rogers, W.L. (1976) The Quality of American Life. New York: Russell Sage Foundation.

Campbell, L.J. and Fiske, D.W. (1959) Convergent and discriminant validation by the multitrait-multimethod matrix. Psychological Bulletin, 56: 81–105.

Campbell, P.B. (1967) School and self concept. Educational Leadership, 24: 510–15.

Campos, B., Schetter, C., Abdou, C. et al. (2008) Familialism, social support, and stress: positive implications for pregnant Latinas. Cultural Diversity and Ethnic Minority Psychology, 14: 155–62.

Cano, S.J., Lamping, D.L., Bamber, L. et al. (2012) The Anti-Clot Treatment Scale (ACTS) in clinical trials: cross-cultural validation in venous thromboembolism patients. Health and QoL Outcomes, 10: 120.

Cantril, H. (1965) The Pattern of Human Concerns. New Brunswick, NJ: Rutgers University Press.

Caplan, G. (1974) Support Systems and Community Mental Health. New York: Behavioral Publications.

Carp, F.M. (1977) What questions are we asking of whom? in C.N. Nydegger (ed.) Measuring Morale: A Guide to Effective Assessment. Washington, DC: Gerontology Society.

Carr-Hill, R. (1989) Assumption of the QALY procedure. Social Science and Medicine, 29: 469–77.

Carr-Hill, R. (1992) A second opinion: Health-related quality of life measurement – Euro style. Health Policy, 20: 321–8.

Carr-Hill, R. and Morris, J. (1991) Current practice in obtaining the 'Q' in QALYS – a cautionary note. British Medical Journal, 303: 699–701.

Carroll, B.J., Fielding, J.M. and Blash, T.G. (1973) Depression rating scales: a critical review. Archives of General Psychiatry, 28: 361–6.

Carroll, B.T., Kathol, R.G., Noyes, R. et al. (1993) Screening for depression and anxiety in cancer patients using the Hospital Anxiety and Depression Scale. Journal of General Hospital Psychiatry, 15: 69–74.

Carter, W., Bobbitt, R.A., Bergner, M. et al. (1976) Validation of an interval scaling: the Sickness Impact Profile. Health Services Research, 11: 516–28.

Cartwright, A. and Anderson, R. (1981) General Practice Revisited: A Second Study of Patients and Their Doctors. London: Tavistock Press.

Casellas, F., Lopez-Vivancos, J., Badia, X. et al. (2000) Impact of surgery for Crohn's disease on health-related quality of life. American Journal of Gastroenterology, 95: 177–82.

Cassel, J. (1976) The contribution of the social environment to host resistance. American Journal of Epidemiology, 104: 107–23.

Cavanaugh, S. (1983) The prevalence of emotional and cognitive dysfunction in a general medical population: using the MMSE, GHQ and BDI. General Hospital Psychiatry, 5: 15–24.

Celiker, R. and Borman, P. (2001) Fibromyalgia versus rheumatoid arthritis: a comparison of psychological disturbance and life satisfaction. Journal of Musculoskeletal Pain, 9: 35–45.

Chambers, L.W. (1984) The McMaster Health Index Questionnaire, in N.K. Wenger, M.E. Mattson, C.D. Furberg et al. (eds) Assessment of Quality of Life in Clinical Trials of Cardiovascular Therapies. New York: Le Jacq.

Chambers, L.W. (1993) The McMaster Health Index Questionnaire: an update, in S.R. Walker and R.M. Rosser (eds) *Quality of Life Assessment: Key Issues in the 1990s*. The Netherlands: Kluwer Academic Publishers.

Chambers, L.W. (1998) McMaster Health Index Questionnaire. Emotional Function Index scoring method, in S. Salek, *Compendium on Quality of Life Instruments*. Chichester: Wiley & Sons.

Chambers, L.W., Sackett, D.L., Goldsmith, C.H. *et al.* (1976) Development and application of an index of social function. *Health Services Research*, 11: 430–41.

Chambers, L.W., MacDonald, L.A., Tugwell, P. *et al.* (1982) The McMaster Health Index Questionnaire as a measure of quality of life for patients with rheumatoid disease. *Journal of Rheumatology*, 9: 780–4.

Chambers, L.W., Haight, M., Norman, G. *et al.* (1987) Sensitivity to change and the effect of mode of administration on health status measurement. *Medical Care*, 25: 470–9.

Chaplin, W.F. (1984) State–trait anxiety inventory, in D.J. Keyser and R.C. Sweetland (eds) *Test Critiques*, Vol. 1. Kansas City, MO: Test Corporation of America.

Chapman, P.L. and Mullis, A.K. (2002) Readdressing gender bias in the Coopersmith Self-Esteem Investory – Short Form. *Journal of Genetic Psychology*, 163: 403–9.

Charles, S.T., Reynolds, C.A. and Gatz, M. (2001) Age-related differences and change in positive and negative affect over 23 years. *Journal of Personality and Social Psychology*, 80: 136–51.

Charlton, J.R.H., Patrick, D.L. and Peach, H. (1983) Use of multivariate measures of disability in health surveys. *Journal of Epidemiology and Community Health*, 37: 296–304.

Chassany, O., Dimenäs, E., Dubois, D. and Wu, A. (2004) *The Psychological General Well-Being Index (PGWBI) User Manual*. Lyon: MAPI Research Institute, www: 178.23.156.107:8085/Instruments_ files/USERS/pgwbi.pdf, accessed 27 November 2015.

Chaturvedi, S.K. (1990) Asian patients and the HAD scale. *British Journal of Psychiatry*, 156: 133.

Cella, D. (1995) Methods and problems in measuring quality of life. *Support Care Cancer*, 3: 11–22.

Chen, Y., Hicks, A., While, A.E. (2014) Validity and reliability of the modified Chinese version of the Older People's Quality of Life Questionnaire (OPQOL) in older people living alone in China. *International Journal of Older People Nursing*, 9: 306–16.

Cheng, H. (2003) Personality, self-esteem, and demographic predictions of happiness and depression. *Journal of Personality and Individual Differences*, 34: 921–42.

Cherlin, A. and Reeder, L.G. (1975) The dimensions of psychological well being: a critical review. *Sociological Methods Research*, 4: 189–214.

Chiange, C.L. (1965) *An Index of Health: Mathematical Models*. Washington, DC: US Government Printing Office, PHS Publication no. 1000, Series 2, no. 5.

Chlan, L., Savik, K. and Weinert, C. (2003) Development of a shortened state anxiety scale from the Spielberger State–Trait Anxiety Inventory (STAI) for patients receiving mechanical ventilatory support. *Journal of Nursing and Measurement*, 11: 283–93.

Choi , M., Mesa-Frias M., Nuesch E., *et al.* (2014) Social capital, mortality, cardiovascular events and cancer: a systematic review of prospective studies. *International Journal of Epidemiology*, 43: 1895–920.

Chou, K.L. and Chi, I. (1999) Determinants of life satisfaction among Chinese older adults: a longitudinal study. *Ageing and Mental Health*, 3: 327–34.

Chou, K.L. and Chi, I. (2001) Stressful life events and depressive symptoms: social support and sense of control as mediators or moderators? *International Journal of Aging and Human Development*, 52: 155–71.

Christakou, A., Papadopoulos, E., Patsaki, I. *et al.* (2013) Functional assessment scales in a general intensive care unit. A review. *Hospital Chronicles*, 8: 164–70.

Clark, K.K., Borman, C.A., Cropanzano, R.S. and James, K. (1995) Validation evidence for three coping measures. *Journal of Personality Assessment*, 65: 434–55.

Clarke, P.J., Marshall, V.W., Ryff, C.D. and Wheaton, B. (2001) Measuring psychological well-being in the Canadian Study of Health and Aging. *International Psychogeriatrics*, 13: 79–90.

Cleary, P.D., Goldberg, D.M., Kessler, L.G. *et al.* (1982) Screening for mental disorder among primary care physicians: usefulness of the General Health Questionnaire. *Archives of General Psychiatry*, 39: 837–40.

Clinton, M., Lunney, P., Edwards, H. *et al.* (1998) Perceived social support and community adaptation in schizophrenia. *Journal of Advanced Nursing*, 27: 955–65.

Coates, A., Gebski, V., Stat, M. *et al.* (1987) Improving the quality of life during chemotherapy for advanced breast cancer. *New England Journal of Medicine*, 317: 1490–5.

Coates, A.K. and Wilkin, D. (1992) Comparing the Nottingham Health Profile with the Dartmouth COOP Charts, in J.H.G. Scholten (ed.) *Functional Status Assessment in Family Practice*. Lelystad: Meditekst.

Cobb, S. (1976) Social support as a moderator of life stress. *Psychosomatic Medicine*, 38: 300–14.

Cochrane, A.L. and Holland, W.W. (1971) Validation of screening procedures. *British Medical Bulletin*, 27: 3–8.

Cockerham, W.C. (1995) *Medical Sociology* (6th edn). Englewood Cliffs, NJ: Prentice Hall.

Coen, R., O'Mahony, D., O'Boyle, C.A. *et al.* (1993) Measuring the quality of life of dementia patients using the Schedule for the Evaluation of Individualised Quality of Life. *Irish Journal of Psychology*, 14: 154–63.

Coen, R.F., Swanwick, G.R., O'Boyle, C.A. and Coakley, D. (1997) Behaviour disturbance and other predictors of carer burden in Alzheimer's disease. *International Journal of Geriatric Psychiatry*, 12: 331–6.

Coen, R.F., O'Boyle, C.A., Swanwick, G.R.J. and Coakley, D. (1999) Measuring the impact on relatives of caring for people with Alzheimer's Disease: quality of life, burden and well-being. *Psychology and Health*, 14: 253–61.

Cohen, S., Mermelstein, R., Karmack, T. and Hoberman, H.M. (1985) Measuring the functional components of social support, in I.S. Saronson and B.R. Saronson (eds) *Social Support: Theory, Research and Applications*. Boston, MA: Martinus Nijhoff.

Cohen, C.I., Teresi, J. and Holmes, D. (1987) Social networks and mortality in an inner-city elderly population. *International Journal of Ageing and Human Development*, 24: 257–69.

Cohen, S., Underwood, L.G. and Gottlieb, B.H. (2000) Social relationships and health, in *Social Support Measurement and Intervention. A Guide for Health and Social Scientists*. New York: Oxford University Press.

Coleman, P. (1984) Assessing self-esteem and its sources in elderly people. *Ageing and Society*, 4: 117–35.

Collen, F.M., Wade, D.T. and Bradshaw, C.M. (1990) Mobility after stroke: reliability of measures of impairment and disability. *International Disability Studies*, 12: 6–9.

Collin, C., Wade, D.T., Davies, D. *et al.* (1988) The Barthel ADL Index: a reliability study. *International Disability Studies*, 10: 61–3.

Conner, K.A., Powers, E. and Bultena, G.L. (1979) Social interaction and life satisfaction: an empirical assessment of late life patterns. *Journal of Gerontology*, 34: 116–21.

Contreras, J., Mangelsdorf, S., Rhodes, J. *et al.* (1999) Parent-child interaction among Latino adolescent mothers: the role of family and social support. *Journal of Research on Adolescent*, 9: 417–39.

Convery, F.R., Minteer, M.A., Amiel, D. and Connett, K.L. (1977) Polyarticular disability: a functional assessment. *Archives of Physical Medicine and Rehabilitation*, 58: 494–9.

Cook, E.A. (1998) Effects of reminiscence on life satisfaction of elderly female nursing home residents. *Health Care Women International*, 19: 109–18.

Cooper, C.L. and Kasl, S.V. (1995) *Research Methods for Stress and Health Psychology*. Chichester: John Wiley.

Cooper, K., Arber, S., Fee, L. and Ginn, J. (1999) *The Influence of Social Support and Social Capital on Health: A Review and Analysis of British Data*. London: Health Education Authority.

Cooper, P.J. and Fairburn, C.G. (1986) The depressive symptoms of bulimia nervosa. *British Journal of Psychiatry*, 148: 268–74.

Coopersmith, S. (1967) *The Antecedents of Self-Esteem*. San Francisco, CA: W.H. Freeman, reprinted 1981.

Coopersmith, S. (1975) *Developing Motivation in Young Children*. San Francisco, CA: Albion Publishing.

Coopersmith, S. (1981a) *The Antecedents of Self-Esteem*. Palo Alto, CA: Consulting Psychologists Press.

Coopersmith, S. (1981b) *Self-esteem Inventories*. Palo Alto, CA: Consulting Psychologists Press.

Copeland, J.R.M., Kelleher, M.J., Kellet, J.M. *et al.* (1976) A semi-structured clinical interview for the assessment of diagnosis and mental state in the elderly: the Geriatric Mental State: Schedule 1. Development and reliability. *Psychological Medicine*, 6: 439–49.

Corcoran, J., Franklin, C. and Bennett, P. (1998) The use of the Social Support Behaviors Scale with adolescents. *Research on Social Work Practice*, 8: 302–14.

Costa, P.T., Zonderman, A.B., McRae, R.R. *et al.* (1987) Longitudinal analysis of psychological well-being in national samples: stability of mean levels. *Journal of Gerontology*, 42: 50–5.

Coulthard, M., Walker, A. and Morgan, A. (2001) *People's Perceptions of their Neighbourhood and Community Involvement. Results from the Social Capital Module of the General Household Survey 2000*. London: The Stationery Office.

Cox, B.D., Blaxter, M., Buckle, A.L.J. *et al.* (1987) *The Health and Lifestyle Survey*. London: Health Promotion Research Trust.

Cox, B.D., Huppert, F.A. and Whichelow, M.J. (1993) *The Health and Lifestyle Survey: Seven Years on*. London: Health Promotion Research Trust.

Crandall, R.C. (1973) The measurement of self esteem and related constructs, in J. Robinson and P. Shaver (eds) *Measures of Social Psychological Attitudes*. Ann Arbor, MI: Institute for Social Research.

Craven, P. and Wellman, B. (1974) The network city, in M.P. Effrat (ed.) *The Community: Approaches and Applications*. New York: Free Press.

Crawford-Little, J. and McPhail, N.I. (1973) Measures of depressive mood at monthly intervals. *British Journal of Psychiatry*, 122: 447–52.

Cronbach, L.J. (1951) Coefficient alpha and the internal structure of tests. *Psychometrika*, 22: 293–6.

Crooks, V.C., Lubben, J., Petitti, D.B. *et al.* (2008) Social network, cognitive function, and dementia incidence among elderly women. *American Journal of Public Health*, 98: 1221–7.

Crossley, T.F. and Kennedy, S. (2000) The stability of self-assessed health status. Social and Economic Dimensions of an Aging Population. SEDAP Research Paper no. 26. Canberra, ACT: SEDAP, Australian National University.

Crowne, D.P. and Marlowe, D. (1964) *The Approval Motive: Studies in Evaluation Dependence*. New York: John Wiley & Son.

Cuffel, B.J. and Akamatsu, T.J. (1989) The structure of loneliness: a factor-analytic investigation. *Cognitive Therapy and Research*, 13: 459–74.

Cummins, R. (2010) Subjective wellbeing, homeostatically protected mood and depression: a synthesis. *Journal of Happiness Studies*, 11: 1–17.

Dalton, D.S., Cruickshanks, K.J., Klein, B.E. *et al.* (2003) The impact of hearing loss on quality of life in older adults. *The Gerontologist*, 43: 661–8.

Dantas, R.A., Motzer, S.A. and Ciol, M.A. (2002) The relationship between quality of life, sense of coherence and self-esteem in persons after coronary artery bypass graft surgery. *International Journal of Nursing Studies*, 39: 745–55.

Davies, A.R. and Ware, J.E. (1981) *Measuring Health Perceptions in the Health Insurance Program*. Santa Monica, CA: RAND Corporation: R-2711-HHS.

Davies, B., Burrows, G. and Poynton, C.A. (1975) Comparative study of four depression rating scales. *Australian and New Zealand Journal of Psychiatry*, 9: 21–4.

Davies, A.R., Sherbourne, C.D., Peterson, J.R. and Ware, J.E. (1988) *Scoring Manual: Adult Health Status and Patient Satisfaction Measures Used in RAND's Health Insurance Experiment*. Publication No. N-2190HHS. Santa Monica, CA: RAND Corporation.

Dean, K., Holst, E., Kremer, S. *et al.* (1994) The measurement issues in research on social support and health. *Journal of Epidemiology and Community Health*, 48: 201–6.

Deary, I.J., Watson, R. A., Booth, T. and Gale, C.R. (2013) Does cognitive ability influence responses to the Warwick-Edinburgh Mental Well-Being Scale? *Psychological Assessment*, 25: 313–18.

de Bruin, A.F., de Witte, L.P., Stevens, F.C. and Diederiks, J.P. (1992) Sickness Impact Profile: the state of the art of a generic functional status measure. *Social Science and Medicine*, 8: 1003–14.

de Bruin, A.F., Diederiks, J.P.M., de Witte, L.P. and Stevens, F.C.J. (1993) The first testing of the SIP-68, a short generic version of the Sickness Impact Profile. Paper presented to the Fifth European Health Services Research Conference, Maastricht, December.

Deci, E.L., Ryan, R.M. (2008) Hedonia, eudaimonia, and well-being: an introduction. *Journal of Happiness Studies*, 9, 1–11.

de Girolamo, G., Rucci, P., Scocco, P. *et al.* (2000) Quality of life assessment: validation of the Italian version of the WHOQOL-Brief. *Epidemiol. Psichiatr. Soc.*, 9: 45–55.

de Haan, R., Limburg, M., Schuling, J. *et al.* (1993) Clinimetric evaluation of the Barthel Index, a measure of limitations in daily activities. *Netherlands Tijdschr Geneeskd*, 137: 917–21.

De Jong Gierveld, J. and Van Tilburg, T. (2006) A 6-item scale for overall, emotional, and social loneliness. Confirmatory tests on survey data. *Research on Aging*, 28: 582–98.

de Joode, E.W., van Meeteren, N.L., van den Berg, H.M. *et al.* (2001) Validity of health status measurement with the Dutch Arthritis Impact Measurement Scale 2 in individuals with severe haemophilia. *Haemophilia*, 7: 190–7.

de Leo, D., Diekstra, R.F.W., Lonnqvist, J. *et al.* (1998a) LEIPAD, an internationally applicable instrument to assess quality of life in the elderly. *Behavioural Medicine*, 24: 17–27.

de Leo, D., Diekstra, R.F.W., Lonnqvist, J. et al. (1998b) *LEIPAD Questionnaire. Compendium of Quality of Life Instruments*. Chichester, West Sussex: John Wiley & Sons.

Demetri, G.D., Gabrilove, J.L., Blasi, M.V. et al. (2002) Benefits of epoetin alfa in anemic breast cancer patients receiving chemotherapy. *Clinical Breast Cancer*, 3: 45–51.

Demyttenaere, K. and Fruyt, J. (2003) Getting what you asked for: on the selectivity of depression rating scales. *Psychotherapy Psychosomatics*, 72: 61–70.

Demyttenaere, K. Desaiah, D., Petit, C. et al. (2009) Patient-assessed versus physician-assessed disease severity and outcome in patients with nonspecific pain associated with major depressive disorder. *Journal of Clinical Psychiatry*, 11: 8–15.

Dennerstein, L., Dudley, E., Guthrie, J. and Barrett-Conner, E. (2000) Life satisfaction, symptoms, and the menopausal transition. *Medscape Women's Health*, 5: E4.

Denniston, O.L. and Jette, A.M. (1980) A functional status assessment instrument: validation in an elderly population. *Health Services Research*, 15: 21–4.

DeSalvo, K.B., Bloser, N., Reynolds, K. et al. (2006) Mortality prediction with a single general self-rated health question. *Journal of General Internal Medicine*, 21: 267–75.

Deyo, R.A. (1993) Measuring the quality of life of patients with rheumatoid arthritis, in S.R. Walker and R.M. Rosser (eds) *Quality of Life Assessment: Key Issues in the 1990s*. Dordrecht: Kluwer Academic.

Deyo, R.A., Inui, T.S., Leininger, J.D. et al. (1982) Physical and psychological functions in rheumatoid arthritis: clinical use of a self-administered instrument. *Archives of Internal Medicine*, 142: 879–82.

Deyo, R.A., Inui, T.S., Leininger, J.D. et al. (1983) Measuring functional outcomes in chronic disease: a comparison of traditional scales and a self-administered health status questionnaire in patients with rheumatoid arthritis. *Medical Care*, 21: 180–92.

Dias, R.C., Dias, J.M. and Ramos, L.R. (2003) Impact of an exercise and walking protocol on quality of life in elderly people with OA of the knee. *Physiotherapy Research International*, 8: 121–30.

Diener, E. and Suh, E. (1997) Measuring quality of life: economic, social and subjective indicators. *Social Indicators Research*, 40: 189–216.

Diener, E., Emmons, R.A., Larsen, R.J. and Griffin, S. (1985) The Satisfaction with Life Scale. *Journal of Personality Assessment*, 49: 71–5.

Diener, E., Sandvik, E., Pavot, W. and Gallagher, D. (1991) Response artefacts in the measurement of subjective well-being. *Social Indicators Research*, 24: 35–56.

Diener, E., Oishi, S. and Lucas, R.E. (2003) Personality, culture, and subjective well-being: emotional and cognitive evaluations of life. *Annual Review of Psychology*, 54: 403–25.

Diener, E., Tay, L. and Myers, D. (2011) The religion paradox: if religion makes people happy, why are so many dropping out? *Journal of Personality and Social Psychology*, 101: 1278–90.

Diener, E., Ronald F., Inglehart, R.F. and Tay, L. (2013) Theory and validity of life satisfaction scales. *Social Indicators Research*, 112: 497–527.

Doble, S.E., Fisk, J.D., MacPherson, K.M. et al. (1997) Measuring functional competence in older persons with Alzheimer's disease. *International Psychogeriatics*, 9: 25–38.

Dobson, C., Powers, E.A., Keith, P.M. et al. (1979) Anomie, self-esteem, and life satisfaction: interrelationships amog three scales of well-being. *Journal of Gerontology*, 34: 569–72.

Dodds, T.A., Martin, D.P., Stolov, W.C. et al. (1993) A validation of the Functional Independence measure (FIM). Measurement of its performance among rehabilitation patients. *Archives of Physical Medicine Rehabilitation*, 74: 531–6.

Dodge, R., Daly, A., Huyton, J. and Sanders, L. (2012) The challenge of defining wellbeing. *International Journal of Wellbeing*, 2: 222–35.

Doherty, T., Njegovan, N. and Sandhu, V. (2013) Hospital anxiety and depression scale (HADS) results in ankylosing spondylitis (AS). *Annals of Rheumatic Disorders*, 72, Supplement A962.

Dolan, P. (1997) Modelling valuations for EuroQol health states. *Medical Care*, 35: 1095–108.

Dolan, P., Gudex, C., Kind, P. and Williams, A. (1996) The time-trade-off method: results from a general population study. *Health Economics*, 5: 141–54.

Donald, C.A. and Ware, J.E. (1982) *The Quantification of Social Contacts and Resources*. Santa Monica, CA: RAND Corporation R-2937-HHS.

Donald, C.A., Ware, J.E., Brook, R.H. et al. (1978) *Conceptualization and Measurement of Health for Adults in the Health Insurance Study, vol. IV, Social Health*. Santa Monica, CA: RAND Corporation R-1987/4HEW.

Dorman, P.J., Slattery, J., Farrell, B. *et al.* (1997a) A randomised comparison of the EuroQol and Short Form-36 after stroke. *British Medical Journal*, 315: 416.

Dorman, P.J., Waddell, F., Slattery, J. *et al.* (1997b) Are proxy assessments of health status after stroke with the EuroQol questionnaire feasible, accurate, and unbiased? *Stroke*, 28: 1883–7.

Dozois, D.J. (2003) The psychometric characteristics of the Hamilton Depression Inventory. *Journal of Personality Assessment*, 80: 31–40.

Dubec, N., Haley, S.M., Ni, P. *et al.* (2004) Function and disability in late life: comparison of the Late-Life Function and Disability instrument to the Short-Form-36 and the London Handicap Scale. *Disability and Rehabilitation*, 26: 362–70.

Dubuisson, D. and Melzack, R. (1976) Classification of clinical pain descriptions by multiple group discriminant analysis. *Experimental Neurology*, 51: 480–7.

Dunnell, K. and Cartwright, A. (1972) *Medicine Takers, Prescribers and Hoarders*. London: Routledge & Kegan Paul.

Dupuy, H.J. (1973) *Developmental Rationale, Substantive, Derivable, and Conceptual Relevance of the General Well-Being Schedule*. Fairfax, VA: National Center for Health Statistics.

Dupuy, H.J. (1974) Utility of the National Center for Health Statistics' General Well-Being Schedule in the Assessment of Self-Representations of Subjective Well-Being and Distress, in *Report of The National Conference on Evaluation in Alcohol, Drug Abuse and Mental Health Programs*. Washington, DC: ADA MHA.

Dupuy, H.J. (1978) Self representations of general psychological well-being of American adults. Paper presented at American Public Health Association Meeting. Los Angeles, California, 17 October.

Dupuy, H.J. (1984) The psychological General Well-being Index, in N.K. Wenger, M.E. Mattson, C.D. Furberg *et al.* (eds) *Assessment of Quality of Life in Clinical Trials of Cardiovascular Therapies*. New York: Le Jacq.

Durkheim, E. (1895) *The Rules of Sociological Method* (ed. S. Lukes, trans. W.D. Halls 1938). Free Press, New York, reprinted 1982.

Durkheim, E. (1897) *Suicide: A Study in Sociology* (ed. G. Stimpson, trans. J.A. Spaulding and G. Stimpson 1951). Free Press, New York, reprinted 1997.

Dworkin, R.H., Turk, D.C., Revicki, D.A. *et al.* (2009) Development and initial validation of an expanded and revised version of the Short-form McGill Pain Questionnaire (SF-MPQ). *Pain*, 144: 35–42.

Earl-Slater, A. (2002) *The Handbook of Clinical Trials and other Research*. Oxford: Radcliffe Medical Press.

Edwards, D.W., Yarvis, R.M., Mueller, D.P. *et al.* (1978) Test-taking and the stability of adjustment scales: can we assess patient deterioration? *Evaluation Q*, 2: 275–91.

Edwards, J.N. and Klemmack, D.L. (1973) Correlates of life satisfaction: a re-examination. *Journal of Gerontology*, 28: 479–502.

Eisenberg, E., Damunni, G., Hoffer, E. *et al.* (2003) Lamotrigine for intractable sciatica: correlation between dose plasma concentration and analgesia. *European Journal of Pain*, 7: 485–91.

Eklund, M., Bengtsson-Tops, A. and Lindstedt, H. (2007) Construct and discriminant validity and dimensionality of the Interview Schedule for Social Interaction (ISSI) in three psychiatric samples. Nordic Journal of Psychiatry, 61: 182–8.

Ellwardt, L., Van Tilburg, T.G. and Aartsen, M.J. (2015) The mix matters: complex personal relationships relate to higher cognitive functioning in old age. *Social Science and Medicine*, 125: 107–15.

Emmons, R.A. and Diener, E. (1985) Personality correlates of subjective well-being. *Personality and Social Psychology Bulletin*, 11: 89–97.

Eriksson, M. and Lindström, B. (2005) Validity of Antonovsky's sense of coherence scale: a systematic review. *Journal of Epidemiology and Community Health*, 59: 460–6.

Eriksson, M., Lindström, B. and Lija, J. (2007) A sense of coherence and health. Salutogenesis in a societal context: Åand, a special case? *Journal of Epidemiology and Community Health*, 61: 684–8.

Eskin, M. (1993) Swedish translations of the Suicide Probability Scale, Perceived Social Support from Family and Friends Scales, and the Scale for Interpersonal Behavior: a reliability analysis. *Scandinavian Journal of Psychology*, 34: 276–81.

Espwall, M. and Olofsson, N. (2002) Social networks of women with undefined musculoskeletal disorder. *Social Work in Health Care*, 36: 77–91.

EuroQol Group (1990) EuroQol – a new facility for the measurement of health-related quality of life. *Health Policy*, 16: 199–208.

Evans, D. and Cope, W. (1994) *The Quality of Life Questionnaire– D. Complete Kit*. Northern Tonawanda, New York: Multi-Health Systems.

Evans, K., Tyrer, P., Catalan, J. et al. (1999) Manual assisted cognitive-behavior therapy (MACT): a randomised controlled trial of a brief intervention with bibliotherapy in the treatment of recurrent deliberate self-harm. *Psychological Medicine*, 29: 19–25.

Evans, R.W., Manninen, D.L., Overcast, T.D. et al. (1984) *The National Heart Transplantation Study: Final Report*. Seattle, WA: Battelle Human Affairs Research Centre.

Fallowfield, L.J., Baum, M. and Maguire, G.P. (1987) Do psychological studies upset patients? *Journal of the Royal Society of Medicine*, 80: 59.

Fanshel, S. and Bush, J.W. (1970) A health status index and its applications to health services outcomes. *Operational Research*, 18: 1021–65.

Farmer, M.M. and Ferraro, K.F. (1997) Distress and perceived health: mechanisms of health decline. *Journal of Health and Social Behaviour*, 38: 298–311.

Farquhar, M. (1995a) Definitions of quality of life: a taxonomy. *Journal of Advanced Nursing*, 22: 502–8.

Farquhar, M. (1995b) Elderly people's definitions of quality of life. Special Issue 'Quality of Life' in *Social Science and Medicine*, 10: 1439–46.

Fayers, P.M. and Hand, D.J. (2002) Causal variables, indicator variables and measurement scales: an example from quality of life. *Journal of the Royal Statistical Association*, 165, Part 2: 1–21.

Fazio, A.F. (1977) *A Concurrent Validation Study of the NCHS General Well-Being Schedule*. Vital and Health Statistics Series 2, no. 73 DHEW Publication No. (HRA) 78–1347. Hyattsville, MD: US Department of Health, Education and Welfare, National Center for Health Statistics.

Fillenbaum, G.G. (1978) Multi-dimensional functional assessment: The OARS Methodology – A Manual, 2nd edn. Durham, NC: Center for the Study of Aging and Human Development, Duke University.

Fillenbaum, G.G. (1988) *Multidimensional Functional Assessment of Older Adults: the Duke Older Americans Resources and Services Procedures*. Hillsdale, NJ: Lawrence Erlbaum. Updated 1996 (available only from Center for the Study of Aging and Human Development, Duke University Medical Center, Durham, NC 27710).

Fillenbaum, G.G. and Smyer, M.A. (1981) The development, validity and reliability of the OARS multidimensional functional assessment questionnaire: disability and pain scales. *Journal of Gerontology*, 36: 428–33.

Finch, J. (1989) *Family Obligations and Social Change*. Cambridge: Policy Press.

Finlay Jones, R.A. and Murphy, E. (1979) Severity of psychiatric disorder and the 30-item General Health Questionnaire. *British Journal of Psychiatry*, 134: 609–16.

Fiore, J., Coppel, D.B., Becker, J. et al. (1986) Social support as a multifaceted concept: examination of important dimensions for adjustment. *American Journal of Community Psychology*, 14: 93–111.

Fiori, K.L., Smith, J. and Antonucci, T.C. (2007) Social network types among older adults: a multidimensional approach. *Journal of Gerontology (Psychological Sciences)*, 62B: 322–30.

Firat, S., Byhardt, R.W. and Gore, E. (2002) Comorbidity and Karnofsky performance score are independent prognostic factors in stage III non-small-cell lung cancer: an institutional analysis of patients treated on four RTOG studies. Radiation Therapy Oncology Group. *International Journal of Radiation Oncology Biology Physiology*, 54: 357–64.

Fitts, W.H. (1965) *Tennessee Self-Concept Scale Manual*. Nashville, TN: Counselor Recordings and Tests.

Fitts, W.H. (1972) *The Self-Concept and Performance*, Research Monograph no. 5. Nashville, TN: Social and Rehabilitation Service.

Fitts, W.H. and Warren, W.L. (1996) *Tennessee Self-Concept Scale* (4th edn). Los Angeles, CA: Western Psychological Corporation.

Fitzpatrick, R. (1999) Assessment of quality of life as an outcome: finding measurements that reflect individual's priorities (editorial). *Quality in Health Care*, 8: 1–2.

Fitzpatrick, R., Newman, S., Lamb, R. and Shipley, M. (1988) Social relationships and psychological wellbeing in rheumatoid arthritis. *Social Science and Medicine*, 27: 399–403.

Fitzpatrick, R., Newman, S., Lamb, R. and Shipley, M. (1989) A comparison of measures of health status in rheumatoid arthritis. *British Journal of Rheumatology*, 28: 201–6.

Fitzpatrick, R., Ziebland, S., Jenkinson, C. and Mowat, A. (1992) A generic health status instrument in the assessment of rheumatoid arthritis. *British Journal of Rheumatology*, 31: 87–90.

Fjartoft, H., Indredavik, B. and Lydersen, S. (2003) Stroke unit care combined with early supported discharge. Long-term follow-up of a randomised controlled trial. *Stroke*, 34: 2691–2.

Flax, M.J. (1972) *A Study in Comparative Urban Indicators: Conditions in 18 Large Metropolitan Areas.* Washington, DC: The Urban Institute.

Fleck, M.P., Louzada, S., Xavier, M. *et al.* (2000) Application of the Portugese version of the abbreviated instrument of quality of life WHOQOL-BREF. *Rev Saude Publica*, 34: 178–83.

Fletcher, A., McLoone, P. and Bulpitt, C. (1988) Quality of life on angina therapy: a randomized controlled trial of transdermal glyceryl trinitrate against placebo. *Lancet*, 2: 4–8.

Folstein, M.F., Folstein, S.E. and McHugh, P.R. (1975) 'Mini-Mental State': A practical method for grading the cognitive state of patients for the clinician. *Journal of Psychiatric Research*, 12: 189–98.

Forsberg, C. and Bjorvell, H. (1993) Swedish population norms for the GHRI, HI and STAI-state. *Quality of Life Research*, 2: 349–56.

Fortinsky, R.H., Granger, C.V. and Selzer, G.B. (1981) The use of functional assessment in understanding home care needs. *Medical Care*, 19: 489–97.

Fountoulakis, K.N., Lacovides, A., Samolis, S. *et al.* (2001) Reliability, validity and psychometric properties of the Greek translation of the Zung depression rating scale. *BMC Psychiatry*, 1: 6.

Francis, D. (1984) *Will You Still Need Me, Will You Still Feed Me, When I'm 84?* Bloomington, IN: Indiana University Press.

Franke, G.H., Reimer, J., Philipp, T. and Heemann, U. (2003) Aspects of quality of life through end-stage renal disease. *Quality of Life Research*, 12: 103–15.

Freedland, K.E., Skala, J.A., Carney, R.M. *et al.* (2002) The Depression Interview and Structured Hamilton (DISH): rationale, development, characteristics, and clinical validity. *Psychosomatic Medicine*, 64: 897–905.

Freemantle, N., Long, A., Mason, J. *et al.* (1993) The treatment of depression in primary care. *Effective Health Care*, 5 (whole issue).

Fries, J.F. (1983) The assessment of disability: from first to future principles. Paper presented at conference, Advances in Assessing Arthritis, held at the London Hospital, March (mimeo).

Fries, J.F., Hess, E.V. and Klinenberg, J. (1974) A standard database for rheumatic disease. *Arthritis and Rheumatism*, 17: 327–36.

Fries, J.F., Spitz, P.W., Kraines, R.G. and Holman, H.R. (1980) Measurement of patient outcome in arthritis. *Arthritis and Rheumatism*, 23: 137–45.

Fries, J.F., Spitz, P.W. and Young, D.Y. (1982) The dimensions of health outcomes: the Health Assessment Questionnaire, disability and pain scales. *Journal of Rheumatology*, 9: 789–93.

Frisch, M.B., Cornell, J., Villanueva, M. and Retzlaff, P.J. (1992) Clinical validation of the Quality of Life Inventory. A measure of life satisfaction for use in treatment planning and outcome assessment. *Psychological Assessment*, 4: 92–101.

Frosch, D.L., Kaplan, R.M., Ganiats, T.G. *et al.* (2004) Validity of self-administered Quality of Well-being Scale in musculoskeletal disease. *Arthritis & Rheumatism*, 51: 28–33.

Fry, P.S. (2000) Whose quality of life is it anyway? Why not ask seniors to tell us about it? *International Journal of Aging and Human Development*, 50: 361–83.

Fryback, D.G., Dunham, N.C., Palta, M. *et al.* (2007) US norms for six generic health-related quality of life indexes from the National Health Measurement study. *Medical Care*, 45: 1162–70.

Gallagher, D., Nies, G. and Thompson, L.W. (1982) Reliability of the Beck Depression Inventory with older adults. *Journal of Consulting and Clinical Psychology*, 50: 152–3.

Gallegos-Orozco, J.F., Fuentes, A.P., Gerardo Argueta, J. *et al.* (2003) Health-related quality of life and depression in patients with chronic hepatitis C. *Archives Medical Research*, 34: 124–9.

Gana, K. and Garnier, S. (2001) Latent structure of the sense of coherence scale in a French sample. *Journal of Personality and Individual Differences*, 31: 1079–90.

Gandek, B. and Ware, J.E. (eds) (1998) Translating functional health and well-being: International quality of life assessment (IQOLA) project studies of the SF-36 Health Survey. *Journal of Clinical Epidemiology*, 51: 891–1214.

Garratt, A.M. and Ruta, D.A. (1999) The Patient Generated Index, in C.R.B. Joyce, C.A. O'Boyle and H. McGee, *Individual Quality of Life. Approaches to Conceptualisation and Assessment.* Amsterdam: Harwood Academic Publishers.

Garratt, A.M., Ruta, D.A., Abdalla, M.I. *et al.* (1993) The SF-36 health survey questionnaire: an outcome measure suitable for routine use within the NHS? *British Medical Journal*, 306: 1440–4.

Garratt, A.M., Ruta, D.A., Abdalla, M.I. and Russell, I.T. (1994) SF-36 health survey questionnaire: II. Responsiveness to changes in health status in four common clinical conditions. *Quality in Health Care*, 3: 186–92.

Garratt, A.M., Schmidt, L., Mackintosh, A. and Fitzpatrick, R. (2002) Quality of life measurement: bibliographic study of patient assessed health outcome measures. *British Medical Journal*, 324: 1417.

Gatz, M., Pederson, N.L. and Harris, J. (1987) Measurement characteristics of the mental health scale from the OARS. *Journal of Gerontology*, 42: 332–5.

Gavazzi, S.M. (1994) Perceived social support from family and friends in a clinical sample of adolescents. *Journal of Personality Assessment*, 62: 465–71.

Gee, C. and Rhodes, J. (2008) A social support and strain measure for minority adolescent mothers: a confirmatory factor analytic study. *Child: Care, Health and Development*, 34: 87–97.

George, L.K. (1979) The happiness syndrome: methodological and substantive issues in the study of psychological well-being in adulthood. *Gerontologist*, 19: 210–16.

George, L.K. and Bearon, L.B. (1980) *Quality of Life in Older Persons: Meaning and Measurement*. New York: Human Sciences Press.

George, L.K., Blazer, D.G., Hughes, D.C. *et al.* (1989) Social support and the outcome of major depression. *British Journal of Psychiatry*, 154: 478–85.

Gibbons, R.D., Clark, D.C. and Kupfer, D.J. (1993) Exactly what does the Hamilton Depression Rating Scale measure? *Journal of Psychiatric Research*, 27: 259–73.

Gilson, B.S., Bergner, M., Bobbitt, R.A. *et al.* (1979) *The Sickness Impact Profile: Final Development and Testing: 1975–1978*. Seattle, WA: University of Washington Press.

Gjesfjeld, C., Greeno, C., Kim, K. and Anderson, C. (2010) Economic stress, social support, and maternal depression: is social support deterioration occurring? *Social Work Research*, 34: 135–3.

Glass, T.A. and Maddox, G.L. (1992) The quality and quantity of social support: stroke recovery as psychosocial transition. *Social Science and Medicine*, 34: 1249–61.

Goldberg, D.P. (1978) *Manual of the General Health Questionnaire*. Windsor: NFER-Nelson.

Goldberg, D.P. (1985) Identifying psychiatric illness among general medical patients. *British Medical Journal*, 291: 161–3.

Goldberg, D.P. and Hillier, V.F. (1979) A scaled version of the General Health Questionnaire. *Psychological Medicine*, 9: 139–45.

Goldberg, D.P. and Huxley, P. (1980) *Mental Illness in the Community: The Pathway to Psychiatric Care*. London: Tavistock.

Goldberg, D.P. and Williams, P. (1988) *A User's Guide to the General Health Questionnaire*. Windsor: NFERNelson.

Golden, J., Conroy, R.M., Bruce, I. *et al.* (2009) Loneliness, social support networks, mood and wellbeing in community-dwelling elderly. *International Journal of Geriatric Psychiatry*, 24: 694–700.

Goldstein, M.S., Siegel, J.M. and Boyer, R. (1984) Predicting changes in perceived health status. *American Journal of Public Health*, 74: 611–15.

Gompertz, P., Pound, P. and Ebrahim, S. (1993a) The reliability of stroke outcome measurement. *Clinical Rehabilitation*, 7: 290–6.

Gompertz, P., Pound, P. and Ebrahim, S. (1993b) *Kudos: A Kit for Describing the Outcome of Stroke*. London: Department of Public Health, Royal Free Hospital Medical School.

Goodchild, M.E. and Duncan Jones, P. (1985) Chronicity and the General Health Questionnaire. *British Journal of Psychiatry*, 146: 55–61.

Goodrick, G.K., Pendleton, V.R., Kimball, K.T. *et al.* (1999) Binge eating severity, self-concept, dieting self-efficiency and social support during treatment of binge eating disorder. *International Journal of Eating Disorders*, 26: 295–300.

Gough, I.R., Furnival, C.M., Schilder, L. *et al.* (1983) Assessment of the quality of life of patients with advanced cancer. *European Journal of Cancer and Clinical Oncology*, 19: 1161–5.

Grady, K.L., Meyer, P.M., Dressler, D. *et al.* (2003) Change in quality of life from after left ventricular assist device implantation to after heart transplantation. *Journal of Heart and Lung Transplantation*, 22: 1254–67.

Grafton, K.V., Foster, N.E. and Wright, C.C. (2005) Test-retest reliability of the Short-Form McGill Pain Questionnaire: assessment of intraclass correlation coefficients and limits of agreement in patients with osteoarthritis. *Clinical Journal of Pain*, 21: 73–82.

Granger, C.V. (1982) Health accounting-functional assessment of the long-term patient, in F.J. Kottke, G.K. Stillwell and J.F. Lehmann (eds) *Krusen's Handbook of Physical Medicine and Rehabilitation*, 3rd edn. Philadelphia, PA: W.B. Saunders.

Granger, C.V. and McNamara, M.A. (1984) Functional assessment utilization: the long-range evaluation system (LRES), in C.V. Granger and G.E. Gresham (eds) *Functional Assessment in*

Rehabilitation Medicine. Baltimore, MD: Williams & Williams.

Granger, C.V., Albrecht, G.L. and Hamilton, B.B. (1979) Outcome of comprehensive medical rehabilitation: measurement by PULSES profile and the Barthel Index. *Archives of Physical Medicine and Rehabilitation*, 60: 145–54.

Grant, C.R.H. (1966) Age differences in self-concept from early adulthood through old age. Dissertation from the University of Nebraska.

Grasbeck, R. and Saris, N.E. (1969) Establishment and use of normal values. *Scandinavian Journal of Clinical and Laboratory Investigation*, Supplement no. 110: 62–3.

Greenberger, E., Chen, C., Dmitrieva, J. and Farruggia, S.P. (2003) Item-wording and the dimensionality of the Rosenberg Self-Esteem Scale: do they matter? *Journal of Personality and Individual Differences*, 35: 1241–54.

Greenblatt, H.N. (1975) *Measurement of Social Well-being in a General Population Survey*. Berkeley, CA: Human Population Laboratory, California State Department of Health.

Greenwald, H.P. (1987) The specificity of quality of life measures among the seriously ill. *Medical Care*, 25: 642–51.

Greiner, P.A., Snowdon, D.A. and Greiner, L.H. (1999) Self-rated function, self-rated health, and postmortem evidence of brain infarcts: findings from the Nun study. *Journal of Gerontology (B)*, 54: S219–22.

Griffiths, R.A., Beaumont, P.J., Giannakopoulos, E. et al. (1999) Measuring self-esteem in dieting disordered patients: the validity of the Rosenberg and Coopersmith contrasted. *International Journal of Eating Disorders*, 25: 227–31.

Groessl, E.J., Kaplan, R.M. and Cronan, T.A. (2003) Quality of well-being in older people with osteoarthritis. *Arthritis and Rheumatism*, 49: 23–8.

Grossi, E., Groth, N., Mosconi, P. et al. (2006) Development and validation of the short version of the Psychological General Well-Being Index (PGWB-S). *Health and Quality of Life Outcomes*, 4: 88.

Groth-Marnat, G. (1990) *The Handbook of Psychological Assessment*, 2nd edn. New York: John Wiley and Sons.

Grummon, K., Rigby, E.D., Orr, D. et al. (1994) Psychosocial variables that affect the psychological adjustment of IVDU patients with AIDS. *Journal of Clinical Psychology*, 50: 488–502.

Grundy, E. and Bowling, A. (1999) Enhancing the quality of extended life years. Identification of the oldest old with a very good and very poor quality of life. *Ageing and Mental Health*, 3: 199–212.

Grundy, E., Bowling, A. and Farquhar, M. (1996) Social support, life satisfaction and survival at older ages, in G. Casselli and A. Lopez (eds) *Health and Mortality among Elderly Populations*. Oxford: Clarendon Press.

Guillemin, F., Coste, J., Pouchot. J. et al. (1997) The AIMS2-SF: a short form of the Arthritis Impact Measurement Scales-2 – French quality of life in rheumatology group. *Arthritis and Rheumatism*, 40: 1267–74.

Guillon, M.S., Crocq, M.A. and Bailey, P.E. (2003) The relationship between self-esteem and psychiatric disorders in adolescents. *European Psychiatry*, 18: 59–62.

Guralnik, J.M., Simonsick, E.M., Ferrucci, L. et al. (1994) A short physical performance battery assessing lower extremity function: associations with self-reported disability and prediction of mortality and nursing home admission. *Journals of Gerontology*, 49: M85–94.

Gurin, G., Vero., J. and Feld, S. (1960) *Americans View their Mental Health*. New York: Basic Books.

Gurtman, M.B. (1985) Self-rating Depression Scale, in D.J. Keyser and R.C. Sweetland (eds) *Test Critiques*, Vol. III. Kansas City, MO: Test Corporation of America.

Guttman, L. (1944) A basis for scaling qualitative data. *American Sociological Review*, 9: 139.

Guyatt, G.H., Berman, L.B., Townsend, M. et al. (1987) A measure of quality of life for clinical trials in chronic lung disease. *Thorax*, 42: 773–8.

Guyatt, G.H., Nogradi, S., Halcrow, S. et al. (1989) Development and testing of a new measure of health status for clinical trials in heart failure. *Journal of General Internal Medicine*, 4: 101–7.

Guyatt, G.H., Eagle, D.J., Sackett, B. et al. (1993) Measuring quality of life in the frail elderly. *Journal of Clinical Epidemiology*, 46: 1433–44.

Haavardsholm, E.A., Kvien, T.K., Uhlig, T. et al. (2000) A comparison of agreement and sensitivity to change between AIMS2 and a short form of AIMS2 (AIMS2-SF) in more than 1,000 rheumatoid arthritis patients. *Journal of Rheumatology*, 27: 2810–16.

Haber, L.D. (1968) *Prevalence of Disability among Noninstitutionalized Adults under Age 65: 1966 Survey of Disabled Adults*, Research and Statistics Note no. 4. US Department of Health Education and Welfare, Office of Research and Statistics.

Hagerty M.R., Cummins, R.A., Ferriss, A.L. *et al.* (2001) Quality of life indexes for national policy: review and agenda for research. *Social Indicators Research,* 55: 1–96.

Hagg, O., Fritzell, P., Nordwall, A. and the Swedish Lumbar Spine Study Group (2003) The clinical importance of changes in outcome scores after treatment for low back pain. *European Spine Journal,* 12: 12–20.

Haley, S.M., McHorney, C.A. and Ware, J.E. (1994) Evaluation of the MOS SF-36 Physical Functioning Scale (PF-10): I. Unidimensionality and reproducibility of the Rasch item scale. *Journal of Clinical Epidemiology,* 47: 671–84.

Hall, J., Hall, N., Fisher, E. *et al.* (1987) Measurement of outcomes of general practice: comparison of three health status measures. *Family Practice,* 4: 117–23.

Hall, K.M. (1992) Overview of functional assessment scales in brain injury rehabilitation. *Neuro Rehabilitation,* 2: 97–112.

Hall, K.M. (1997) The Functional Assessment Measure (FAM). *Journal of Rehabilitation Outcome Measures,* 1: 63–5.

Hall, K.M., Mann, N., High, W. *et al.* (1996). Functional measures after traumatic brain injury: ceiling effects of FIM, FIM+FAM, DRS and CIQ. *Journal of Head Trauma Rehabilitation,* 11: 27–39.

Hall, R., Horrocks, J.C., Clamp, S.E. *et al.* (1976) Observer variation in assessment of results of surgery for peptic ulceration. *British Medical Journal,* i: 814–16.

Hamer, D., Sanjeev, D., Butterworth, E. and Barzak, P. (1991) Using the Hospital Anxiety and Depression Scale to screen for psychiatric disorders in people presenting with deliberate self-harm. *British Journal of Psychiatry,* 158: 782–4.

Hamilton, B.B., Laughlin, J.A., Granger, C.V. *et al.* (1991) Interrater agreement of the seven level Functional Independence Measure (FIM). *Archives of Physical Medical Rehabilitation,* 72: 790.

Hamilton, M. (1959) The assessment of anxiety states by rating. *British Journal of Medical Psychology,* 32: 50–5.

Hamilton, M. (1960) Rating scale for depression. *Journal of Neurology, Neurosurgery and Psychiatry,* 23: 56–62.

Hamilton, M. (1967) Development of a rating scale for primary depressive illness. *British Journal of Social and Clinical Psychology,* 6: 278–96.

Hamilton, M. (1976) Clinical evaluation of depression: clinical criteria and rating scales, including a Guttman Scale, in M. Gallant and G.M. Simpson (eds) *Depression: Behavioral, Biochemical Diagnostic and Treatment Concepts.* New York: Spectrum Publications.

Hammen, C.L. (1981) Assessment: a clinical and cognitive emphasis, in L.P. Rehm (ed.) *Behaviour Therapy for Depression: Present Status and Future Directions.* New York: Academic Press.

Hamrén, K., Chungkham, H.S. and Hyde, M. (2015) Religion, spirituality, social support and quality of life: measurement and predictors CASP-12 (v2) amongst older Ethiopians living in Addis Ababa. *Aging and Mental Health,* 19: 610–21.

Hankins, M. (2008) The factor structure of the twelve item General Health Questionnaire (GHQ-12): the result of negative phrasing? *Clinical Practice and Epidemiology in Mental Health,* 4: 10.

Hanley, J.A. and McNeil, B.J. (1982) The meaning and use of the area under a Receiver Operating Characteristic (ROC) curve. *Radiology,* 143: 29–36.

Harman, H.H. (1976) *Modern Factor Analysis.* Chicago, IL: University of Chicago Press.

Harrington, R. and Loffredo, D.A. (2001) The relationship between life satisfaction, self-consciousness, and the Myers-Briggs type inventory dimensions. *Journal of Psychology,* 135: 439–50.

Harris, L. (1975) *The Myth and Reality of Ageing in America.* Washington, DC: National Council on the Ageing.

Hart, G.L. and Evans, R.W. (1987) The functional status of ESRD patients as measured by the Sickness Impact Profile. *Journal of Chronic Diseases,* 40: 117S–130S (Supplement).

Harvey, I., Nelson, S.J., Lyons, R.A. *et al.* (1998) A randomised controlled trial and economic evaluation of counselling in primary care. *British Journal of General Practice,* 48: 1043–8.

Harwood, R.H. and Ebrahim, S. (1995) *Manual of the London Handicap Scale.* Nottingham: University of Nottingham, Department of Health Care of the Elderly.

Harwood, R.H., Rogers, A., Dickinson, E. and Ebrahim, S. (1994) Measuring handicap: the London Handicap Scale, a new outcome measure for chronic disease. *Quality in Health Care,* 3: 11–16.

Harwood, R.H., Carr, A.J., Thompson, P.W. and Ebrahim, S. (1996) Handicap in inflammatory arthritis. *British Journal of Rheumatology,* 35: 891–7.

Harwood, R.H., Gompertz, P., Pound, P. and Ebrahim, E. (1997) Determinants of handicap 1 and 3 years after stroke. *Disability and Rehabilitation*, 19: 205–11.

Harwood, R.H., Prince, M., Mann, A. and Ebrahim, S. (1998a) Associations between diagnoses, impairments, disability and handicap in a population of elderly people. *Journal of Epidemiology*, 27: 261–8.

Harwood, R.H., Prince, M., Mann, A. and Ebrahim, S. (1998b) The prevalence of diagnoses, impairments, disabilities and handicaps in a population of elderly people living in a defined geographical area: the Gospel Oak project. *Age and Ageing*, 27: 707–14.

Hauser, K. and Walsh, D. (2008) Visual analogue scales and assessment of quality of life in cancer. *Journal of Supportive Oncology*, 6: 277–82.

Hawker, G.A., Mian, S., Kendzerska, T. and French, M. (2011) Measures of adult pain. *Arthritis Care and Research*, 63, S11: S240–52.

Hayes, R.D. and Morales, L.S. (2001) The RAND-36 measure of health-related quality of life. The Finnish Medical Society Duodecim. *Annals of Medicine,* 33: 350–57.

Hays, R., Siu, A., Keeler, E. *et al.* (1996) Long term care residents' preferences on the QWB scale. *Medical Decision Making*, 16: 254–61.

Haywood, K.L., Garratt, A.M., Dziedzic, K. and Dawes, P.T. (2003) Patient centred assessment of ankylosing spondylitis-specific health-related quality of life: evaluation of the Patient Generated Index. *Journal of Rheumatology*, 30: 764–73.

Haywood, K.L., Garratt, A.M. and Fitzpatrick, R. (2005) Older people specific health status and quality of life: a structured review of self-assessed instruments. *Journal of Evaluation in Clinical Practice*, 11: 315–27.

Headey, B.W. and Wearing, A.J. (1989) Personality, life events and subjective well-being: toward a dynamic equilibrium model. *Journal of Personality and Social Psychology*, 57: 731–9.

Headey, B.W., Glowacki, T., Holstrom, E.L. and Wearing, A.J. (1985) Modelling change in perceived quality of life. *Social Indicators Research*, 17: 276–98.

Health Outcomes Institute (1990) *Report on a Survey of Elderly Rural Residents: Health Status, Use of Health Care Services and Satisfaction with Quality of Care*. Bloomington, IN: HOI.

Heasman, M.A. and Lipworth, L. (1966) *Accuracy of Certification of Cause of Death*. Studies on Medical and Population Subjects no. 20. London: General Register Office.

Hedley, M.M., Oza, D., Feld, R. *et al.* (2002) The palliative benefit of irinotecan in 5-fluorouracil-refractory colorectal cancer: its prospective evaluation by a multicenter Canadian Trial. *Clinical Colorectal Cancer*, 2: 93–101.

Helmes, E., Goffin, R.D. and Chrisjohn, R.D. (2010) Confirmatory analysis of the Bradburn Affect Balance Scale and its relationship with morale in older Canadian adults. Canadian Journal on Aging/La Revue canadienne du vieillissement, 29: 259–66.

Hemingway, H., Stafford, M., Stansfeld, S. *et al.* (1997) Is the SF-36 a valid measure of change in population health? Results from the Whitehall Study. *British Medical Journal*, 315: 1273–9.

Henderson, S., Duncan-Jones, P., Byrne, D.G. and Scott, R. (1980) Measuring social relationships: the Interview Schedule for Social Interaction. *Psychological Medicine*, 10: 723–34.

Henderson, S., Byrne, D.G. and Duncan-Jones, P. (1981a) *Neurosis and the Social Environment*. London: Academic Press.

Henderson, S., Lewis, I.C., Howell, R.H. *et al.* (1981b) Mental health and the use of alcohol, tobacco, analgesics and vitamins in a secondary school population. *Acta Psychiatrica Scandinavica*, 63: 186–9.

Herron, M.K., Michaux, W.W., Katz, M.M. *et al.* (1964) *Supplemental Instructions for the Administration of the Katz Adjustment Scales*. Baltimore, MD: Spring Grove State Hospital, Research Department.

Heylighten, F. and Bernheim, J. (2000) Global progress I: empirical evidence for ongoing increase in quality of life. *Journal of Happiness Studies*, I: 323–49.

Hickey, A.M., Bury, G., O'Boyle, C.A. *et al.* (1996) A new short form individual quality of life measure (SEIQoL-DW): application in a cohort of individuals with HIV/AIDS. *British Medical Journal*, 313: 29–33.

Hickey, A., O'Boyle, C.A., McGee, H.M. and McDonald, N.J. (1997) The relationship between post-trauma problem reporting and carer quality of life after severe head injury. *Psychology and Health*, 12: 827–38.

Higgs, P., Hyde, M., Wiggins, R. and Blane, D. (2003) Researching quality of life in early old age: the importance of the sociological dimension. *Social Policy and Administration*, 37: 239–52.

Hill, S. and Harries, U. (1994) Assessing the outcome of health care for the older person in community settings: should we use the SF-36? Outcomes Briefing. *UK Clearing House for Health Outcomes*, 4: 26–7.

Hill, S., Harries, U. and Popay, J. (1995) Is the SF-36 suitable for routine health outcomes assessment in health care for older people? Evidence from preliminary work in community-based health services in England. *Journal of Epidemiology and Community Health*, 50: 94–8.

Hinterberger, W., Gadner, H., Hocker, P. *et al.* (1987) Survival and quality of life in 23 patients with severe aplastic anaemia treated with BMT. *Blut*, 54: 137–46.

Hirsch, B.J. (1980) Natural support systems and coping with major life changes. *American Journal of Community Psychology*, 8: 159–72.

Hirsch, B.J. (1981) Social networks and the coping process: creating personal communities, in B.H. Gottlieb (ed.) *Social Networks and Social Support*. Beverly Hills, CA: Sage Publications.

Hobart, J.C., Lamping, D.L., Freeman, J.A. *et al.* (2001) Evidence-based measurement: which disability scale for neurologic rehabilitation? *Neurology*, 57: 639–44.

Hobbs, P., Ballinger, C.B. and Smith, A.H.W. (1983) Factor analysis and validation of the General Health Questionnaire in women: a general practice survey. *British Journal of Psychiatry*, 142: 257–64.

Hobbs, P., Ballinger, C.B., Greenwood, C. *et al.* (1984) Factor analysis and validation of the General Health Questionnaire in men: a general practice survey. *British Journal of Psychiatry*, 144: 270–5.

Hodkinson, H.M. (1972) Evaluation of a mental test score for the assessment of mental impairment in the elderly. *Age and Ageing*, 1: 233–8.

Hoffmeister, J.K. (1976) *Some Information Regarding the Characteristics of the Two Measures Developed from the Self-Esteem Questionnaire (SEQ-3)*. Boulder, CO: Test Analysis and Development Corporation.

Holt-Lunstad, J., Smith, T.B., and Layton, J.B. (2010) Social relationships and mortality risk: a meta-analytic review. *PLoS Medicine*, 7: e1000316.

Holt-Lunstad, J., Smith, T.B., Baker, M. *et al.* (2015) Loneliness and social isolation as risk factors for mortality: a meta-analytic review. *Perspectives on Psychological Science*, 10: 227–37.

Hörnquist, J.O. (1982) The concept of quality of life. *Scandinavian Journal of Social Medicine*, 10: 57–61.

House, J.S. (1981) *Work, Stress and Social Support*. Reading, MA: Addison-Wesley.

House, J.S. and Kahn, R.L. (1985) Measures and concepts of social support, in S. Cohen and S.L. Syme (eds) *Social Support and Health*. Orlando, FL: Academic Press.

House, J.S., Robbins, C. and Metzner, H.L. (1982) The association of social relationships and activities with mortality: prospective evidence from the Tecumseh Community Health Study. *American Journal of Epidemiology*, 116: 123–40.

Hoyt, D.R. and Creech, J.C. (1983) The life satisfaction index: a methodological and theoretical critique. *Journal of Gerontology*, 38: 111–16.

Hsueh, I.P., Lin, J.H., Jeng, J.S. *et al.* (2002) Comparison of the psychometric properties of the functional independence measure 5 item Barthel Index, and 10 item Barthel index in patients with stroke. *Journal of Neurology, Neurosurgery, Psychiatry*, 73: 188–90.

Hughes, T.E., Kaplan, R.M., Cons, S.J. *et al.* (1997) Construct validities of the Quality of Well-Being Scale and the MOS-HIV-34 Health Survey for HIV-infected patients. *Medical Decision Making*, 17: 439–46.

Hunt, S.M. (1984) Nottingham Health Profile, in N.K. Wenger, M.E. Mattson, C.D. Furberg *et al.* (eds) *Assessment of Quality of Life in Clinical Trials of Cardiovascular Therapies*. New York: Le Jacq.

Hunt, S.M. (1988) Subjective health indicators and health promotion. *Health Promotion*, 3: 23–34.

Hunt, S.M. (1999) The researcher's tale: a story of virtue lost and regained, in C.R.B. Joyce, H.M. McGee and C.A. O'Boyle (eds) *Individual Quality of Life. Approaches to Conceptualisation and Assessment*. The Netherlands: Harwood Academic Publishers.

Hunt, S.M. and McKenna, S.P. (1992) British adaptation of the General Well-Being Index: a new tool for clinical research. *British Journal of Medical Economics*, 2: 49–60.

Hunt, S.M. and McKenna, S.P. (1993) Measuring patients' views of their health. SF-36 misses the mark (letter). *British Medical Journal*, 307: 125.

Hunt, S.M., McKenna, S.P., McEwan, J. *et al.* (1980) A quantitative approach to perceived health status: a validation study. *Journal of Epidemiology and Community Health*, 34: 281–6.

Hunt, S.M., McKenna, S.P. and Williams, J. (1981) Reliability of a population survey tool for measuring perceived health problems: a study of patients with osteoarthritis. *Journal of Epidemiology and Community Health*, 35: 297–300.

Hunt, S.M., McEwan, J., McKenna, S.P. *et al.* (1984a) Subjective health assessments and the perceived outcome of minor surgery. *Journal of Psychosomatic Research*, 28: 105–14.

Hunt, S.M., McEwan, J. and McKenna, S.P. (1984b) Perceived health: age and sex comparisons in a community. *Journal of Epidemiology and Community Health*, 34: 281–6.

Hunt, S.M., McEwan, J. and McKenna, S.P. (1986) *Measuring Health Status*. London: Croom Helm.

Huppert, F.A. and Garcia, A.W. (1991) Qualitative differences in psychiatric symptoms between high risk groups assessed on a screening test (GHQ–30). *Social Psychiatry and Psychiatric Epidemiology*, 26: 252–8.

Huppert, F.A., Walters, D.E., Day, N.E. and Elliott, B.J. (1989) The factor structure of the General Health Questionnaire (GHQ–30). A reliability study on 6317 community residents. *British Journal of Psychiatry*, 155: 178–85.

Huskisson, E.C. (1974) Measurement of pain. *Lancet*, ii: 1127–31.

Hutchinson, T.A., Boyd, N.F. and Feinstein, A.R. (1979) Scientific problems in clinical scales as demonstrated in the Karnofsky index of performance status. *Journal of Chronic Diseases*, 32: 661–6.

Hwang, S.S., Chang, V.T., Rue, M. and Kasimis, B. (2003) Multi-dimensional independent predictors of cancer-related fatigue. *Journal of Pain Symptom Management*, 26: 604–14.

Hyde, M., Wiggins, R.D., Higgs, P. and Blane, D. (2003) A measure of quality of life in early old age: the theory, development and properties of a needs satisfaction model (CASP-19). *Ageing and Mental Health*, 7: 186–94.

Hyde, M., Higgs, P., Wiggins, R.D. and Blane, D. (2015) A decade of research using the CASP scale: key findings and future directions. *Aging and Mental Health*, 19(7): 571–5.

Hyland, M.E. and Kenyon, P. (1992) A measure of positive health-related quality of life: the Satisfaction with Illness Scale. *Psychological Reports*, 71: 1137–8.

Hyler, S.E. and Rieder, R.O. (1987) Personality Diagnostic Questionnaire-Revised. New York: New York State Psychiatric Institute.

Hyyppa, M.T. and Maki, J. (2003) Social participation and health in a community rich in stock of social capital. *Health Education Research*, 18: 770–9.

Idler, E.I. and Kasl, S.V. (1995) Self-ratings of health: do they also predict change in functional ability? *Journal of Gerontology (B)*, 50: S344–53.

Iliffe, S., Harari, D., Swift, C. *et al.* (2007) Health risk appraisal in older people 2: the implications for clinicians and commissioners of social isolation risk in older people. *British Journal of General Practice*, 57: 277–83.

Iliffe, S., Kendrick, D., Morris. R., *et al.* (2014) Multi-centre cluster randomised trial comparing a community group exercise programme with home based exercise with usual care for people aged 65 and over in primary care. *Health Technology Assessment*, 18(49).

Inglehart, R. and Rabier, J.R. (1986) Aspirations adapt to situations – but why are the Belgians so much happier than the French? A cross-cultural analysis of the subjective quality of life, in F.M. Andrews (ed.) *Research on the Quality of Life*. Ann Arbor, MI: Survey Research Center, Institute for Social Research, University of Michigan.

Insinga, R.P. and Fryback, D.G. (2003) Understanding differences between self-ratings and population ratings for health in the EuroQol. *Quality of Life Research*, 12: 611–19.

Jachuck, S.J., Brierly, H., Jachuk, S. *et al.* (1982) The effect of hypotensive drugs on the quality of life. *Journal of the Royal College of General Practitioners*, 32: 103–5.

Jalenques, I., Auclair, C., Roblin, J. *et al.* (2013) Cross-cultural evaluation of the French version of the LEIPAD, a health-related quality of life instrument for use in the elderly living at home. *Quality of Life Research*: 509–20.

Janssens, A., Thompson Coon, J., Rogers, M. *et al.* (2015) A systematic review of generic multidimensional patient-reported outcome measures for children, Part 1: Descriptive characteristics. *Value in Health*, 18: 315–33.

Jenkinson, C. and Layte, R. (1997) Development and testing of the UK SF-12 (short form health survey). *Journal of Health Services Research and Policy*, 2: 14–18.

Jenkinson, C. and McGee, H. (1998) *Health Status Measurement: A Brief but Critical Introduction*. Oxford: Radcliffe Medical Press.

Jenkinson, C., Fitzpatrick, R. and Argyle, M. (1988) The Nottingham Health Profile: an analysis of its sensitivity in differentiating illness groups. *Social Science and Medicine*, 27: 1411–14.

Jenkinson, C., Ziebland, S., Fitzpatrick, R. *et al.* (1991) Sensitivity to change of weighted and unweighted versions of two health status measures. *International Journal of Health Sciences*, 2: 189–94.

Jenkinson, C., Coulter, A. and Wright, L. (1993) Short Form-36 (SF-36) health survey questionnaire: Normative data for adults of working age. *British Medical Journal*, 306: 1437–40.

Jenkinson, C., Carroll, D., Egerton, M. *et al.* (1995) Comparison of the sensitivity to change of long and short form pain measures. *Quality of Life Research*, 4: 353–57.

Jenkinson C., Layte, R., Wright, L. and Coulter, A. (1996) *The UK SF-36: An Analysis and Interpretation Manual*. Oxford: University of Oxford, Health Services Research Unit, Department of Public Health and Primary Care.

Jenkinson, C., Layte, R. and Lawrence, K. (1997) Development and testing of the SF-36 summary scale scores in the United Kingdon: results from a large scale survey and clinical trial. *Medical Care*, 35: 410–16.

Jenkinson, C., Stewart-Brown, S., Petersen, S. and Paice, C. (1999) Assessment of the SF-36 Mark 2 in the United Kingdom. *Journal of Epidemiology and Community Health*, 53: 46–50.

Jenkinson, C., Mant, J., Carter, J. *et al.* (2000) The London handicap scale: a re-evaluation of its validity using standard scoring and simple summation. *Journal of Neurology, Neurosurgery and Psychiatry*, 68: 365–7.

Jenkinson, C., Mayou, R., Day, A. *et al.* (2002) Evaluation of the Dartmouth COOP Charts in a large-scale community survey in the United Kingdom. *Journal of Public Health Medicine,* 24: 106–11.

Jette, A.M. (1980) The Functional Status Index: Reliability of a chronic disease evaluation instrument. *Archives of Physical Medicine and Rehabilitation*, 61: 395–401.

Jirik-Babb, P. and Geliebter, A. (2003) Comparison of psychological characteristics of binging and nonbinging obese, adult, female outpatients. *Eating and Weight Disorders*, 8: 173–7.

Johnson, J.A. and Maddigan, S.L. (2004) Performance of the RAND-12 and SF-12 summary scores in type 2 diabetes. *Quality of Life Research*, 13: 449–56.

Jones, D.A., Victor, C.R. and Vetter, N.J. (1985) The problem of loneliness in the elderly in the community: characteristics of those who are lonely and the factors related to the loneliness. *Journal of the Royal College of General Practitioners*, 35: 136–9.

Joore, M.A., Potjewijd, J. Timmerman, A.A. *et al.* (2002) Response shift in the measurement of quality of life in hearing impaired adults after hearing aid fitting. *Quality of Life Research*, 11: 299–307.

Joyce, C.R., McGee, H.M. and O'Boyle, C.A. (1999) Individual quality of life: review and outlook, in C.R.B. Joyce, C.A. O'Boyle and H. McGee, *Individual Quality of Life. Approaches to Conceptualisation and Assessment*. Amsterdam: Harwood Academic Publishers.

Joyce, C.R., Hickey, A., McGee, H.M. and O'Boyle, C.A. (2003) A theory-based method for the evaluation of individual quality of life: the SEIQoL. *Quality of Life Research*, 12: 275–80.

Julian, L.J. (2011) Measures of anxiety: State-Trait Anxiety Inventory (STAI), Beck Anxiety Inventory (BAI), and Hospital Anxiety and Depression Scale-Anxiety (HADS-A). *Arthritis Care Research*, 63: Supplement S11: S467–72.

Julious, S.A., George, S. and Campbell, J. (1995) Sample sizes for studies using the short form 36 (SF-36). *Journal of Epidemiology and Community Health*, 49: 642–4.

Juniper, E.F., Guyatt, G.H., Streiner, D.L. and King, D.R. (1997) Clinical impact versus factor analysis for quality of life questionnaire construction. *Journal of Clinical Epidemiology*, 50: 233–8.

Kaambwa, B., Gill, L., McCaffrey, N. *et al.* (2015) An empirical comparison of the OPQoL-Brief, EQ-5D-3 L and ASCOT in a community dwelling population of older people. *Health and Quality of Life Outcomes*, 13: 164.

Kabacoff, R.I., Segal, D.L., Hersen, M. and Van Hasselt, V.B. (1997) Psychometric properties and diagnostic utility of the Beck Anxiety Inventory and the State-Trait Inventory with older adult psychiatric outpatients. *Journal of Anxiety Disorders*, 11: 33–47.

Kafonek, S., Ettinger, W.H., Roca, R. *et al.* (1989) Instruments for screening for depression and dementia in a long-term care facility. *Journal of the American Geriatrics Society*, 37: 29–34.

Kahn, R.L., Goldfarb, A.I., Pollack, M. *et al.* (1960a) The relationship of mental and physical status in institutionalized aged persons. *American Journal of Psychiatry*, 117: 120–4.

Kahn, R.L., Goldfarb, A.I., Pollack, M. *et al.* (1960b) Brief objective measures for the determination of mental status in the aged. *American Journal of Psychiatry*, 117: 326–8.

Kaipper, M.B., Chachamovich, E., Hidalgo, M.P. *et al.* (2010) Evaluation of the structure of the Brazilian State-Trait Anxiety Inventory using a Rasch psychometric approach. *Journal of Psychosomatic Research*, 68: 223–33.

Kalra, L. and Crome, P. (1993) The role of prognostic scores in targeting stroke rehabilitation in elderly patients. *Journal of the American Geriatrics Society*, 41: 396–400.

Kalson, C. (1976) MASH – a program of social interaction between institutionalised aged and adult mentally retarded persons. *The Gerontologist*, 16: 340–8.

Kammann, R. and Flett, R. (1983) Affectometer 2: a scale to measure current level of general happiness. *Australian Journal of Psychology*, 35: 259–65.

Kane, R.L., Rockwood, T., Philp, I. and Finch, M. (1998) Differences in valuation of functional status components among consumers and professionals in Europe and the United States. *Journal of Clinical Epidemiology*, 51: 657–66.

Kaplan, B.H. (1975) An epilogue: toward further research on family and health, in B.H. Kaplan and J.C. Cassel (eds) *Family and Health: An Epidemiological Approach*. Chapel Hill, NC: University of North Carolina, Institute for Research and Social Science.

Kaplan, G.A. and Camacho, T. (1983) Perceived health and mortality: a nine-year follow-up of the Human Population Laboratory Cohort. *American Journal of Epidemiology*, 117: 292–8.

Kaplan, G.A., Salonen, J.T., Cohen, R.D. *et al.* (1988) Social connections and mortality from all causes and cardio-vascular disease: prospective evidence from eastern Finland. *American Journal of Epidemiology*, 128: 370–80.

Kaplan, H.B. and Porkorny, A.D. (1969) Self derogation and psychosocial adjustment. *Journal of Nervous and Mental Disease*, 149: 421–34.

Kaplan, R.M. (1988) New health promotion indicators: the general health policy model. *Health Promotion*, 3: 35–48.

Kaplan, R.M. (1994) Using quality of life information to set priorities in health policy. *Social Indicators Research*, 33: 121–63.

Kaplan, R.M. and Anderson, J.P. (1988) The quality of well-being scale. Rationale for a single quality of life index, in S.R. Walker and R. Rosser (eds) *Quality of Life: Assessment and Application*. London: MTP Press.

Kaplan, R.M. and Bush, J.W. (1982) Health-related quality of life measurement for evaluation research analysis. *Health Psychology*, 1: 61–80.

Kaplan, R.M. and Ernst, J.A. (1983) Do category rating scales produce biased preference weights for a health index? *Medical Care*, 21: 193–207.

Kaplan, R.M., Bush, J.W. and Berry, C.C. (1976) Health status: types of validity and the Index of Wellbeing. *Health Services Research*, 11: 478–507.

Kaplan, R.M., Bush, J.W. and Berry, C.C. (1978) The reliability, stability and generalizability of a health status index. American Statistical Association. *Proceedings of the Social Statistics Section*, 704–9.

Kaplan, R.M., Bush, J.W. and Berry, C.C. (1979) Health Status Index: category rating versus magnitude estimation for measuring levels of well-being. *Medical Care*, 17: 501–23.

Kaplan, R.M., McCutchan, J.A., Navarro, A.M. *et al.* (1994) Quality adjusted survival analysis: a neglected application of the quality of well-being scale. *Psychology and Health*, 9: 131–41.

Kaplan, R.M., Anderson, J.P., Patterson, T.L. *et al.* (1995) Validity of the Quality of Well-Being Scale for persons with human immunodeficiency virus infection. *Psychosomatic Medicine*, 57: 138–47.

Karnofsky, D.A. and Burchenal, J.H. (1949) The clinical evaluation of chemotherapeutic agents in cancer, in C.M. McLeod (ed.) *Evaluation of Chemotherapeutic Agents*. Columbia: Columbia University Press.

Karnofsky, D.A., Abelmann, W.H., Craver, L.F. *et al.* (1948) The use of nitrogen mustards in the palliative treatment of carcinoma. *Cancer*, I: 634–56.

Kasl, S. and Cobb, S. (1966) Health behavior, illness behavior and sick role behavior. *Archives of Environmental Health*, 12: 246–66.

Kasl, S.V. and Cooper, C.L. (1987) *Stress and Health Issues in Research Methodology*. Chichester: John Wiley.

Kaszmak, A.W. and Allender, J. (1985) Psychological assessment of depression in older adults, in G.M. Chaisson-Stewart (ed.) *Depression in the Elderly: An Interdisciplinary Approach*. New York: John Wiley.

Katschnig, H. (2005) Quality of life in mental disorders: challenges for research and clinical practice. *World Psychiatry (Journal of the World Psychiatric Association)*, 5: 139–45.

Katz, J.N., Larson, M.G., Phillips, C.B. *et al.* (1992) Comparative measurement sensitivity of short and longer health status instruments. *Medical Care*, 30: 917–25.

Katz, S. and Akpom, C.A. (1976) Index of ADL. *Medical Care*, 14: 116–18.

Katz, S., Ford, A.B., Moskowitz, R.W. *et al.* (1963) Studies of illness in the aged: the index of ADL – a standardized measure of biological and psychosocial function. *Journal of the American Medical Association*, 185: 914–19.

Katz, S., Ford, A.B., Chinn, A.B. *et al.* (1966) Prognosis after strokes: long-term course of 159 patients with stroke. *Medicine*, 45: 236–46.

Katz, S., Vignos, P.J., Moskowitz, R.W. *et al.* (1968) Comprehensive outpatient care in rheumatoid arthritis: a controlled study. *Journal of the American Medicine Association*, 206: 1249.

Katz, S., Downs, T.D., Cash, H.R., Grotz, R.C. (1970) Progress in the development of and index of ADL. *Gerontologist*, 10: 20–30.

Katz, S., Akpom, C.A., Papsidero, J.A. *et al.* (1973) Measuring the health status of populations, in R.L. Berg (ed.) *Health Status of Populations*. Chicago, IL: Hospital Research and Educational Trust.

Kaufman, A.V. (1990) Social network assessment: a critical component in case management for functionally impaired older persons. *International Journal of Ageing and Human Development*, 30: 63–75.

Kawachi, I. and Berkman, L. (2000) Social cohesion, social capital and health, in L.F. Berkman and I. Kawachi (eds) *Social Epidemiology*. Oxford: Oxford University Press.

Kawachi, I., Kennedy, B.P., Lochner, K. and Prothrow-Stith, D. (1997a) Social capital, income inequality and mortality. *American Journal of Public Health*, 87, 1491–8.

Kawachi, I., Kennedy, B.P. and Lochner, K. (1997b) Long live community: social capital as public health. *The American Prospect*, November/December: 56–9.

Kawachi, I., Kennedy, B.P. and Glass, R. (1999) Social capital and self-rated health: a contextual analysis. *American Journal of Public Health*, 89, 1187–93.

Kearns, N.P., Cruickshank, C.A., McGuigan, K.J. *et al.* (1982) A comparison of depression rating scales. *British Journal of Psychiatry*, 141: 45–9.

Keith, R.A., Granger, C.V. and Hamilton, B.B. (1987) The functional independence measure: a new tool for rehabilitation, in M.G. Eisenberg and R.C. Grzesiak (eds) *Advances in Clinical Rehabilitation*, Vol 1. New York: Springer.

Keyes, C.L. (2002) The mental health continuum: from languishing to flourishing in life. *Journal of Health and Social Behavior*, 43: 207–22.

Keyes, C.L., Shmotkin, D. and Ryff, C.D. (2002) Optimizing well-being: the empirical encounter of two traditions. *Journal of Personality and Social Psychology*, 82: 1007–22.

Khan, A., Khan, S.R., Shankles, E.B. and Polissar, N.L. (2002) Relative sensitivity of the Montgomery-Asberg Depression Rating Scale, the Hamilton Depression rating scale and the Clinical Global Impressions rating scale in antidepressant clinical trials. *International Clinical Psychopharmacology*, 17: 281–5.

Kharroubi, S., Brazier, J.E., Roberts, J.R. *et al.* (2007) Modelling SF-6D health state preference data using a nonparametric Bayesian method. *Journal of Health Economics*, 26: 597–612.

Kidd, D., Stewart, G., Baldry, J. *et al.* (1995) The Functional Independence Measure: a comparative validity and reliability study. *Disability and Rehabilitation*, 17: 10–14.

Kim, D., Subramanian, S.V. and Kawachi, I. (2006) Bonding versus bridging social capital and their associations with self rated health: a multi-level analysis of 40 US communities. *Journal of Epidemiology and Community Health*, 60: 116–22.

Kim, G.R., Netuvelli, G., Blane, D. *et al.* (2015) Psychometric properties and confirmatory factor analysis of the CASP-19, a measure of quality of life in early old age: the HAPIEE study. *Aging and Mental Health*, 19: 595–609.

Kind, P. (undated) *Scaling the Nottingham Health Profile*. Mimeo. York: University of York, Centre for Health Economics.

Kind, P. (1996) The EuroQol instrument: an index of health-related quality of life, in B. Spilker (ed.) *Quality of Life and Pharmacoeconomics in Clinical Trials* (2nd edn). Philadelphia, PA: Lippincott-Raven.

Kind, P. and Carr-Hill, R. (1987) The Nottingham Health Profile: a useful tool for epidemiologists? *Social Science and Medicine*, 25: 905–10.

Kind, P., Hardman, G. and Macran, S. (1999) Population norms for EQ-5D. York: University of York: Centre for Health Economics, Discussion Paper no. 172, November.

King, J.T. and Roberts, M.S. (2002) Validity and reliability of the Short form-36 in cervical spondylotic myelopathy. *Journal of Neurosurgery*, 97: 180–5.

Kiran, R.P., Delaney, C.P., Senagore, A.J. *et al.* (2003) Prospective assessment of Cleveland Global Quality of Life (CGQL) as a novel marker of quality of life and disease activity in Crohn's disease. *American Journal of Gastroenterology*, 98: 1783–9.

Kirby, M., Denihan, A., Bruce, I. *et al.* (2000) The pattern of support networks among the community dwelling elderly in urban Ireland: variations with mental disorder. *Irish Journal of Psychological Medicine*, 17: 43–9.

Kirwan, R.J. and Reeback, J.S. (1983) Using a modified Stanford Health Assessment Questionnaire to assess disability in UK patients with rheumatoid arthritis. *Annals of the Rheumatic Diseases*, 42: 219–20.

Knapp, M.R.J. (1976) Predicting the dimensions of life satisfaction. *Journal of Gerontology*, 31: 595–604.

Knesevich, J.W., Biggs, J.T., Clayton, P.J. and Ziegler, V.E. (1977) Validity of the Hamilton rating scale for depression. *British Journal of Psychiatry*, 131: 49–52.

Knight, R.G., Waal-Manning, H.J. and Spears, G.F. (1983) Some norms and reliability data for the State-Trait Anxiety Inventory and the Zung Self-Rating Depression Scale. *British Journal of Clinical Psychology*, 22: 245–9.

Koenig, H.G., Meador, K.G., Cohen, H.J. *et al.* (1988) Self-rated depression scales and screening for major depression in the older hospitalized patient with medical illness. *Journal of the American Geriatrics Society*, 36: 699–706.

Kohn, M.L. (1969) *Class and Conformity: A Study in Values*. Homewood, IL: Dorsey.

Kokenes, B. (1974) Grade level differences in factors of self esteem. *Development Psychology*, 10: 954–8.

Korner, A., Nielsen, B.M., Eschen, F. *et al.* (1990) Quantifying depressive symptomatology: inter-rater and inter-item correlations. *Journal of Affective Disorders*, 20: 140–9.

Kovacs, M. and Beck, A.T. (1977) An empirical-clinical approach toward a definition of childhood depression, in J.G. Schulterbrandt and A. Raskin (eds) *Depression in Childhood: Diagnosis, Treatment and Conceptual Models*. New York: Raven Press.

Kozma, A. and Stones, M.J. (1987) Social desirability in measures of subjective well-being: a systematic evaluation. *Journal of Gerontology*, 42: 56–9.

Krefetz, D.G., Steer, R.A., Gulab, N.A. and Beck, A.T. (2002) Convergent validity of the Beck depression inventory-II with the Reynolds Adolescent Depression Scale in psychiatric in-patients. *Journal of Personality Assessment*, 78: 451–60.

Kritz-Silverstein, D., Wingard, D.L. and Barrett-Connor, E. (2002) Hysterectomy status and life satisfaction in older women. *Journal of Women's Health and Gender Based Medicine*, 11: 181–90.

Kuijpers, P.M., Denollet, J., Lousberg, R. *et al.* (2003) Validity of the hospital anxiety and depression scale for use with patients with noncardiac chest pain. *Psychosomatics*, 44: 329–35.

Kurtin, P.S., Davies, A.R., Meyer, K.B. *et al.* (1992) Patient-based health status measurements in outpatient dialysis: Early experiences in developing an outcomes assessment program. *Medical Care*, 30: MS136–49 (suppl. 5).

Kushman, J. and Lane, S. (1980) A multivariate analysis of factors affecting perceived life satisfaction and psychological well-being among the elderly. *Social Science Quarterly*, 61: 264–77.

Kuspinar, A. and Mayo, N.E. (2014) A review of the psychometric properties of generic utility measures in multiple sclerosis. *Pharmacoeconomics*, 32: 759–73.

Kutlay, S., Nergizoglu, G., Kutlay, S. *et al.* (2003) General or disease specific questionnaire? A comparative study in hemodialysis patients. *Renal Failure*, 25: 95–103.

Kutner, B., Fansel, D., Togo, A.M. *et al.* (1956) *Five Hundred Over 60*. New York: Russell Sage.

Kutner, N.G., Fair, P.L. and Kutner, M.H. (1985) Assessing depression and anxiety in chronic dialysis patients. *Journal of Psychosomatic Research*, 29: 23–31.

Kvaal, K., Laake, K. and Engedal, K. (2001) Psychometric properties of the state part of the Spielberger State-Trait Anxiety Inventory (STAI) in geriatric patients. *International Journal of Geriatric Psychiatry*, 16: 980–6.

Lamb, K.L., Brodie, D.A. and Roberts, K. (1988) Physical fitness and health-related fitness as indicators of a positive health state. *Health Promotion*, 3: 171–82.

Land, K.C. (1975) Social indicators models: an overview, in K.C. Land and S. Spilerman (eds) *Social Indicator Models*. New York: Russell Sage Foundation.

Landgraf, J.M. and Nelson, E.C. (1992) Summary of the WONCA/COOP international health assessment field trial. *Australian Family Physician*, 21: 255–69.

Landgraf, J.M., Nelson, E.C., Hays, R.D. *et al.* (1990) Assessing function: does it really make a difference? A preliminary evaluation of the acceptability and utility of the COOP function charts, in M. Lipkin (ed.) *Functional Status Measurement in Primary Care*. New York: Springer-Verlag.

Langius, A. (1995) Quality of life in a group of patients with oral and pharyngeal cancer. Sense of coherence, functional status and well-being. Stockholm: Department of Medicine, Centre of Caring Sciences North, Karolinska Institute.

Langius, A., Björvell, H. and Antonovsky, A. (1992) The sense of coherence concept and its relation to personality traits in Swedish samples. *Scandinavian Journal of Caring Science*, 6: 165–71.

Langius, A., Björvell, H. and Lind, M. (1994) Functional status and coping in patients with oral and pharyngeal cancer before and after surgery. *Head and Neck*, 16: 559–68.

LaPlante, M.P. (2010) The classic measure of disability in activities of daily living is biased by age but an expanded IADL/ADL measure is not. *J. Gerontol. B Phychol. Sci. Soc. Sci.* 65B: 720–32.

Larson, R. (1978) Thirty years of research on the subjective well-being of older Americans. *Journal of Gerontology*, 33: 109–25.

Lasgaard, M. (2007) Reliability and validity of the Danish version of the UCLA loneliness scale. *Personality and Individual Differences*, 42: 1359–66.

Lawton, M.P. (1972) The dimensions of morale, in D. Kent, R. Kastenbaum and S. Sherwood (eds) *Research, Planning and Action for the Elderly*. New York: Behavioral Publications.

Lawton, M.P. (1975) The Philadelphia Geriatric Center Morale Scale: a revision. *Journal of Gerontology*, 30: 85–9.

Lawton, M.P. (1991) Background. A multidimensional view of quality of life in frail elders, in J.E. Birren, J. Lubben, J. Rowe and D. Deutchman (eds) *The Concept and Measurement of Quality of Life in the Frail Elderly*. San Diego, CA: Academic Press.

Lefante, J.J., Harmon, G.N., Ashby, K.M. et al. (2005) Use of the SF-8 to assess health-related quality of life for a chronically ill, low-income population participating in the Central Louisiana medication Access Program (CMAP). *Quality of Life Research*, 14: 665–73.

Le Fevre, P., Devereaux, J., Smith, J. et al. (1999) Screening for psychiatric illness in the palliative care inpatient setting: a comparison between the Hospital Anxiety and Depresion Scale and the General Health Questionnaire. *Palliative Medicine*, 12: 399–407.

Leff, J. (ed.) (1993) The TAPS project: evaluating community placement of long stay psychiatric patients. *British Journal of Psychiatry*, 162: 1–56 (suppl. 19).

Leff, J., O'Driscoll, C., Dayson, D. et al. (1990) The TAPS project: V. The structure of social network data obtained from long-stay patients. *British Journal of Psychiatry*, 157: 848–52.

Lehman, A. (1983) The well-being of chronic mental patients. *Archives of General Psychiatry*, 40: 369–73.

Lehman, A. (1988) A quality of life interview for the chronically mentally ill. *Evaluation and Program Planning*, 11: 51–62.

Leighton Read, J., Quinn, R.J. and Hoefer, M.A. (1987) Measuring overall health: an evaluation of three important approaches. *Journal of Chronic Diseases*, 40 (Supplement 1): 7S–21S.

Leonardson, G.R., Daniels, M.C. and Ness, F.K. (2003) Validity and reliability of the general well-being schedule with northern plains American Indians diagnosed with type 2 diabetes mellitus. *Psychology Reports*, 93: 49–58.

Leplege, A., Reveilere, C., Ecosse, E. et al. (2000) Psychometric properties of a new instrument for evaluating quality of life, the WHOQOL-26, in a population of patients with neuromuscular diseases. *Encephale*, 26: 13–22.

Lerner, M. (1973) Conceptualization of health and wellbeing. *Health Services Research*, 8: 6–12.

Lesher, E.L. (1986) Validation of the Geriatric Depression Scale among nursing home residents. *Clinical Gerontology*, 4: 21–8.

Levine, M.N., Guyatt, G.H., Gent, M. et al. (1988) Quality of life in stage 11 breast cancer: An instrument for clinical trials. *Journal of Clinical Oncology*, 6: 1798–810.

Lewis, C.A., Shevlin, M.E., Bunting, B.P. and Joseph, S. (1995) Confirmatory factor analysis of the Satisfaction with Life Scale: replication and methodological refinement. *Journal of Perceptual and Motor Skills*, 80: 304–6.

Lewis, G. and Wessely, S. (1990) Comparison of the General Health Questionnaire and the Hospital Anxiety and Depression Scale. *British Journal of Psychiatry*, 157: 860–4.

Li, Y. (2003) Social capital and social exclusion in England and Wales (1972–1999). *British Journal of Sociology*, 54: 497–526.

Liang, J. (1984) Dimensions of the life satisfaction Index A: a structural formation. *Journal of Gerontology*, 39: 613–22.

Liang, J. and Bollen, K.A. (1983) The structure of the Philadelphia Center Morale Scale: a reinterpretation. *Journal of Gerontology*, 30: 77–84.

Liang, J. and Bollen, K.A. (1985) Sex differences in the structure of the Philadelphia Geriatric

Center Morale Scale. *Journal of Gerontology*, 40: 468–77.

Liang, J., Bennett, J., Akiyama, H. and Maeda, D. (1992) The structure of the PGC Morale Scale in American and Japanese aged: a further note. *Journal of Cross Cultural Gerontology*, 7: 45–68.

Liang, M.H., Larson, M., Cullen, K. and Schwartz, J. (1985) Comparative measurement efficiency and sensitivity of five health status instruments for arthritis research. *Arthritis and Rheumatism*, 28: 524–47.

Liddle, J., Gilleard, C. and Neil, A. (1993) Elderly patients' and their relatives' views on CPR (letter). *Lancet*, 342: 1055.

Liem, G.R. and Liem, J.H. (1978) Social support and stress. Some general issues and their application to the problems of unemployment. Unpublished manuscript. Boston College and University of Massachusetts.

Likert, R. (1952) A technique for the development of attitude scales. *Educational and Psychological Measurement*, 12: 313–15.

Lim, L.L. and Fisher, J.D. (1999) Use of the 12-item short form (SF-12) health survey in an Australian heart and stroke population. *Quality of Life Research*, 8: 1–8.

Lim, T.O. and Morad, Z. (1998) Reliability, validity and discriminatory ability of Spitzer's QL-index in dialysis patients. *Medical Journal of Malaysia*, 53: 392–400.

Lin, J., Thompson, M.P. and Kaslow, N.J. (2009) The mediating role of social support in the community environment – psychological distress link among low-income African American women. *Journal of Community Psychology*, 27: 459–70.

Lin, N., Simeone, R., Ensel, W. *et al.* (1979) Social support, stressful life events and illness, a model and an empirical test. *Journal of Health and Social Behaviour*, 20: 108–19.

Lin, Y.L. (2002) The role of perceived social support and dysfunctional attitudes in predicting Taiwanese adolescents' depressive tendency. *Adolescence*, 37: 823–34.

Lindfors, P. (2002) Positive health in a group of Swedish white-collar workers. *Psychological Reports*, 91: 839–45.

Lintern, T.C., Beaumont, J.C., Kenealy, P.M. and Murrell, R.C. (2001) Quality of life (QoL) in severely disabled multiple sclerosis patients: comparison of three QoL measures using multidimensional scaling. *Quality of Life Research*, 10: 371–8.

Linzer, M., Pontinen, M., Gold, D. *et al.* (1991) Impairment of physical and psychological function in recurrent syncope. *Journal of Clinical Epidemiology*, 44: 1037–43.

Litwin, H. (2001) Social network type and morale in old age. *The Gerontologist*, 41: 516–24.

Litwin, H. and Shiovitz-Ezra, S. (2011) Social network type and subjective well-being in a national sample of older Americans. *The Gerontologist*, 51: 379–88.

Llobera, J., Esteva, M., Benito, E. *et al.* (2003) Quality of life for oncology patients during the terminal period. Validation of the HRCA-QL index. *Support Care Cancer*, 11: 294–303.

Lloyd-Williams, M., Friedman, T. and Rudd, N. (2001) An analysis of the validity of the Hospital Anxiety and Depression Scale as a screening tool in patients with advanced metastatic cancer. *Journal of Pain Symptom Management*, 22: 990–6.

Locke, D.E.C., Decker, P.A., Sloan, J.A. *et al.* (2007) Validation of single-item linear analog scale assessment of quality of life in neuro-oncology patients. *Journal of Pain and Symptom Management*, 34: 628–38.

Lohmann, N. (1977) Correlations of life satisfaction, morale and adjustment measures. *Journal of Gerontology*, 32: 73–5.

López, M.L. and Cooper, L. (2011) Social support measures review. National Centre for Latino Child and Family Research, Laytonsville, MD, www.first5la.org/.../SSMS_LopezCooper_LiteratureReviewandTable_02, accessed 1 September 2009.

Lorig, K.R., Sobel, D.S., Ritter, P.L. *et al.* (2001) Effect of a self-management program on patients with chronic disease. *Effective Clinical Practice*, 4: 256–62.

Louks, J., Hayne, C. and Smith, J. (1989) Replicated factor structure of the Beck Depression Inventory. *Journal of Nervous Mental Disease*, 177: 473–9.

Lovas, K., Kalo, Z., McKenna, S.P. *et al.* (2003) Establishing a standard for patient-completed instrument adaptations in eastern Europe: experience with the Nottingham Health Profile in Hungary. *Health Policy*, 63: 49–61.

Love, A., Loeboeuf, D.C. and Crisp, T.C. (1989) Chiropractic chronic low back pain sufferers and self-report assessment methods. Part 1. A reliability study of the Visual Analogue Scale, the pain drawing and the McGill Pain Questionnaire. *Journal of Manipulative and Physiological Therapeutics*, 12: 21–5.

Lowe, N.K., Walker, S.N. and McCallum, R.C. (1991) Confirming the theoretical structure of the McGill Pain Questionnaire in acute clinical pain. *Pain*, 46: 53–60.

Lowenthal, M.F. and Haven, C. (1968) Interaction and adaptation: intimacy as a critical variable. *American Sociological Review*, 33: 20–30.

Lowrie, E.G., Curtain, R.B., Lepain, N. and Schatell, D. (2003) Medical outcomes study short form-36: a consistent and powerful predictor of morbidity and mortality in dialysis patients. *American Journal of Kidney Disease*, 41: 1286–92.

Lubben, J.E. (1985) Health and psychological assessment instruments of community-based long-term care: the California Multipurpose Senior Services Project (MSSP) experience. Dissertation, Berkeley, CA: University of California.

Lubben, J.E. (1988) Assessing social networks among elderly populations. *Family and Community Health*, 11: 42–52.

Lubben, J.E. and Gironda, M. (2003) Centrality of social ties to the health and well-being of older adults, in B. Berkman and L.K. Harooytoan (eds) *Social Work and Health Care in an Aging World*. New York: Springer.

Lubben, J. and Gironda, M. (2004) Measuring social networks and assessing their benefits, in C. Phillipson, G. Allan and D. Morgan (eds) *Social Networks and Social Exclusion: Sociological and Policy Perspectives*. Aldershot: Ashgate.

Lubben, J.E., Blozik, E., Gillmann, G. et al. (2006) Performance of an abbreviated version of the Lubben Social Network Scale among three European community-dwelling older adult populations. *Gerontologist*, 46: 503–13.

Lubeck, D.P. (2002) Health-related quality of life measurements and studies in rheumatoid arthritis. *American Journal of Managed Care*, 8: 811–20.

Lubeck, D.P. and Fries, J.F. (1992) Changes in quality of life among persons with HIV infection. *Quality of Life Research*, 1: 359–66.

Lundberg, O. and Nystrom, M. (1995) A simplified way of measuring sense of coherence. Experience from a population survey in Sweden. *European Journal of Public Health*, 5: 56–9.

Lundgren-Nilsson, A., Jonsdottir, I.H., Ahlborg, G. et al. (2013) Construct validity of the psychological general well being index (PGWBI) in a sample of patients undergoing treatment for stress-related exhaustion: a Rasch analysis. *Health and Quality of Life Outcomes*, 11: 2.

Luo, N., Chew, L.H., Fong, K.Y. et al. (2003) A comparison of the EuroQol-dD and the Health Utilities Index mark 3 in patients with rheumatic disease. *Journal of Rheumatology*, 30: 2268–74.

Lyons, J., Strain, J.J., Hammer, J.S. et al. (1989) Reliability, validity, and temporal stability of the Geriatric Depression Scale in hospitalized elderly. *International Journal of Psychiatry and Medicine*, 19: 203–9.

Lyons, J., Perrota, P. and Hancher-Kvam, S. (1998) Perceived social support from family and friends: measurement across disparate samples. *Journal of Personality Assessment*, 52: 42–7.

Lyons, R.A., Perry, H.M. and Littlepage, B.N.C. (1994) Evidence for the validity of the short-form 36 questionnaire (SF-36) in an elderly population. *Age and Ageing*, 23: 182–4.

Lyons, R.A., Crome, P., Monaghan, S. et al. (1997) Health status and disability among elderly people in three UK districts. *Age and Ageing*, 26: 203–9.

Lyons, R.A., Wareham, K., Lucas, M. et al. (1999) SF-36 scores vary by method of administration: implications for study design. *Journal of Public Health Medicine*, 21: 41–5.

Macduff, C. and Russell, E. (1998) The problem of measuring change in individual health-related quality of life by postal questionnaire: use of the patient generated index in a disabled population. *Quality of Life Research*, 7: 761–9.

Maes, S., Vingerhoets, A. and Van Heck, G. (1987) The study of stress and disease: some developments and requirements. *Social Science and Medicine*, 25: 567–78.

Magne, I.U., Ojehagen, A. and Traskman, B.L. (1992) The social network of people who attempt suicide. *Acta Psychiatrica Scandinavica*, 86: 153–8.

Maheswaran, H., Weich, S., Powell, J. and Stewart-Brown, S. (2012) Evaluating the responsiveness of the Warwick-Edinburgh Mental Well-Being Scale (WEMWBS): group and individual level analysis. *Health and Quality of Life Outcomes*, 10: 156.

Mahon, N.E. and Yarcheski, A. (1990) The dimensionality of the UCLA Loneliness Scale in early adolescents. *Research in Nursing and Health*, 13: 45–52.

Mahon, N.E., Yarcheski, T.J. and Yarcheski, A. (1995) Validation of the revised UCLA Loneliness Scale for adolescents. *Research in Nursing and Health*, 18: 263–70.

Mahoney, F.I. and Barthel, D.W. (1965) Functional evaluation: the Barthel Index. *Maryland State Medical Journal*, 14: 61–5.

Maitland, S.B., Dixon, R.A., Hultsch, D.F. and Hertzog, C. (2001) Well-being as a moving target: measurement equivalence of the Bradburn Affect Balance Scale. *Journal of Gerontology (B)*, 56: 69–77.

Makowska, Z. and Merecz, D. (2000) The usefulness of the Health Status Questionnaire: D. Goldberg's GHQ-12 and GHQ-28 for diagnosis of mental disorders in workers. *Medycyny Pracy*, 51: 589–601.

Malley, J. and Netten, A. (2009) Measuring outcomes of social care. *Research Policy and Planning*, 27: 85–96.

Malley, J.N., Towers, A-M., Netten, A.P. *et al.* (2012) An assessment of the construct validity of the ASCOT measure of social care-related QoL with older people. *Health and QoL Outcomes,* 10: 21.

Mangione, C.M., Marcantonio, E.R., Goldman, L. *et al.* (1993) Influence of age on measurement of health status in patients undergoing elective surgery. *Journal of the American Geriatrics Society*, 41: 377–83.

Manne, S. and Schnoll, R. (2001) Measuring supportive and unsupportive responses during cancer treatment; a factor analytic assessment of the Partner Responses to Cancer Inventory. *Journal of Behavioral Medicine*, 24: 297–321.

Marks, N.F. and Lambert, J.D. (1999) Transitions to caregiving, gender, and psychological well-being: prospective evidence from the National Survey of Families and Households. NSFH Working Paper No. 82. Wisconsin: Center for Demography and Ecology, University of Wisconsin-Madison.

Marl, J.D.J. and Williams, P. (1985) A comparison of the validity of two psychiatric screening questionnaires (GHQ-12 and SRQ-20) in Brazil, using relative operating characteristics (ROC) analysis. *Psychological Medicine*, 15: 651–9.

Marteau, T.M. and Bekker, H. (1992) The development of a six-item short-form of the state scale of the Spielberger State-Trait Anxiety Inventory (STAI). *British Journal of Clinical Psychology*, 31: 301–6.

Martin, A.J. (1987) Patients and presentation: a profile from general practice. *Modern Medicine*, April: 14–18.

Martin, C.R., Lewin, R.J., Thompson, D.R. *et al.* (2003) A confirmatory factor analysis of the Hospital Anxiety and Depression Scale in coronary care patients following acute myocardial infarction. *Psychiatry Research*, 30: 85–94.

Martin, F., Camfield, L., Rodham, K. *et al.* (2007) Twelve years' experience with the Patient Generated Index (PGI) of quality of life: a graded structured review. *Quality of Life Research*, 16: 705–15.

Maslow, A.H. (1954) *Motivation and Personality*. New York: Harper.

Maslow, A.H. (1962) *Toward a Psychology of Being* (2nd edn). Princeton, NJ: Van Nostrand.

Matsuura, E., Ohta, A., Kanegae, F. *et al.* (2003) Frequency and analysis of factors closely associated with the development of depressive symptoms in patients with scleroderma. *Journal of Rheumatology*, 30: 1782–7.

Mattison, P.G., Aitken, R.C.B. and Prescot, R.J. (1991) Rehabilitation status – the relationship between the Edinburgh Rehabilitation Status Scale (ERSS), Barthel Index and PULSES Profile. *International Disability Studies*, 13: 9–11.

Mauskopf, J., Austin, R., Dix, L. *et al.* (1994) The Nottingham Health Profile as a measure of quality of life in zoster patients: convergent and discriminant validity. *Quality of Life Research*, 3: 431–5.

McColl, E., Steen, I.N., Meadows, K.A. *et al.* (1995) Developing outcome measures for ambulatory care – an application to asthma and diabetes. Special Issue 'Quality of Life' in *Social Science and Medicine*, 10: 1339–48.

McDowell, I. (2006) *Measuring Health: A Guide to Rating Scales and Questionnaires* (43rd edn). New York: Oxford University Press.

McDowell, I. and Newell, C. (1996) *Measuring Health: A Guide to Rating Scales and Questionnaires*, 2nd edn. New York: Oxford University Press.

McGee, H.M., O'Boyle, C.A., Hickey, A. *et al.* (1991) Assessing the quality of life of the individual: The SEIQoL with a healthy and a gastroenterology unit population. *Psychological Medicine*, 21: 749–59.

McGee, M., Johnson, A.L., Kay, D.W.K. and MRC CFAS Analysis subcommittee (1998) The description of activities of daily living in five centres in England and Wales. The Medical Research Council Cognitive Function and Ageing Study (1998). *Age and Ageing*, 27: 605–13.

McGuire, B. and Tinsley, H.E.A. (1981) A contribution to the construct validity of the Tennessee Self-Concept Scale: a confirmatory factor analysis. *Applied Psychological Measurement*, 5: 449–57.

McHorney, C.A., Ware, J.E., Rogers, W. *et al.* (1992) The validity and relative precision of MOS short- and long-form health status scales and Dartmouth COOP Charts: results from the medical outcomes study. *Medical Care*, 30: MS253-MS265.

McHorney, C.A., Ware, J.E. and Raczek, A.E. (1993) The MOS 36-Item Short Form Health Survey (SF–36): II. Psychometric and clinical tests of validity in measuring physical and mental health constructs. *Medical Care*, 31: 247–63.

McHorney, C.A., Kosinski, M. and Ware, J.E. (1994) Comparisons of the costs and quality of norms for the SF-36 Health Survey collected by mail versus telephone interview: results from a national survey. *Medical Care*, 32: 551–67.

McHorney, C.A., Haley, S.M. and Ware, J.E. (1997) Evaluation of the MOS SF-36 Physical Functioning Scale (PF-10): II. Comparison of relative precision using Likert and Rasch scoring methods. *Journal of Clinical Epidemiology*, 50: 451–61.

McKenna, S.P., Hunt, S.M. and McEwan, J. (1981) Weighting the seriousness of perceived health problems using Thurstone's method of paired comparisons. *International Journal of Epidemiology*, 10: 93–7.

McKenna, S.P., McEwan, J., Hunt, S.M. *et al.* (1984) Changes in the perceived health of patients recovering from fractures. *Public Health*, 98: 97–102.

McMillan, S.C. (1996) Quality-of-life assessment in palliative care. *Cancer Control*, 3: 223–9.

McMurdo, M.E.T. and Rennie, L. (1993) A controlled trail of exercise by residents of old people's homes. *Age and Ageing*, 22: 11–15.

McNeil, B.J., Weichselbaum, R. and Pauker, S.G. (1978) Fallacy of the five year survival in lung cancer. *New England Journal of Medicine*, 299: 1397–401.

McNeil, B.J., Weichselbaum, R. and Pauker, S.G. (1981) Speech and Survival: tradeoffs between quality and quantity of life in laryngeal cancer. *New England Journal of Medicine*, 305: 982–7.

McPherson, F.M., Gamsu, C.V., Kiemle, G. *et al.* (1985) The concurrent validity of the survey version of the Clifton Assessment Procedures for the Elderly (CAPE). *British Journal of Clinical Psychology*, 24: 83–91.

McQuay, H.J. (1990) Assessment of pain, and effectiveness of treatment, in A. Hopkins and D. Costain (eds) *Measuring the Outcomes of Medical Care*. London: Royal College of Physicians.

McWhirter, B.T. (1990) Factor analysis of the Revised UCLA Loneliness Scale. *Current Psychology Research and Reviews*, 9: 56–68.

Mechanic, D. (1962) The concept of illness behaviour. *Journal of Chronic Diseases*, 15: 189–94.

Mechanic, D. (1978) Medical Sociology (2nd edn). New York: The Free Press.

Medical Outcomes Trust (1993) *How to Score the SF-36 Health Survey*. Boston, MA: Medical Outcomes Trust.

Meenan, R.F. (1982) The AIMS approach to health status measurement: conceptual background and measurement properties. *Journal of Rheumatology*, 9: 785–8.

Meenan, R.F. (1985) New approaches to outcome assessment: the AIMS questionnaire for arthritis, in G.H. Stollerman (ed.) *Advances in Internal Medicine*, vol. 31. New York: Year Book Medical Publishers.

Meenan, R.F. and Mason, J.H. (1990) *AIMS2 users' guide*. Boston, MA: Boston University School of Medicine, Boston University Arthritis Center and Department of Public Health.

Meenan, R.F. and Mason, J.H. (1994) *AIMS2 users' guide* (revised). Boston, MA: Boston University School of Medicine, Boston University Arthritis Center and Department of Public Health.

Meenan, R.F., Gertman, P.M. and Mason, J.H. (1980) Measuring health status in arthritis: the arthritis impact measurement scales. *Arthritis and Rheumatism*, 23: 146–52.

Meenan, R.F., Gertman, P.M., Mason, J.H. *et al.* (1982) The arthritis impact measurement scales: further investigations of a health status measure. *Arthritis and Rheumatism*, 25: 1048–53.

Meenan, R.F., Anderson, J.J., Kazis, L.E. *et al.* (1984) Outcome assessment in clinical trials: evidence for the sensitivity of a health status measure. *Arthritis and Rheumatism*, 27: 1344–52.

Meenan, R.F., Mason, J.H., Anderson, J.J. *et al.* (1992) AIMS2. The content and properties of a revised and expanded Arthritis Impact Measurement Scales Health Status Questionnaires. *Arthritis and Rheumatism*, 35: 1–10.

Mellor, K.S. and Edelmann, R.J. (1988) Mobility, social support, loneliness and well-being amongst two groups of older adults. *Journal of Personality and Individual Differences*, 9: 1–5.

Melzack, R. (1975) The McGill pain questionnaire: major properties and scoring methods. *Pain*, 1: 277–99.

Melzack, R. (1983) *Pain Measurement and Assessment*. New York: Raven Press.

Melzack, R. (1987) The short-form McGill Pain Questionnaire. *Pain*, 30: 191–7.

Melzack, R. and Katz, J. (1992) The McGill Pain Questionnaire: appraisal and current status, in D.C. Turk and R. Melzack (eds) *Handbook of Pain Assessment*. New York: The Guilford Press.

Melzack, R. and Torgerson, W.S. (1971) On the language of pain. *Anesthesiology*, 34: 50.

Melzack, R., Terrence, C., Fromm, G. and Amsel, R. (1986) Trigeminal neuralgia and atypical face pain: use of the McGill Pain Questionnaire for discrimination and diagnosis. *Pain*, 27: 297–302.

Melzer, D., McWilliams, B., Brayne, C. *et al.* (2000) The Medical Research Council Cognitive Function and Ageing Study (MRC CFAS) writing committee (2000): Socioeconomic status and the expectation of disability in old age: estimates for England. *Journal of Epidemiology and Community Health*, 54: 286–92.

Merrell, M. and Reed, L.J. (1949) *The Epidemiology of Health, Social Medicine, its Deviations and Objectives*. New York: The Commonwealth Fund.

Messick, S. (1980) Test validity and the ethics of assessment. *American Psychologist*, 35: 1012–27.

Metcalfe, M. and Goldman, E. (1965) Validation of an inventory for measuring depression. *British Journal of Psychiatry*, 111: 240–2.

Meyboom-de Jong, B. and Smith, R.J.A. (1990) Studies with the Dartmouth COOP Charts in general practice: comparison with the Nottingham Health Profile and the General Health Questionnaire, in M. Lipkin (ed.) *Functional Status Measurement in Primary Care*. New York: Springer-Verlag.

Meyer-Rosenberg, K., Burckhardt, C.S., Huizar, K. *et al.* (2001) A comparison of the SF-36 and Nottingham Health Profile in patients with chronic neuropathic pain. *European Journal of Pain*, 5: 391–403.

Michalos, A.C. (1986) Job satisfaction, marital satisfaction and the quality of life: a review and preview, in F.M. Andrews (ed.) *Research on the Quality of Life*. Ann Arbor, MI: Survey Research Center, Institute for Social Research, University of Michigan.

Michalos, A.C., Hubley, A.M., Zumbo, B.D. *et al.* (2001) Health and other aspects of the quality of life of older people. *Social Indicators Research*, 54: 239–74.

Michaud, K., Messer, J., Choi, H.K. and Wolfe, F. (2003) Direct medical costs and their predictors in patients with rheumatoid arthritis: a three year study of 7,527 patients. *Arthritis and Rheumatism*, 48: 2750–62.

Michopoulos, I., Douzenis, A. Kalkavoura, C. *et al.* (2008) Hospital Anxiety and Depression Scale (HADS): validation in a Greek general hospital; sample. *Annals of General Phychiatry*, 7: 4.

Mikołajewska, E. (2013) Changes in Barthel Index outcomes as result of poststroke rehabilitation using NDT-Bobath method. *International Journal on Disability and Human Development*, 12: 363–7.

Milte, C.M., Walker. R., Luszcz, M.A. *et al.* (2014) How important is health status in defining quality of life for older people? An exploratory study of the views of older South Australians. *Applied Health Economics and Health Policy*, 12: 73–84.

Mitchell, J.C. (1969) The concept and use of social networks, in J.C. Mitchell (ed.) *Social Networks in Urban Situations: Analysis of Personal Relationships in Central African Towns*. Manchester: Manchester University Press.

Mitchell, R.E. and Trickett, E.J. (1980) Social networks as mediators of social support: an analysis of the effects and determinants of social networks. *Community Mental Health Journal*, 16: 27–44.

Moinpour, C.M., Lyons, B., Schmidt, S.P. *et al.* (2000) Substituting proxy ratings for patient ratings in cancer clinical trials: an analysis based on Southwest Oncology Group trial patients with brain metastases. *Quality of Life Research*, 9: 219–31.

Mokken, R.J. (1971) *A Theory and Procedure of Scale Analysis*. Berlin, Germany: De Gruyter.

Monk, M. (1981) Blood pressure awareness and psychological well-being in the Health and Nutrition Examination Survey. *Clinical Investigative Medicine*, 4: 183–9.

Montgomery, S.A. and Asberg, M. (1979) A new depression scale designed to be sensitive to change. *British Journal of Psychiatry*, 134: 382–9.

Montgomery, S.A., Asberg, M., Traskman, L. and Montgomery, D. (1978) Cross cultural studies on the use of the CPRS in English and Swedish depressed patients. *Acta Psychiatrica Scandinavica*, 271: 3–37 (suppl.).

Moorey, S., Greer, S., Watson, M. *et al.* (1991) The factor structure and factor stability of the Hospital Anxiety and Depression Scale in patients with cancer. *British Journal of Psychiatry*, 158: 255–9.

Moos, R.H. and Moos, B.S. (1981) *Manual for Family Environment Scale*. Palo Alto, CA: Consulting Psychologists Press.

Moos, R.H. and Moos, B.S. (1994) *Family Environment Scale (FES) and Manual*, 3rd edn. Palo Alto, CA: Consulting Psychologists Press.

Mor, V. (1987) Cancer patients' quality of life over the disease course: lessons from the real world. *Journal of Chronic Disease*, 40: 535–44.

Mor, V., Laliberte, L., Morris, J.N. *et al.* (1984) The Karnofsky performance status scale: an examination of its reliability and validity in a research setting. *Cancer*, 53: 2002–7.

Moran, S.M., Cockram, L.L., Walker, B. and McPherson, F.M. (1990) Prediction of survival by the Clifton Assessment Procedures for the Elderly (CAPE). *British Journal of Clinical Psychology*, 29: 225–6.

Moreno, J.K., Fuhriman, A. and Selby, M.J. (1993) Measurement of hostility, anger, and depression in depressed and non-depressed subjects. *Journal of Personality Assessment*, 61: 511–23.

Morgan, K., Dallosso, H.M., Arie, T. *et al.* (1987) Mental health and psychological well-being among the old and the very old living at home. *British Journal of Psychiatry*, 150: 801–7.

Morris, J.C.D., Suissa, A., Sherwood, S. *et al.* (1986) Last days: a study of the quality of life of terminally ill cancer patients. *Journal of Chronic Disease*, 39: 47–62.

Morris, J.N. (1975) Changes in morale experienced by the elderly institutionalized applicants along the institutional path. *Gerontologist*, 15: 345–9.

Morris, J.N. and Sherwood, S. (1975) A re-testing and modification of the Philadelphia Geriatric Center Morale Scale. *Journal of Gerontology*, 30: 77–84.

Morris, J.N. and Sherwood, S. (1987) Quality of life of cancer patients at different stages in the disease trajectory. *Journal of Chronic Disease*, 40: 545–53.

Morris, J.N., Wolf, R.S. and Klerman, L.V. (1975) Common themes among morale and depression scales. *Journal of Gerontology*, 30: 209–15.

Morris, L.W., Morris, R.G. and Britton, P.G. (1989) Social support networks and formal support as factors influencing the psychological adjustment of spouse caregivers of dementia sufferers. *International Journal of Geriatric Psychiatry*, 4: 47–51.

Morton-Williams, J. (1979) Alternative patterns of care for the elderly: Methodological report. London. *Social and Community Planning Research*.

Motzer, S.A., Hertig, V., Jarrett, M. *et al.* (2003) Sense of coherence and quality of life in women with and without irritable bowel syndrome. *Nursing Research*, 52: 329–37.

Mowbray, R.M. (1972) The Hamilton Rating Scale for Depression: A factor analysis. *Psychological Medicine*, 2: 272.

Mulder, R.T., Joyce, P.R. and Frampton, C. (2003) Relationships among measures of treatment outcome in depressed patients. *Journal of Affective Disorder*, 76: 127–35.

Mulgrave, N.W. (1985) Clifton Assessment Procedures for the elderly, in D.J. Keyser and R.C. Sweetland (eds) *Test Critiques*, vol. II. Kansas City, MI: Test Corporation of America.

Muller, M.J. and Dragicevic, A. (2003) Standardized rater training for the Hamilton Depression Rating Scale (HAMD-17) in psychiatric novices. *Journal of Affective Disorders*, 77: 65–9.

Mumford, D.B., Tareen, I.A., Bajwa, M.A. *et al.* (1991) The translation and evaluation of an Urdu version of the Hospital Anxiety and Depression Scale. *Acta Psychiatrica Scandinavica*, 83: 81–5.

Nagi, S. (1965) Some conceptual issues in disability and rehabilitation, in M. Sussman (ed.) *Sociology and Rehabilitation*. Washington, DC: American Sociological Society.

Nagi, S. (1991) Disability concepts revisited: implications for prevention, in A. Pope and A. Tarlor (eds) *Disability in America: Towards a National Agenda for Prevention*. Washington, DC: National Academy Press.

Nakayama, T., Toyoda, H., Ohno, K. *et al.* (2000) Validity, reliability and acceptability of the Japanese version of the General Well-Being Schedule. *Quality of Life Research*, 9: 529–39.

Nanda, U., McLendon, P.M., Andresen, E.M. and Armbrecht, E. (2003) The SIP68: an abbreviated Sickness Impact Profile for disability outcomes research. *Quality of Life Research*, 12: 583–95.

National Heart and Lung Institute (1976) Report of a task group on cardiac rehabilitation, in *Proceedings of the Heart and Lung Institute Working Conference on Health Behaviour*. Bethesda, MD: US Department of Health, Education and Welfare.

Naughton, M.J. and Wiklund, I. (1993) A critical review of dimension-specific measures of health related quality of life in cross-cultural research. *Quality of Life Research*, 2: 397–432.

Nayani, S. (1989) The evaluation of psychiatric illness in Asian patients by the HAD scale. *British Journal of Psychiatry*, 155: 545–7.

Nelson, E.C. and Berwick, D.M. (1989) The measurement of health status in clinical practice. *Medical Care*, 27 (Supplement to no. 3): S77–90.

Nelson, E.C., Conger, R., Douglas, D. *et al.* (1983) Functional health status levels of primary care patients. *Journal of the American Medical Association*, 249: 3331–8.

Nelson, E.C., Landgraf, J.M., Hays, R.D. *et al.* (1990a) The functional status of patients: how can it be measured in physicians' offices? *Medical Care*, 28: 1111–26.

Nelson, E.C., Landgraf, R.D., Hays, J.W. *et al.* (1990b) The COOP Function Charts: a system to measure patient function in physician's office, in *WONCA Classification Committee: Functional status measurement in primary care*. New York: Springer-Verlag.

Nelson, E.J., Wasson, J., Kirk, A. *et al.* (1987) Assessment of function in routine clinical practice: description of the COOP Chart method and preliminary findings. *Journal of Chronic Diseases*, 40 (Supplement 1): 55S–63S.

Nemeth, K.A., Graham, I.D. and Harrison, M.B. (2003) The measurement of leg ulcer pain: identification and appraisal of pain assessment tools. *Advanced Skin Wound Care*, 16: 260–7.

Neto, F. and Barros, J. (2000) Psychosocial concomitants of loneliness among students of Cape Verde and Portugal. *Journal of Psychology*, 134: 503–14.

Netten, A. (2011) *Overview of Outcome Measurement for Adults Using Social Care Services and Support.* London: NIHR School for Social Care Research, London School of Economics.

Netten, A., Beadle Brown, J., Caiels, J. *et al.* (2011) ASCOT adult social care outcomes toolkit. Main guidance v2.1. PSSRU Discussion Paper 2716/3.

Netten, A., Burge, P., Malley, J. *et al.* (2012) Outcomes of social care for adults: developing a preference-weighted measure. *Health Technol. Assess.* 16: 16.

Neudert, C., Wasner, M. and Borasio, G.D. (2001) Patients' assesment of quality of life instruments: a randomized study of SIP, SF-36 and SEIQoL-DW in patients with amyotropic lateral sclerosis. *Journal of Neurological Science*, 191: 103–9.

Neugarten, B.L., Havighurst, R.J. and Tobin, S.S. (1961) The measurement of life satisfaction. *Journal of Gerontology*, 16: 134–43.

Noelker, L. and Harel, Z. (1978) Predictors of well-being and survival among institutionalized aged. *Gerontologist*, 18: 562–7.

Noll, H.H. (2004) Social indicators and quality of life research. Background, achievements and current trends, in N. Genov (ed.) *Advances in Sociological Knowledge over Half a Century.* Wiesbaden: VS Verlag für Sozialwissenschaften.

Norris, J.T., Gallagher, D., Wilson, A. *et al.* (1987) Assessment of depression in geriatric medical outpatients: the validity of two screening measures. *Journal of the American Geriatrics Society*, 35: 989–95.

Nou, E. and Aberg, T. (1980) Quality of survival in patients with surgically treated bronchial carcinoma. *Thorax*, 35: 255–63.

Nouri, F.M. and Lincoln, N.B. (1987) An extended activities of daily living scale for stroke patients. *Clinical Rehabilitation*, 1: 301–5.

Novy, D.M., Nelson, D.V., Goodwin, J. and Rowze, R.D. (1993) Psychometric comparability of the State-Trait Anxiety Inventory for different ethnic subpopulations. *Psychological Assessment*, 5: 343–9.

Nunnally, J. (1978) *Psychometric Theory* (2nd edn). New York: McGraw-Hill.

Nybo, H., Gaist, D., Jeune, B., McGue, M. *et al.* (2001) Functional status and self-rated health in 2,262 nonagenarians: the Danish 1905 cohort survey. *Journal of the American Geriatrics Society*, 49: 601–9.

Nydegger, C. (1986) Measuring morale and life satisfaction, in C.L. Fry and J. Keith (eds) *New Methods for Old Age Research: Strategies for Studying Diversity*. Boston, MA: Bergin and Garvey.

O'Boyle, C.A. (1996) Quality of life in palliative care, in G. Ford and I. Lewin (eds) *Managing Terminal Illness*. London: Royal College of Physicians Publications.

O'Boyle, C.A. (1997a) Measuring the quality of later life. Philosophy Transactions of the Royal Society of London, 352: 1871–9.

O'Boyle, C.A. (1997b) Quality of life assessment: a paradigm shift in healthcare? *Irish Journal of Psychology*, 18: 51–66.

O'Boyle, C.A., McGee, H., Hickey, A. *et al.* (1992) Individual quality of life in patients undergoing hip replacement. *Lancet*, 339: 1088–91.

O'Boyle, C.A., McGee, H.M., Hickey, A. *et al.* (1993) *The Schedule for the Evaluation of Individual Quality of Life (SEIQoL). Administration Manual*. Dublin: Royal College of Surgeons in Ireland.

O'Brien, B.J. (1988) Assessment of treatment in heart disease, in G. Teeling Smith (ed.) *Measuring Health: A Practical Approach*. Chichester: John Wiley.

O'Brien, B.J., Banner, N.R., Gibson, S. *et al.* (1988) The Nottingham Health Profile as a measure of quality of life following combined heart and lung transplantation. *Journal of Epidemiology and Community Health*, 42: 232–4.

O'Brien, B.J., Spath, M., Blackhouse, G. *et al.* (2003) A view from the bridge: agreement between the SF-6D utility algorithm and the Health Utilities Index. *Health Economics*, 12: 975–81.

Office for National Statistics (2002) Living in Britain: Results from the 2000 General Household Survey. London: ONS web-based publication: www.ons.gov.uk/ons/rel/ghs/general-household-survey/index.html (accessed 8 August 2016).

Office for National Statistics (2015) *Harmonised Concepts and Questions for Social Data Sources Primary Principles Long-lasting Health Conditions and Illnesses: Impairments and Disability*, http://www.ons.gov.uk/ons/guide-method/harmonisation/primary-set-of-harmonised-concepts-and-questions/index.html (accessed 8 August 2016)

Office of Population Censuses and Surveys (1987) *General Household Survey* (1985). London: HMSO.

Oga, T., Nishimura, K., Tsukino, M. *et al.* (2003) A comparison of the responsiveness of different generic health status measures in patients with asthma. *Quality of Life Research*, 12: 555–63.

Ohta, Y., Kawasaki, N., Araki, K. *et al.* (1995) The factor structure of the General Health Questionnaire (GHQ-30) in Japanese middle aged and elderly residents. *International Journal of Social Psychiatry*, 41: 268–75.

Oken, M.M., Creech, R.H., Tormey, D.C. *et al.* (1982) Toxicity and response criteria of the Eastern Cooperative Oncology Group. *American Journal of Clinical Oncology*, 5: 649–55.

Oliver, J.P., Huxley, P.J., Priebe, S. and Kaiser, W. (1997) Measuring the quality of life of severely mentally ill people using the Lancashire Quality of Life Profile. *Social Psychiatry and Psychiatric Epidemiology*, 32: 76–83.

Olsen, O. (1992) Impact of social network on cardiovascular mortality in middle-aged Danish men. *Journal of Epidemiology and Community Health*, 47: 176–80.

Oman, D. and Reed, D. (1998) Religion and mortality among the community-dwelling elderly. *American Journal of Public Health*, 88: 1469.

O'Reilly, P. (1988) Methodological issues in social support and social network research. *Social Science and Medicine*, 26: 863–73.

O'Riordan, T.G., Haynes, J.P. and O'Neil, D. (1990) The effect of mild to moderate dementia on the Geriatric Depression Scale and on the General Health Questionnaire. *Age and Ageing*, 19: 57–61.

Orth-Gomér, K. and Johnson, J. (1987a) Social network interaction and mortality. A six-year follow-up study of a random sample of the Swedish population. *Journal of Chronic Diseases*, 40: 949–57.

Orth-Gomér, K. and Unden, A.L. (1987b) The measurement of social support in population surveys. *Social Science and Medicine*, 24: 83–94.

Orth-Gomér, K., Britton, M. and Rehnqvist, N. (1979) Quality of care in an out-patient department: the patient's view. *Social Science and Medicine*, 13A: 347–57.

Osborn, D.P., Fletcher, A.E., Smeeth, S. *et al.* (2002) Geriatric Depression Scale scores in a representative sample of 14,545 people aged 75 and over in the United Kingdom: results from the MRC trial of assessment and management of older people in the community. *International Journal of Geriatric Psychiatry*, 17: 592.

Ott, C.R., Sivarajan, E.S., Newton, K.M. *et al.* (1983) A controlled randomized study of early cardiac rehabilitation: the Sickness Impact Profile as an assessment tool. *Heart and Lung*, 12: 162–70.

Ottenbacher, K.S., Mann, W.G., Granger, C.V. *et al.* (1994) Inter-rater agreement and stability of functional assessment in the community-based elderly. *Archives of Physical Medicine and Rehabilitation*, 75: 1297–301.

Oxman, T.E. and Berkman, L.F. (1990) Assessment of social relationships in elderly patients. *International Journal of Psychiatry in Medicine*, 20: 65–84.

Pallant, J.F. and Lae, L. (2002) Sense of coherence, well-being, coping and personality factors: further evaluation of the sense of coherence scale. *Journal of Personality and Individual Differences*, 33: 39–48.

Pandey, M., Singh, S.P., Behere, P.B. *et al.* (2000) Quality of life in patients with early and advanced carcinoma of the breast. *European Journal of Surgical Oncology*, 26: 20–4.

Parker, R.D., Flint, E.P., Bosworth, H.B. *et al.* (2003) A three-factor analytic model of the MADRS in geriatric depression. *International Journal of Geriatric Psychiatry*, 18: 73–7.

Parker, S.G., Du, X., Bardsley, M.J. *et al.* (1994) Measuring outcomes in care of the elderly. *Journal of the Royal College of Physicians of London*, 28: 428–33.

Parker, S.G., Bechinger-English, D., Jagger, C. *et al.* (2006) Factors affecting completion of the SF-36 in older people. *Age and Ageing*, 35: 376–81.

Patrick, D.L. (ed.) (1982) *Health and Care of the Physically Disabled in Lambeth*. Report of Phase II of the Longitudinal Disability Interview Survey. London: St Thomas's Hospital Medical School, Department of Community Medicine.

Patrick, D.L. (2003) Patient-reported outcomes (PROs). An organizing tool for concepts, measures and applications. *Quality of Life Newsletter*, 31: 1–5.

Patrick, D.L. and Erickson, P. (1993) *Health Status and Health Policy. Quality of Life in Health Care Evaluation and Resource Allocation.* New York: Oxford University Press.

Patrick, D.L., Bush, J.W. and Chen, M.M. (1973a) Methods for measuring levels of well-being for a health status index. *Health Services Research*, 11: 516.

Patrick, D.L., Bush, J.W. and Chen, M.M. (1973b) Toward an operational definition of health. *Journal of Health and Social Behaviour*, 14: 6–23.

Pattie, A.H. (1981) A survey version of the Clifton Assessment procedures for the Elderly (CAPE). *British Journal of Clinical Psychology*, 20: 173–8.

Pattie, A.H. and Gilleard, C.J. (1975) A brief psychogeriatric assessment schedule. Validation against psychiatric diagnosis and discharge from hospital. *British Journal of Psychiatry*, 127: 489–93.

Pattie, A.H. and Gilleard, C.J. (1979) *Manual of the Clifton Assessment Procedures for the Elderly.* Sevenoaks: Hodder & Stoughton.

Pavot, W. and Diener, E. (1993) Review of the Satisfaction with Life Scale. *Psychological Assessment*, 5: 164–72.

Pavot, W., Diener, E., Colvin, C.R. and Sandvik, E. (1991) Further validation of the satisfaction with Life Scale: evidence for the cross-method convergence of well-being measures. *Journal of Personality Assessment*, 57: 149–61.

Paykel, E.S. (1985) Clinical interview for depression, development, reliability and validity. *Journal of Affective Disorders*, 9: 85–96.

Payne, R.L. and Graham Jones, J. (1987) Measurement and methodological issues in social support, in S.V. Kasl and C.L. Cooper (eds) *Stress and Health: Issues in Research Methodology.* Chichester: John Wiley.

Pearlin, L.I. and Schooler, C. (1978) The structure of coping. *Journal of Health and Social Behavior*, 19: 2–21.

Penley, J.A., Wiebe, J.S. and Nwosu, A. (2003) Psychometric properties of the Spanish Beck Depression Inventory-II in a medical sample. *Psychological Assessment*, 15: 569–77.

Perlman, D. and Peplau, L.A. (1981) Toward a social psychology of loneliness, in R. Gilmour and S. Duck (eds) *Personal Relationships: 3. Personal Relationships in Disorder.* London: Academic Press.

Perlman, R.A. (1987) Development of a functional assessment questionnaire for geriatric patients: the comprehensive older persons' evaluation (COPE). *Journal of Chronic Diseases*, 40: 85S–94S, Supplement.

Perloff, J.M. and Persons, J.B. (1988) Biases resulting from the use of indexes: an application to attributional style and depression. *Psychological Bulletin*, 103: 95–104.

Permanyer-Miralda, G., Alonso, J., Anto, J.M. *et al.* (1991) Comparison of perceived health status and conventional functional evaluation in stable patients with coronary artery disease. *Journal of Clinical Epidemiology*, 44: 779–86.

Persson, R. and Orbaek, P. (2003) The influence of personality traits on neuropsychological test performance and self-reported health and social contacts in women. *Journal of Personality and Individual Differences*, 34: 295–313.

Pettit, T., Livingstone, G., Manela, M. *et al.* (2001) Validation and normative data of health status measures in older people: the Islington study. *International Journal of Geriatric Psychiatry*, 16: 1061–70.

Péus, D., Newcomb, N. and Hofer, S. (2013) Appraisal of the Karnofsky Performance Status and proposal of a simple algorithmic system for its evaluation. *BMC Medicine, Informatics Decision Making*, 13: 72.

Pfeiffer, B.A., McClelland, T. and Lawson, J. (1989) Use of the Functional Assessment Inventory to distinguish among the rural elderly in five service settings. *Journal of the American Geriatrics Society*, 37: 243–8.

Pfeiffer, E. (1975) A short portable mental status questionnaire for the assessment of organic brain deficit in elderly patients. *Journal of American Geriatrics Society*, 23: 433–41.

Pibernik-Okanovic, M. (2001) Psychometric properties of the World Health Organization quality of life questionnaire (WHOQOL-100) in diabetic patients in Croatia. *Diabetes Research in Clinical Practice*, 51: 133–43.

Pierce, G.R., Sarason, I.G. and Sarason, B.R. (1991) General and relationship-based perceptions of social support: are two constructs better than one? *Journal of Personality and Social Psychology*, 61: 1028–39.

Pincus, T., Summey, J.A., Soraci, S.A. *et al.* (1983) Assessment of patient satisfaction in activities of daily living using a modified Stanford Health Assessment Questionnaire. *Arthritis and Rheumatism*, 26: 1346–53.

Pincus, T., Yazici, Y. and Bergman, M. (2005) Development of a multi-dimensional health assessment questionnaire (MDHAQ) for the infrastructure of standard clinical care. *Clinical and Experimental Rheumatology*, 23 (suppl. 39): S19–28.

Pollard, W.E., Bobbitt, R.A., Bergner, M. *et al.* (1976) The Sickness Impact Profile: reliability of a health status measure. *Medical Care*, 14: 57–67.

Pollard, W.E., Bobbitt, R.A. and Bergner, M. (1978) Examination of variable errors of measurement in a survey-based social indicator. *Social Indicators Research*, 5: 279–301.

Pomeroy, E., Cook, B. and Benjafield, J. (1992) Perceived social support in three residential contexts. *Canadian Journal of Community Mental Health*, 11: 101–7.

Post, M.W., de Bruin, A., De Witte, L. and Schrijvers, A. (1996) The SIP68: a measure of health-related functional status in rehabilitation medicine. *Archives of Physical Medicine and Rehabilitation*, 77: 440–5.

Post, M.W., Gerritsen, J., Diederikst, J.P. and DeWittet, L.P. (2001) Measuring health status of people who are wheelchair-dependent: validity of the Sickness Impact Profile 68 and the Nottingham Health Profile. *Disability and Rehabilitation*, 23: 245–53.

Potts, M.K., Daniels, M., Burnam, A. and Wells, K.B. (1990) A structured interview version of the Hamilton Depression Rating Scale: Evidence of reliability and versatility of administration. *Journal of Psychiatric Research*, 24: 335–50.

Power, M., Harper, A. and Bullinger, M. and the WHO Quality of Life Group (1999) The World Health Organization WHOQOL-100: tests of the universality of quality of life in 15 different cultural groups worldwide. *Health Psychology*, 18: 495–505.

Power, M., Quinn, K., Schmidt, S. and WHOQOL-OLD Group (2005) Development of WHOQOL-OLD module. *Quality of Life Research*, 14: 2197–214.

Pretorius, T.B. and Diedricks, M. (1993) A factorial investigation of the dimensions of social support. *South African Journal of Psychology*, 23: 32–5.

Priestman, T.J. and Baum, M. (1976) Evaluation of quality of life in patients receiving treatment for advanced breast cancer. *Lancet*, 1: 899–901.

Prieto, E.J. and Geisinger, K.F. (1983) Factor analytic studies of the McGill Pain Questionnaire, in R. Melzack (ed.) *Pain Measurement and Assessment*. New York: Raven Press.

Prince, M.J., Harwood, R.H., Blizzard, R.A. *et al.* (1997) Impairment, disability and handicap as risk factors for depression in old age. The Gospel Oak Project. *Psychological Medicine*, 27: 311–21.

Prince, M.J., Harwood, R.H., Thomas, A. *et al.* (1998) A prospective population-based cohort study of the effects of disablement and social milieu on the onset and maintenance of late life depression. The Gospel Oak Project. *Psychological Medicine*, 28: 337–50.

Procidano, M.E. and Heller, K. (1983) Measures of perceived social support from friends and from family: three validation studies. *American Journal of Community Psychology*, 11: 1–24.

Putnam, M. (2002) Linking aging theory and disability models: increasing the potential to explore aging with physical impairment. *The Gerontologist*, 42: 799–806.

Putnam, R.D. (1995) Bowling alone: America's declining social capital. *Journal of Democracy*, 6: 65–78.

Putnam, R.D. (2000) *Bowling Alone. The Collapse and Revival of American Community*. New York: Simon & Schuster.

Pyne, J.M., Sieber, W.J., David, K. *et al.* (2003) Use of the quality of well-being self administered version (QWB-SA) in assessing health-related quality of life in depressed patients. *Journal of Affective Disorders*, 76: 237–47.

Quinn, T.J., Langhorne, P. and Stott, D.J. (2011) Barthel Index for Stroke Trials. Development, Properties, and Application. *Stroke*, 242: 1146–51.

Quintana, J.M., Padierna, A., Esteban, C. *et al.* (2003) Evaluation of the psychometric characteristics of the Spanish version of the Hospital Anxiety and Depression Scale. *Acta Psychiatrica Scandinavica*, 107: 216–21.

Raczek, A.E., Ware, J.E., Bjorner, J.B. *et al.* (1998) Comparison of Rasch and summated rating scales constructed from SF-36 physical functioning items in seven countries. Result from the IQOLA project. *Journal of Clinical Epidemiology*, 51: 1203–14.

Radloff, L.S. (1977) Sex differences in depression: the effects of occupation and marital status. *Sex Roles*, 1: 249–65.

Radosevich, D.M. and Husnik, M.J. (1995) An abbreviated health status questionnaire: the HSQ-12. Update. Bloomington, IN: Newsletter of the Health Outcomes Institute, 2: 1–4.

Radosevich, D.M. and Pruitt, M.J.H. (1995) HSQ-12 Cooperative validation project: phase 1 reliability, validity and comparability. Update. Bloomington, IN: Newsletter of the Health Outcomes Institute, 2: 3.

Ramey, D.R., Raynauld, J.P. and Fries, J.F. (1992) The Health Assessment Questionnaire 1992. *Arthritis Care and Research*, 5: 119–29.

Ramey, D.R., Fries, J.F. and Singh, G. (1996) The Health Assessment Questionnaire 1995 – Status and review, in B. Spilker (ed.) *Pharmacoeconomics and Quality of Life in Clinical Trials* (2nd edn). Philadelphia: Lippincott-Raven.

Rand, S.E., Malley, J.N., Netten, A.P. and Forder, J.E. (2015) Factor structure and construct validity of the Adult Social Care Outcomes Toolkit for Carers (ASCOT-Carer). *Quality of Life Research*, 24: 2601–14.

Ranhoff, A.H. and Laake, K. (1993) The Barthel ADL Index: scoring by the physician from patient interview is not reliable. *Age and Ageing*, 22: 171–4.

Rankin, J. (1957) Cerebral vascular accidents in people over the age of 60. II. Prognosis. *Scottish Medical Journal*, 2: 200–15.

Ranzijn, R. and Luszcz, M. (2000) Measurement of subjective quality of life in elders. *International Journal of Aging and Human Development*, 50: 263–78.

Raskin, A. (1986) Sensitivity to treatment effects of evaluation instruments completed by psychiatrists, psychologists, nurses, and patients, in N. Sartorius and T. Ban (eds) *Assessment of Depression*. Berlin: Springer.

Read, L.J., Quinn, R.J. and Hoefer, M.A. (1987) Measuring overall health: an evaluation of three important approaches. *Journal of Chronic Diseases*, 40: 7S–21S.

Reading, A.E. (1979) The internal structure of the McGill Pain Questionnaire in dysmenorrhoea patients. *Pain*, 7: 353–8.

Reading, A.E., Everitt, B.S. and Sledmere, C.M. (1982) The McGill Pain Questionnaire: a replication of its construction. *British Journal of Clinical Psychology*, 21: 339–49.

Reed, P.F., Fitts, W.H. and Boehm, L. (1980) *Tennessee Self Concept Scale: Bibliography of Research Studies*. Nashville, TN: Councillor Recordings and Tests.

Rehm, L.P. (1981) *Behaviour Therapy for Depression*. New York: Academic Press.

Renne, K.S. (1974) Measurement of social health in a general population survey. *Social Sciences Research*, 3: 25–44.

Rettig, K.D. and Leichtentritt, R.D. (1999) A general theory for perceptual indicators of family life quality. *Social Indicators Research*, 47: 307–42.

Revicki, D.A. and Kaplan, R.M. (1993) Relationship between psychometric and utility-based approaches to the measurement of health-related quality of life. *Quality of Life Research*, 2: 477–87.

Reynolds, W.M. and Gould, J.W. (1981) A psychometric investigation of the standard and short form Beck Depression Inventory. *Journal of Consulting and Clinical Psychology*, 49: 306–7.

Riazi, A., Hobart, J.C., Lamping, D.L. et al. (2003a) Evidence-based measurement in multiple sclerosis: the psychometric properties of the physical and psychological dimensions of three quality of life rating scales. *Multiple Sclerosis*, 9: 411–19.

Riazi, A., Hobart, J.C., Lamping, J.C. et al. (2003b) Using the SF-36 measure to compare the health impact of multiple sclerosis and Parkinson's disease with normal population health profiles. *Journal of Neurology and Neurosurgical Psychiatry*, 74: 710–14.

Richardson, C.A. and Hammond, S.M. (1996) A psychometric analysis of a short device for assessing depression in elderly people. *British Journal of Clinical Psychology*, 35: 543–51.

Richter, P., Werner, J., Heerlien, A. et al. (1998) On the validity of the Beck Depression Inventory. A review. *Psychopathology*, 46: 34–43.

Riggio, R.E., Watring, K.P. and Throckmorton, B. (1993) Social skills, social support, and psychosocial adjustment. *Journal of Personality and Individual Differences*, 15: 275–80.

Rivera, P.A., Rose, J.M., Futterman, A. et al. (1991) Dimensions of perceived support in clinically depressed and non-depressed female caregivers. *Psychology of Aging*, 6: 232–7.

Roberts, B., Browne, J. and Ocaka, K.F. (2008) The reliability and validity of the SF-8 with a conflict-affected population in northern Uganda. *Health and Quality of Life Outcomes*, 6: 108.

Robins, L.N., Helzer, J.E., Croughan, J.L. and Ratcliff, K. (1981) The NIMH diagnostic interview schedule: Its history, characteristics and validity, in J.K. Wing, P. Bebbington and L.N. Robins (eds) *What is a Case? The Problem of Definition in Psychiatric Community Surveys*. London: Grant MacIntyre.

Robinson, J.P. and Shaver, P.R. (1973) *Measures of Social Psychological Attitudes*. Ann Arbor, MI: Survey Research Centre, Institute for Social Research.

Robinson, R.A. (1968) The organisation of a diagnostic and treatment unit for the aged, in UK Giegy, *Psychiatric Disorders in the Aged*. Manchester: World Psychiatric Association.

Rockwood, K., Stolee, P. and Fox, R.A. (1993) Use of goal attainment scaling in measuring clinically important change in the frail elderly. *Journal of Clinical Epidemiology*, 46: 1113–18.

Rodgers, H., Curless, R. and James, O.F.W. (1993) Standardized functional assessment scales for elderly patients. *Age and Ageing*, 22: 161–3.

Rodriguez, N., Mira, C., Myers, H. *et al.* (2003) Family or friends: who plays a greater supportive role for Latino college students? *Cultural Diversity and Ethnic Minority Psychology*, 9: 236–50.

Rogerson, R.J. (1995) Environmental and health-related quality of life: conceptual and methodological similarities. *Social Science and Medicine*, 41: 1373–82.

Rogerson, R.J., Findlay, A.M., Coombes, M.G. and Morris, A. (1989) Indicators of quality of life. *Environment and Planning*, 21, 1655–66.

Roid, G.H. and Fitts, W.H. (1988) *Tennessee Self Concept Scale (TSCS)*. Los Angeles, CA: Western Psychological Services.

Romera, I., Delgado-Cohen, H., Perez, T. *et al.* (2008) Factor analysis of the Zung self-rating depression scale in a large sample of patients with major depressive disorder in primary care. *BMC Psychiatry*, 8: 4.

Rosenberg, M. (1965) *Society and the Adolescent Self Image*. Princeton, NJ: Princeton University Press.

Rosenberg, M. (1986) *Conceiving the Self* (2nd edn). Malabar, FL: Krieger.

Rosenberg, R. (1995) Health-related quality of life between naturalism and hermeneutics. Special Issue 'Quality of Life' in *Social Science and Medicine*, 10: 1411–15.

Ross, C.E. and Mirowsky, J. (2001) Neighbourhood disadvantage, disorder and health. *Journal of Health and Social Behavior*, 42: 258–76.

Rosser, R.M. and Watts, V.C. (1971) The sanative outputs of hospitals. Dallas, 39th conference of the Operational Research Society of America.

Rosser, R.M. and Watts, V.C. (1972) The measurement of hospital output. *International Journal of Epidemiology*, 1: 361–8.

Rouhani, S. and Zoleikani, P. (2013) Socioeconomic status and quality of life in elderly people in rural area of Sari-Iran. *Life Science Journal*, 10: 74–8.

Ruini, C., Ottolini, F., Rafanelli, C. *et al.* (2003) The relationship of psychological well-being to distress and personality. *Psychotherapy and Psychosomatics*, 72: 268–75.

Russell, D. (1982) The measurement of loneliness, in L.A. Peplau and D. Perlman (eds) *Loneliness: A Sourcebook of Current Theory, Research and Therapy*. New York: John Wiley.

Russell, D. (1996) UCLA Loneliness Scale (version 3): reliability, validity, and factor structure. *Journal of Personality Assessment*, 66: 20–40.

Russell, D. and Cutrona, C.E. (1991) UCLA Loneliness Scale version 3, in J.P. Robinson, P.R. Shaver and L.S. Wrightsman (eds) *Measures of Personality and Social Psychological Attitudes*. San Diego, CA: Academic Press.

Russell, D., Peplau, L.A. and Ferguson, M.L. (1978) Developing a measure of loneliness. *Journal of Personality Assessment*, 42: 290–4.

Russell, D., Peplau, L.A. and Cutrona, C.E. (1980a) The revised UCLA Loneliness Scale: concurrent and discriminant validity evidence. *Journal of Personality and Social Psychology*, 39: 472–80.

Russell, D., Peplau, L.A. and Cutrona, C.E. (1980b) Revised UCLA Loneliness Scale version 3 (RULS), in K. Corcoran and J. Fischer (eds) *Measures for Clinical Practice: a Sourcebook*, Vol. 2. New York: Free Press.

Russell, D.W., Cutrona, C.E., McRae, C. and Gomez, M. (2012) Is loneliness the same as being alone? *Journal of Psychology*, 146: 7–22.

Ruta, D.A. (1992) A new approach to the measurement of quality of life. The patient generated index. Paper presented to the Workshop on Quality of Life, Society for Social Medicine 36th Annual Conference, Nottingham, September.

Ruta, D.A., Abdalla, M.I., Garratt, A.M. *et al.* (1994a) SF-36 health survey questionnaire: I. Reliability in two patient-based studies. *Quality in Health Care*, 3: 180–5.

Ruta, D.A., Garratt, A.M., Leng, M. *et al.* (1994b) A new approach to the measurement of quality of life: the patient-generated index. *Medical Care*, 32: 1109–26.

Ruta, D.A., Garratt, A.M. and Russell, I.T. (1999) Patient-centred assessment of quality of life for patients with four common conditions. *Quality in Health Care*, 8: 22–9.

Rutledge, T., Matthews, K., Lui, L.Y., *et al.* (2003) Social networks and marital status predict mortality in older women: prospective evidence from the study of osteoporotic fractures (SOF). *Psychosomatic Medicine*, 65: 688–94.

Ryan, J.M., Corry, J.R., Attewell, R. and Smithsen, M.J. (2002) A comparison of the electronic version of the SF-36 General Health Questionnaire to the standard paper version. *Quality of Life Research*, 11: 19–26.

Ryff, C.D. (1989) Beyond Ponce de Leon and Life satisfaction: New directions in quest of successful aging. *International Journal of Behavioral Development*, 12: 35–55.

Ryff, C.D. (1995) Psychological well-being in adult life. *Current Directions in Psychological Science*, 4: 99–104.

Ryff, C.D. and Essex, M.J. (1991) Psychological wellbeing in adulthood and old age: descriptive markers and explanatory processes, in K. Warner Schaie and M. Powell Lawton (eds) *Annual Review of Gerontology and Geriatrics*, vol. 11: 144–71.

Ryff, C.D. and Keyes, C.L.M. (1995) The structure of psychological well-being revisited. *Journal of Personality and Social Psychology*, 69: 719–27.

Ryff, C.D. and Singer, B. (1996) Psychological well-being: meaning, measurement, and implications for psychotherapy research. *Psychotherapy and Psychosomatics*, 65, 14–23.

Sackett, D.L., Spitzer, W.O., Gent, M. *et al.* (1974) The Burlington Randomized Trial of the nurse practitioner: health outcomes of patients. *Annals of Internal Medicine*, 80: 137–42.

Sainsbury, S. (1973) *Measuring Disability*. London: Bell.

Sala, F., Piva, S., Barreca, C. *et al.* (2000) Validation of an Italian version of the arthritis impact measurement scales 2 (ITALIAN-AIMS2) for patients with osteoarthritis of the knee. Gonarthrosis and quality of life assessment (GOQOLA) Study Group. *Rheumatology*, 39: 720–7.

Salyers, M.P., Bosworth, H.B., Swanson, J.W. *et al.* (2000) Reliability and validity of the SF-12 health survey among people with severe mental illness. *Medical Care*, 38: 1141–50.

Sandler, I.N. and Barrera, M. (1984) Towards a multimethod approach to assessing the effects of social support. *American Journal of Community Psychology*, 12: 37–52.

Sarason, I.G., Levine, H.M., Basham, R.B. and Sarason, B.R. (1983) Assessing social support: the social support questionnaire. *Journal of Personality and Social Psychology*, 44: 127–39.

Sarason, B.R., Sarason, I.G., Hacker, T.A. and Basham, R.B. (1985) Concomitants of social support: social skills, physical attractiveness, and gender. *Journal of Personality and Social Psychology*, 49: 469–80.

Sarason, B.R., Shearin, E.N., Pierce, G.R. and Sarason, I.G. (1987a) Interrelationships of social support measures: theoretical and practical implications. *Journal of Personality and Social Psychology*, 52: 813–32.

Sarason, I.G., Sarason, B.R., Shearin, E.N. and Pierce, G.R. (1987b) A brief measure of social support. Practical and theoretical implications. *Journal of Social and Personal Relationships*, 4: 497–510.

Sarason, I.G., Sarason, B.R. and Pierce, G.R. (1994) Social support: global and relationship-based levels of analysis. *Journal of Social and Personal Relationships*, 11: 295–312.

Saronson, S.B., Carroll, C., Maton, K. *et al.* (1977) *Human Services and Resource Networks*. San Francisco, CA: Jossey-Bass.

Sarvimäki, A. (1999) What do we mean by 'quality of life' in our care for people with dementia? *Journal of Dementia Care*, January/February 35–7.

Sarvimäki, A. and Stonbock-Hult, B. (2000) Quality of life in old age described as a sense of well-being, meaning and value. *Journal of Advanced Nursing*, 32: 1025–33.

Sauer, W.J. and Warland, R. (1982) Morale and life satisfaction, in D.J. Mangen and W.A. Peterson (eds) *Research Instruments in Social Gerontology*, Vol. 1. Clinical and social psychology. Minneapolis, MN: University of Minnesota Press.

Sayer, N.A., Sackheim, H.A., Moeller, J.R. *et al.* (1993) The relations between observer-rating and self-report of depressive symptomatology. *Journal of Psychological Assessment*, 5: 350–60.

Schaafsma, J. and Osoba, D. (1994) The Karnofsky Performance Status scale re-examined: a crossvalidation with the EORTC-C30. *Quality of Life Research*, 3: 413–24.

Schag, C.A.C., Heinrich, R.L. and Ganz, P.A. (1984) Karnofsky Performance Status revisited: reliability, validity and guidelines. *Journal of Clinical Oncology*, 2: 187–93.

Scheier, M.F. and Carver, C.S. (1985) Optimism, coping and health: Assessment and implications of generalised outcome expectancies. *Health Psychology*, 4: 219–47.

Schmitz, N., Kugler, J. and Rollnik, J. (2003) On the relation between neuroticism, self-esteem, and depression: results from the National Comorbidity Survey. *Comprehensive Psychiatry*, 44: 169–76.

Schmutte, P.S. and Ryff, C.D. (1997) Personality and well-being: re-examining methods and meanings. *Journal of Personality and Social Psychology*, 73: 549–59.

Schneiderman, L.J., Kaplan, R.M., Pearlman, R.A. et al. (1993) Do physicians' own preferences for life sustaining treatment influence their perceptions of patients' preferences? *Journal of Clinical Ethics*, 4: 28–33.

Schoenbach, V., Kaplan, B.H., Fredman, L. and Kleinbaum, D.G. (1986) Social ties and mortality in Evans County, Georgia. *American Journal of Epidemiology*, 123: 577–91.

Scholten, J.H.G. and van Weel, C. (1992) Manual for the use of the Dartmouth COOP Functional Health Assessment Charts/WONCA in measuring functional status in family practice (Part I), in J.H. Scholten and C. van Weel (eds) *Functional Status Assessment in Family Practice*. Lelystad: Meditekst.

Scholzel-Dorenbos, C.J. (2000) Measurement Ventegodtof quality of life in patients with dementia of Alzheimer type and their caregivers: Schedule for the Evaluation of Individual Quality of Life (SEIQoL). *Tijdschr Gerontology and Geriatrics*, 31: 23–6.

Schuling, J. and Meyboom-de Jong, B. (1992) Change in clinical status in patients with stroke, in J.H. Scholten and C. van Weel (eds) *Functional Status Assessment in Family Practice*. Lelystad: Meditekst.

Schuling, J., Greidanus, J. and Meyboom-de Jong, B. (1993) Measuring functional status of stroke patients with the Sickness Impact Profile. *Disability and Rehabilitation*, 15: 19–23.

Schumaker, J.F., Shea, J.D., Monfries, M.M. and Groth-Marnat, G. (1993) Loneliness and life satisfaction in Japan and Australia. *Journal of Psychology*, 127: 65–71.

Schumann, A., Hapke, U., Meyer, C. et al. (2003) Measuring sense of coherence with only three items: a useful tool for population surveys. *British Journal of Health Psychology*, 8: 409–21.

Schwab, J.J., Brolow, M.R. and Holser, C.E. (1967) A comparison of two rating scales for depression. *Journal of Clinical Psychology*, 23: 94–6.

Schwartz, A.N. (1975) An observation of self-esteem as the linchpin of quality of life for the aged. An essay. *Gerontologist*, 15: 470–2.

Schwartz, N. and Strack, F. (1999) Reports of subjective wellbeing: judgemental processes and their methodological implications, in D. Kanahan, E. Diener and N. Schwartz (eds) *Wellbeing: the Foundations of Hedonistic Psychology*. New York: Russell Sage Foundation.

Schwarzer, R. and Schwarzer, C. (1996) A critical survey of coping instruments, in: M. Zeidner and N.S. Endler (eds) Handbook of Coping. New York: Wiley.

Scott, J. (2013). *Social Network Analysis: A Handbook* (3rd edn). Thousand Oaks, CA: Sage.

Scott, P.J., Ansell, B.M. and Huskisson, E.C. (1977) The measurement of pain in juvenile chronic polyarthritis. *Annals of the Rheumatic Diseases*, 36: 186–7.

Sedrakyan, A., Vaccarino, V., Paltiel, A.D. et al. (2003) Age does not limit quality of life improvement in cardiac valve surgery. *Journal of the American College of Cardiology*, 42: 1215–17.

Seedhouse, D. (1986) *Health: the Foundations of Achievement*. Chichester: John Wiley.

Seeman, T.E. and Berkman, L.F. (1988) Structural characteristics of social networks and their relationship with social support in the elderly: who provides support? *Social Science and Medicine*, 26: 737–49.

Seeman, T.E., Kaplan, G.A., Knudsen, L. et al. (1987) Social network ties and mortality among the elderly in the Alameda County study. *American Journal of Epidemiology*, 126: 714–23.

Selai, C.E., Elstner, K. and Trimble, M.R. (2000) Quality of life pre- and post-epilepsy surgery. *Epilepsy Research*, 38: 67–74.

Seligman, M. (2002) *Authentic Happiness: Using the New Positive Psychology to Realize Potential for Lasting Fulfilment*. New York: Free Press.

Sen, A. (1985) *Commodities and Capabilities*. Oxford: North-Holland.

Sexton, E., King-Kallimanis, B., Conroy, R. and Hickey, A. (2013) Psychometric evaluation of the CASP-19 quality of life scale in an older Irish cohort. *Quality of Life Research*, 22: 2549–59.

Sexton, E., King-Kallimanis, B., Layte, R. and Hickey, A. (2015) CASP-19 special section: how does chronic disease status affect CASP quality of life at older ages? Examining the WHO ICF disability domains as mediators of this relationship. *Aging and Mental Health*, 19: 622–33.

Seymour, D.G., Ball, A.E., Russell, E.M. et al. (2001) Problems in using health survey questionnaires in older patients with physical disabilities. The reliability and validity of the SF-36 and the effect of cognitive impairment. *Journal of the Evaluation of Clinical Practice* 7: 411–18.

Shah, S., Frank, V. and Cooper, V. (1989) Improving the sensitivity of the Barthel Index for stroke rehabilitation. *Journal of Clinical Epidemiology*, 42: 703–9.

Shanas, E., Townsend, P. and Wedderburn, D. et al. (1968) *Old People in Three Industrial Societies*. London: Routledge & Kegan Paul.

Shaver, P.R. and Brennan, K.A. (1991) Measures of depression and loneliness, in J.P. Robinson, P.R. Shaver and L.S. Wrightsman (eds) *Measures of Personality and Social Psychological Attitudes*. San Diego, CA: Academic Press.

Sheikh, R.L. and Yesavage, J.A. (1986) Geriatric Depression Scale (GDS): recent evidence and development of a shorter version. *Clinical Gerontologist*, 5: 165–73.

Sheikh, R.L., Yesavage, J.A., Brooks, J.O. *et al.* (1991) Proposed factor structure of the Geriatric Depression Scale. *International Psychogeriatrics*, 3: 23–8.

Sherbourne, C.D. and Hays, R.D. (1990) Marital status, social support and health transitions in chronic disease patients. *Journal of Health and Social Behaviour*, 31: 328–43.

Sherbourne, C.D. and Stewart, A.L. (1991) The MOS Social Support Survey. *Social Science and Medicine*, 32: 705–14.

Sherbourne, C.D., Meredith, L.S., Rogers, W. and Ware, J.E. (1992) Social support and stressful life events: Age differences in their effects on health-related quality of life among the chronically ill. *Quality of Life Research*, 1: 235–46.

Sherwood, S.J., Morris, J., Mor, V. and Gutkin, C. (1977) *Compendium of Measures for Describing and Assessing Long Term Care Populations*. Boston, MA: Hebrew Rehabilitation Center for the Aged.

Shiely, J.C., Bayliss, M.S., Keller, S.D. *et al.* (1996) SF-36 Health Survey. Annotated bibliography (1988–1995). Boston, MA: New England Medical Center.

Shin, D.C. and Johnson, D.M. (1978) Avowed happiness as an overall assessment of the quality of life. *Social Indicators Research*, 5: 475–92.

Siegel, M., Bradley, E.H. and Kasl, S.V. (2003) Self-rated life expectancy as a predictor of mortality: evidence from the HRS and AHEAD surveys. *Gerontology*, 49: 265–71.

Silber, E. and Tippett, J. (1965) Self esteem: clinical assessment and measurement validation. *Psychological Reports*, 16: 1017–71.

Silverstone, P.H., Entsuah, R. and Hacket, D. (2002) Two items on the Hamilton Depression rating scale are effect predictors of remission: comparison of selective serotonin reuptake inhibitors with the combined serotonin/norepineph reuptake inhibitor, venlafaxine. *International Clinical Psychopharmacology*, 17: 273–80.

Sims, A.C.P. and Salmons, P.H. (1975) Severity of symptoms of psychiatric out-patients: use of the General Health Questionnaire in hospital and general practice patients. *Psychological Medicine*, 5: 62–6.

Singer, E., Garfinkel, R., Cohen, S.M. *et al.* (1976) Mortality and mental health: evidence from the midtown Manhattan re-study. *Social Science and Medicine*, 10: 517–21.

Singh, J.A., Satele, D., Pattabasavaiah, S. *et al.* (2014) Normative data and clinically significant effect sizes for single-item numerical linear analogue self-assesment (LASA) scales. *Health and Quality of Life Outcomes*, 12: 187.

Sinha, S.P., Nayyar, P. and Sinha, S.P. (2002) Social support and self-control as variables in attitude towards life and perceived control among older people in India. *Journal of Social Psychology*, 142: 527–40.

Sitjas, M.E., San Jose, L.A., Armadans, G.L. *et al.* (2003) Predictor factors about functional decline in community-dwelling older persons. *Atencion Primaria*, 32: 282–7.

Sijtsma, J. (2005) Nonparametric item response theory models. *Encyclopedia of Social Measurement*, 2: 875–82.

Sijtsma, K. and Molenaar, I.W. (2002) *Introduction to Nonparametric Item Response Theory*. New York: Sage.

Singh, J.A., Satel, D., Pattabasavaiah, S. *et al.* (2014) Normative data and clinically significant effect sizes for single-item numerical linear analogue self-assessment (LASA) scales. *Health and Quality of Life Outcomes*, 12: 187.

Skevington, S.M. (1999) Measuring quality of life in Britain: introducing the WHOQOL-100. *Psychomatic Research*, 47: 449–59.

Skevington, S.M., Carse, M.S. and Williams, de C. (2001) Validation of the WHOQOL-100: pain management improves quality of life for chronic pain patients. *Clinical Journal of Pain*, 17: 264–75.

Skevington, S.M., Lotfy, M. and O'Connell, K.A. (2004) The World Health Organization's WHOQOL-BREF quality of life assessment: psychometric properties and results of international field trials. A report from the WHOQOL Group. *Quality of Life Research*, 13: 299–310.

Skinner, D.E. and Yett, D.E. (1972) Debility index for long-term care patients, in R.L. Berg (ed.) *Health Status Indexes*. Chicago, IL: Hospital Research and Education Trust.

Slevin, M.L., Plant, H., Lynch, D. *et al.* (1988) Who should measure quality of life, the doctor or the patient? *British Journal of Cancer*, 57: 109–12.

Sloan, J.A., Loprinzi, C.L., Kuross, S.A. *et al.* (1998) Randomized comparison of four tools measuring overall quality of life of patients with advanced cancer. *Journal of Clinical Oncology*, 16: 3662–73.

Slocum-Gori, S., Zumbo, B., Michalos, A. and Diener, E. (2009) A note on the dimensionality of quality of life scales: an illustration with the Satisfaction with Life Scale. *Social Indicators Research*, 92: 489–96.

Smith, A.H.W., Ballinger, B.R. and Presley, A.S. (1981) The reliability and validity of two assessment scales for the elderly mentally handicapped. *British Journal of Psychiatry*, 138: 15–16.

Smith, H.J., Taylor, R. and Mitchell, A. (2000) A comparison of four quality of life instruments in cardiac patients: SF-36, QLI, QLMI, and SEIQoL. *Heart*, 84: 390–4.

Smith, T.W. (1979) Happiness: time trends, seasonal variations, inter-survey differences and other mysteries. *Social Psychology Quarterly*, 42: 18–30.

Snaith, R.P. (1987) The concepts of mild depression. *British Journal of Psychiatry*, 150: 387–93.

Snaith, R.P. (2003) The Hospital Anxiety and Depression Scale. *Health and Quality of Life Outcomes*, 1: 29.

Snaith, R.P. and Taylor, C.M. (1985) Rating scales for depression and anxiety: a current perspective. *British Journal of Clinical Pharmacology*, 19: 17S–20S (suppl.).

Sokolovsky, J. (1986) Network methodologies in the study of ageing, in J. Keith (ed.) *New Methods for Old Age Research*. Westport, CT: Greenwood Press, Bergin & Garvey.

Söderhamn, U., Sundsli, K., Cliffordson, C., and Dale, B. (2015) Psychometric properties of Antonovsky's 29-item Sense of Coherence scale in research on older home-dwelling Norwegians. *Scandinavian Journal of Public Health*, 1–8.

Spatz, K. and Johnson, F. (1973) Internal consistency of the Coopersmith Self Esteem Inventory. *Educational and Psychological Measurements*, 33: 875–6.

Spector, W.D., Katz, S., Murphy, J.B. *et al.* (1987) The hierarchical relationship between activities of daily living and instrumental activities of daily living. *Journal of Chronic Diseases*, 40: 481–9.

Sperduto, P.W., Kased, N., Roberge, D. *et al.* (2012) Summary report on the graded prognostic assessment: an accurate and facile diagnostic-specific tool to estimate survival for patients with brain metasteses. *Journal of Clinical Oncology*, 30: 419–25.

Spielberger, C.D., Gorsuch, R.L. and Luchene, R.E. (1970) *Manual for the State–Trait Anxiety Inventory*. Palo Alto, CA: Consulting Psychologists Press.

Spielberger, C.D., Davidson, K., Lighthall, F. *et al.* (1973) *STAI Preliminary Manual*. Palo Alto, CA: Consulting Psychologists Press.

Spielberger, C.D., Gorsuch, R.L., Luchene, R.E. *et al.* (1983) *Manual for the State–Trait Anxiety Inventory* (revised edition). Palo Alto, CA: Consulting Psychologists Press.

Spiro, A. and Bossè, R. (2000) Relations between health-related quality of life and well-being: the gerontologist's new clothes? *International Journal of Aging and Human Development*, 50: 297–318.

Spitzer, R.L., Burdock, E.I. and Hardesty, A.S. (1964) *Mental Status Schedule*. New York: Department of Psychiatry, College of Physicians and Surgeons, Columbia University and Biometrics Research Section, New York State Department of Mental Hygiene.

Spitzer, R.L., Endicott, J. and Robins, E. (1978) Research Diagnostic Criteria: rationale and reliability. *Archives of General Psychiatry*, 35: 773–82.

Spitzer, W.O., Dobson, A.J., Hall, J. *et al.* (1981) Measuring quality of life of cancer patients: a concise QL-index for use by physicians. *Journal of Chronic Diseases*, 34: 585–97.

Sprangers, M.A.G. and Schwartz, C.E. (1999) Integrating response shift into health-related quality of life research: a theoretical model. *Social Science and Medicine*, 48: 1507–15.

Sprangers, M.A.G., Van Dam, F.S.A.M., Broersen, J. *et al.* (1999) Revealing response shift in longitudinal research on fatigue: the use of the thentest approach. *Acta Oncologica*, 38: 709–18.

Spruytte, N., Verschueren, K. and Marcoen, A. (1999) Grandparents: their experience of the relationship with the oldest grand-child and their psychological well-being. *Tijdschr Gerontology and Geriatrics*, 30: 21–30.

Staniszewska, S. (1999) Patient expectations and health-related quality of life. *Health Expectations*, 2: 93–104.

Stansfeld, S.A. (1999) Social support and social cohesion, in M. Marmot and R.G. Wilkinson (eds) *Social Determinants of Health*. Oxford: Oxford University Press.

Stansfeld, S.A. and Marmot, M.G. (1992) Social class and minor psychiatric disorder in British civil servants: a validated screening survey using the GHQ. *Psychological Medicine*, 22: 739–49.

Stanwyck, D.J. and Garrison, W.M. (1982) Detecting on faking on the Tennessee Self-Concept Scale. *Journal of Personality Assessment*, 46: 426–31.

Steer, R.A., Beck, A.T. and Garrison, B. (1986) Applications of the Beck Depression Inventory, in N. Sartorius and T.A. Ban (eds) *Assessment of Depression*. Berlin: Springer-Verlag.

Steer, R.A., Ball, R., Ranieri, W.F. and Beck, A.T. (1999) Dimensions of the Beck Depression Inventory-II in clinically depressed out-patients. *Journal of Clinical Psychology*, 55: 117–28.

Steer, R.A., Rissmiller, D.J. and Beck, A.T. (2000) Use of the Beck Depression Inventory-II with depressed geriatric inpatients. *Behavioral Research and Therapy*, 38: 311–18.

Steer, R.A., Brown, G.K., Beck, A.T. and Sanderson, W.C. (2001) Mean Beck Depression Inventory-II scores by severity of major depressive episode. *Psychological Reports*, 88: 1075–6.

Stehouwer, R.S. (1985) Beck Depression Inventory, in D.J. Keyser and R.C. Sweetland (eds) *Test Critiques*, vol. II. Kansas City, MI: Test Corporation of America.

Stewart, A.L. and Ware, J.E. (1992) *Measuring Functioning and Well-being: The Medical Outcomes Study Approach*. Durham, NC: Duke University Press.

Stewart, A.L., Ware, J.E., Brook, R.H. *et al.* (1978) *Conceptualization and Measurement of Health for Adults in the Health Insurance Study*: vol. II: *Physical Health in Terms of Functioning*. Santa Monica, CA: RAND Corporation: R-1987/2-HEW.

Stewart, A.L., Ware, J.E. and Brook, R.H. (1981) Advances in the measurement of functional status: construction of aggregate indexes. *Medical Care*, 19: 473–88.

Stewart, A.L., Hays, R.D. and Ware, J.E. (1988) The MOS Short-form General Health Survey. Reliability and validity in a patient population. *Medical Care*, 26: 724–35.

Stewart, A.L., Greenfield, S., Hays, R. D. *et al.* (1989) Functional status and well-being of patients with chronic conditions: results from the medical outcomes study. *Journal of the American Medical Association*, 262: 907–13.

Stewart-Brown, S., Tennant, A., Tennant, R. *et al.* (2009) Internal construct validity of the Warwick-Edinburgh Mental Well-being Scale (WEMWBS): a Rasch analysis using data from the Scottish Health Education Population Survey. *Health and Quality of Life Outcomes*, 7: 15.

Stineman, M.G., Escarce, J.J., Goin, J.E. *et al.* (1994) A case mix classification system for medical rehabilitation. *Medical Care*, 32: 366–79.

Stock, W.A. and Okun, M.A. (1982) The construct validity of life satisfaction among the elderly. *Journal of Gerontology*, 37: 625–7.

Stokes, J.P. (1983) Predicting satisfaction with social support from social network structure. *American Journal of Community Psychology*, 11: 141–52.

Stokes, J.P. (1985) The relation of social network and individual difference variables to loneliness. *Journal of Personality and Social Psychology*, 48: 981–90.

Stokes, J.P. and Wilson, D.G. (1984) The Inventory of Socially Supportive Behaviours: dimensionality, prediction and gender differences. *American Journal of Community Psychology*, 12: 53–70.

Stones, M.L. and Kozma, A. (1980) Issues relating to the usage of conceptualizations of mental constructs employed by gerontologists. *International Journal of Ageing and Human Development*, 11: 269–81.

Strand, L.I., Ljunggren, A.E. and Bogen, B. (2008) The Short-Form McGill Pain Questionnaire as an outcome measure: test-retest reliability and responsiveness to change. *European Journal of Pain*, 12: 917–25.

Streiner, D.L. and Norman, G.R. (2008) *Health Measurement Scales: A Practical Guide to their Development and Use* (4th edn). Oxford: Oxford University Press.

Struttmann, T., Fabro, M., Romieu, G. *et al.* (1999) Quality-of-life assessment in the old using the WHOQOL 100: differences between patients with senile dementia and patients with cancer. *Int. Psychogeriatr.*, 11: 273–9.

Stueve, A. and Lein, L. (1979) Problems in network analysis: the case of the missing person. Paper presented at 32nd annual general meeting of the Gerontological Society of America.

Stull, D.E. (1987) Conceptualization and measurement of well-being: implications for policy evaluation, in E.F. Borgatta and R.J.V. Montgomery (eds) *Critical Issues in Ageing Policy*. Beverly Hills, CA: Sage Publications.

Stummer, C., Verheydena G., Putman, K. *et al.* (2015) Predicting sickness impact profile at six months after stroke: further results from the European multi-center CERISE study. *Disability and Rehabilitation*, 11: 942–50.

Sugisawa, H., Liang, J., Liu, X. *et al.* (1994) Social networks, social support, and mortality among older people in Japan. *Journal of Gerontology*, 49: S3–13.

Suh, E., Diener, E., Oishi, S. and Trandis, H.C. (1998) The shifting basis of life satisfaction judgments across cultures: emotions versus norms. *Journal of Personality and Social Psychology*, 74: 482–93.

Sullivan, M., Ahlmen, M. and Bjelle, A. (1990) Health status assessment in rheumatoid arthritis: 1. Further work on the validity of the Sickness Impact Profile. *Journal of Rheumatology*, 17: 439–47.

Sullivan, M., Karlsson, J. and Ware, J.R. (1995) The Swedish SF-36 Health Survey – 1. Evaluation of data quality, scaling assumptions, reliability and construct validity across general populations in Sweden. Special Issue 'Quality of Life' in *Social Science and Medicine*, 10: 1349–58.

Sultan, N., Pope, J.E. and Clements, P.J. (2004) The Health Assessment Questionnaire (HAQ) is strongly predictive of good outcome in early diffuse scleroderma: results from an analysis of two randomised controlled trials in early diffuse scleroderma. *Rheumatology*, 43: 472–8.

Surtees, P.G. (1987) Psychiatric disorder in the community and the General Health Questionnaire. *British Journal of Psychiatry*, 150: 828–35.

Sutcliffe, C., Cordingley, L., Burns, A. *et al.* (2000) A new version of the Geriatric Depression Scale for nursing and residential home populations: the Geriatric Depression Scale (residential) (GDS-12R). *International Psychogeriatrics*, 12: 173–81.

Swindells, S., Mohr, J., Justis, J.C. *et al.* (1999) Quality of life in patients with human immunodeficiency virus infection: Impact of social support, coping style and hopelessness. *International Journal of STD and AIDS*, 10: 383–91.

Szabo, S. on behalf of the WHOQOL Group (1996) The World Health Organization Quality of Life (WHOQOL) assessment instrument, in B. Spilker (ed.) *Quality of Life and Pharmacoeconomics in Clinical Trials* (2nd edn). Philadelphia, PA: Lippincox- Raven.

Tabachnick, B.G. and Fidell, L.S. (1996) *Using Multivariate Statistics* (3rd edn). New York: HarperCollins.

Tabali, M., Jeschke, E., Dassen, T. *et al.* (2012) The Nottingham Health Profile: a feasible questionnaire for nursing home residents? *International Psychogeriatrics*, 24: 416–24.

Tamaklo, W., Schubert, D.S., Mentari, A. *et al.* (1992) Assessing depression in the medical patient using the MADRS, a sensitive screening scale. *Journal of Integrative Psychiatry*, 8: 264–70.

Tang, J.A., Oh, T., Scheer, J.K. and Parsa, A.T. (2014) The current trend of administering a patient-generated index in the oncological setting: a systematic review. *Oncology Reviews*, 8: 245.

Tardy, C.H. (1985) Social support measurement. *American Journal of Community Psychiatry*, 13: 187–202.

Tarnopolsky, A., Hand, D.J., McLean, E.K. *et al.* (1979) Validity and uses of a screening questionnaire (GHQ) in the community. *British Journal of Psychiatry*, 134: 508–15.

Tavernier, S.S., Beck, S.L., Clayton, M.F. *et al.* (2011) Validity of the Patient Generated Index as a quality-of-life measure in radiation oncology. *Oncology Nursing Forum*, 38: 319–29.

Taylor, J. and Reitz, W. (1968) *The Three Faces of Self-esteem*. London: University of Western Ontario, Department of Psychology. Research Bulletin no. 80.

Taylor, J.E., Carlos Poston, W.S., Blackburn, G.L. *et al.* (2003) Psychometric characteristics of the General Well-Being Schedule (GWB) with African-American women. *Quality of Life Research*, 12: 31–9.

Teeling Smith, G. (1988) *Measuring Health: A Practical Approach*. Chichester: John Wiley.

Tennant, C. (1977) The General Health Questionnaire: a valid index of psychological impairment in Australian populations. *Medical Journal of Australia*, 2: 392–4.

Tennant, R., Hiller, L., Fishwick, R. *et al.* (2007) The Warwick-Edinburgh Mental Well-being Scale (WEMWBS): development and UK validation. *Health and Quality of Life Outcomes*, 5: 63–75.

Tentes, A.A., Tripsiannis, G., Markakidis, S.K. *et al.* (2003) Peritoneal cancer index: a prognostic indicator of survival in advanced ovarian cancer, 29: 69–73.

Thoits, P.A. (1982) Conceptual, methodological and theoretical problems in studying social support as a buffer against life stress. *Journal of Health and Social Behaviour*, 23: 145–59.

Thomas, M.R. and Lyttle, D. (1980) Patient expectations about success of treatment and reported relief from low back pain. *Journal of Psychosomatic Research*, 24: 297–301.

Thompson, P. (1989) Affective disorders, in P. Thompson (ed.) *The Instruments of Psychiatric Research*. Chichester: John Wiley.

Thompson, P. and Blessed, G. (1987) Correlation between the 37-item Mental Test Score and abbreviated 10-item Mental Test Score by psychogeriatric day patients. *British Journal of Psychiatry*, 151: 206–9.

Thompson, W. (1972) *Correlates of the Self Concept*. Nashville, TN: Counselor Recordings and Tests.

Timmermann, C. (2012) Just give me the best quality of life questionnaire: the Karnofsky scale and the history of quality of life measurements in cancer trials. *Chronic Illness*, 9: 179–90.

Tluczek, A., Henriques, J.B. and Brown, R.L. (2009) Support for the reliability and validity of a six-item State anxiety scale derived From the State-Trait Anxiety Inventory. *Journal of Nursing Measurement*, 17: 19–28.

Toevs, C.D., Kaplan, R.M. and Atkins, C.J. (1984) The costs and effects of behavioral programs in chronic obstructive pulmonary disease. *Medical Care*, 22: 1088–100.

Togari, T., Yamazaki, Y., Nakayama, K. and Shimizu, J. (2007) Development of a short version of the sense of coherence scale for population survey. *Journal of Epidemiology and Community Health*, 61: 921–2.

Tollefson, G.D. and Holman, S.L. (1993) Analysis of the Hamilton Depression Rating Scale factors from a double-blind, placebo-controlled trial of fluoxetine in geriatric major depression. *International Journal of Clinical Psychopharmacology*, 8: 253–9.

Tolsdorf, C.C. (1976) Social networks, support and coping: an exploratory study. *Family Process*, 15: 407–17.

Toner, J., Gurland, B. and Teresi, J. (1988) Comparison of self-administered and rater-administered methods of assessing levels of severity of depression in elderly patients. *Journal of Gerontology*, 43: 136–40.

Torrance, G.W. (1986) Measurement of health state utilities for economic appraisal. *Journal of Health Economics*, 5: 1–30.

Torrance, G.W. (1987) Utility approach to measuring health-related quality of life. *Journal of Chronic Diseases*, 40: 593–600.

Torrance, G.W., Thomas, W.H. and Sackett, D.L. (1972) A utility maximisation model for the evaluation of health care programs. *Health Services Research*, 7: 118–33.

Torrance, G.W., Boyle, M.H. and Horwood, S.P. (1982) Application of multiattribute utility theory to measure social preferences for health states. *Operations Research*, 30: 1043–69.

Tovbin, D., Gidron, Y., Jean, T. *et al.* (2003) Relative importance and interrelations between psychosocial factors and individualized quality of life of hemodialysis patients. *Quality of Life Research*, 12: 709–17.

Townsend, P. (1962) *The Last Refuge*. London: Routledge and Kegan Paul.

Townsend, P. (1979) *Poverty in the United Kingdom*. Harmondsworth: Pelican.

Trowbridge, N. (1970) Effects of socio-economic class on self-concept of children. *Psychology in the Schools*, 7: 304–6.

Trueman, P. and Duthie, T. (1998) Use of the Hospital Anxiety and Depression Scale (HAD) in a large, general population survey of epilepsy. *Quality of Life Newsletter*, 19: 9–10.

Tugwell, P., Bombardier, C., Buchanan, W.W. *et al.* (1987) The MACTAR patient preference disability questionnaire: an individualised functional priority approach for assessing improvement in physical disability in clinical trials in rheumatoid arthritis. *Journal of Rheumatology*, 14: 446–51.

Tugwell, P., Bombardier, C., Buchanan, W.W. *et al.* (1990) Methotrexate in rheumatoid arthritis: Impact on quality of life assessed by traditional standard-item and individualised patient preference health status questionnaire. *Archives of Internal Medicine*, 150: 59–62.

Tully, M. and Cantrill, J. (2000) The validity of the modified Patient Generated Index – a quantitative and qualitative approach. *Quality of Life Research*, 9: 509–20.

Turner-Bowker, D.M., Bayliss, M.S., Ware, J.E. and Kosinski, M. (2003) Usefulness of the SF-8 Health Survey for comparing the impact of migraine and other conditions. *Quality of Life Research*, 12: S10031012.

Turner-Stokes, L., Nyein, K., Turner-Stokes, T. and Gatehouse, C. (1999) The FIM and FAM: development and evaluation. *Clinical Rehabilitation*, 13: 277–87.

Twining, T.C. and Allen, D.G. (1981) Disability factors among residents in old people's homes. *Journal of Epidemiology and Community Health*, 36: 303–5.

Tyrer, P., Seivewright, N., Murphy, S. *et al.* (1988) The Nottingham study of neurotic disorder:

comparison of drug and psychological treatments. *Lancet*, 2: 235–40.

Tzeng, O.C., Maxey, W.A., Fortier, R. and Landis, D. (1985) Construct evaluation of the Tennessee Self Concept Scale. *Educational and Psychological Measurement*, 45: 63–78.

Unden, A.L. and Orth-Gomer, K. (1989) Development of a social support instrument for use in population surveys. *Social Science and Medicine*, 29: 1387–92.

Usui, W.M., Keil, T.J. and Durig, K.R. (1985) Socioeconomic comparisons and life satisfaction of elderly adults. *Journal of Gerontology*, 40: 110–14.

Uutela, T., Hakala, M. and Kautiainen, H. (2003) Validity of the Nottingham Health Profile in a Finnish out-patient population with rheumatoid arthritis. *Rheumatology*, 42: 841–5.

Uyl-de-Groot, C.A., Rutten, F.F.H. and Bonsel, G.J. (1994) Measurement and valuation of quality of life in economic appraisal of cancer treatment. *European Journal of Cancer*, 30A: 111–17.

Vacchiano, R.B. and Strauss, P.S. (1968) The construct validity of the Tennessee Self Concept Scale. *Journal of Clinical Psychology*, 24: 323–6.

Vahedi, S. (2010) World Health Organization Quality-of-Life Scale (WHOQOL-BREF): analyses of their item response theory properties based on the graded responses model, *Iran J Psychiatry*, 5: 140–53.

Valdenegro, J. and Barrera, M. (1983) Social support as a moderator of life stress: a longitudinal study using a multi-method analysis. Paper presented at the meeting of the Western Psychological Association, San Francisco, California.

Valtysdottir, S.T., Gudbjörnsson, B., Lindqvist, U. et al. (2000) Anxiety and depression in patients with primary Sjögren's syndrome. *Journal of Rheumatology*, 27: 165–9.

Van Agt, H.M.E., Esssink-Bot, M.L., van der Meer, J.B.W. and Bonsel, G.J. (1993) The NHP (Dutch version) in general and specified populations. Paper presented to the Fifth European *Health Services Research* Conference, Maastricht, December.

Van Agt, H.M.E., Essinck-Bot, M.L., Krabbe, P.F.M. et al. (1994) Test-retest reliability of health state evaluations collected with the EuroQol questionnaire. *Social Science and Medicine*, 39: 1537–44.

Van de Lisdonk, E.H. and van Weel, C. (1992) Cataract and functional status, in J.H. Scholten and C. van Weel (eds) *Functional Status Assessment in Family Practice*. Lelystad: Meditekst.

Van-Marwijk, H.W., Wallace, P., de-Bock, G.H. et al. (1995) Evaluation of the feasibility, reliability and diagnostic value of shortened versions of the geriatric depression scale. *British Journal of General Practice*, 45: 195–9.

van Weel, C. and Scholten, J.H.G. (1992) Report of an international workshop of the WONCA Research and Classification committee, in J.H. Scholten and C. van Weel (eds) *Functional Status Assessment in Family Practice*. Lelystad: Meditekst.

van Weel, C., König-Zahn, C., Touw-Otten, F.W.M.M. et al. (1995) *COOP/WONCA Charts. A Manual*. The Netherlands: World Organization of Family Doctors, European Research Group on Health Outcomes, Northern Centre for Health Care Research: University of Groningen.

Vaux, A. and Wood, J. (1985) Social support resources, behaviors and appraisals: a path analysis. Paper presented at the meeting of the Midwestern Psychological Association, Chicago.

Vaux, A., Burda, P. and Stewart, D. (1986a) Orientation toward utilizing support resources. *Journal of Community Psychology*, 14: 159–70.

Vaux, A., Phillips, J., Holly, L. et al. (1986b) The social support appraisals (SS-A) scale: studies of reliability and validity. *American Journal of Community Psychology*, 14: 195–219.

Vaux, A., Riedel, S. and Stewart, D. (1987) Modes of social support: the social support behaviours (SS-B) scale. *American Journal of Community Psychology*, 15: 209–337.

Veenhoven, R. (1991) Is happiness relative? *Social Indicators Research*, 24: 1–34.

Veenhoven, R. (1993) *Happiness in Nations: Subjective Appreciation of Life in 56 Nations 1946–1992*. Rotterdam, Netherlands: RISBO, Erasmus University of Rotterdam.

Veenhoven, R. (2000) The four qualities of life. Ordering concepts and measures of the good life. *Journal of Happiness Studies*, 1: 1–39.

Veenhoven, R. (2002) Why social policy needs subjective indicators. *Social Indicators Research*, 58: 33–45.

Ventegodt, S., Merrick, J. and Andersen, N.J. (2003) Measurement of quality of life III. From the IQOL theory: the global generic SEIQoL questionnaire. *Scientific World Journal*, 3: 972–91.

Vetter, N. and Ford, D. (1989) Anxiety and depression scores in elderly fallers. *International Journal of Geriatric Psychiatry*, 4: 159–63.

Vetter, N., Jones, D.A. and Victor, C.R. (1982) The importance of mental disabilities for the use of services by the elderly. *Journal of Psychosomatic Research*, 26: 607–12.

Vetter, N., Smith, A., Sastry, D. and Tinker, G. (1989) *Day Hospital – Pilot Study Report*. Cardiff, S. Wales: Research Team for the Care of Elderly People, Department of Geriatrics, St David's Hospital.

Vieweg, B.W. and Hedlund, J.L. (1983) The General Health Questionnaire: a comprehensive review. *Journal of Operational Psychiatry*, 14: 74–81.

Vincent, J. (1968) An explanatory factor analysis relating to the construct validity of self concept labels. *Educational and Psychological Measurement*, 28: 915–21.

von Strauss, E., Aguero-Torres, H., Kareholt, I. et al. (2003) Women are more disabled in basic activities of daily living than men in very advanced ages: a study on disability, morbidity, and mortality from the Kungsholmen Project. *Journal of Clinical Epidemiology*, 56: 669–77.

Wade, D.T. (1992) *Measurement in Neurological Rehabilitation*. Oxford: Oxford University Press.

Wade, D.T. and Collin, C. (1988) The Barthel ADL Index: a standard measure of physical disability. *International Disability Studies*, 10: 64–7.

Wade, D.T. and Langton-Hewer, R. (1987) Functional abilities after stroke: Measurement, natural history and prognosis. *Journal of Neurology, Neurosurgery and Psychiatry*, 50: 177–82.

Wade, D.T., Legh-Smith, G.L. and Langton-Hewer, R. (1985) Social activities after stroke: Measurement and natural history using the Frenchay Activities Index. *International Rehabilitation Medicine*, 7: 176–81.

Wade, D.T., Collen, F.M., Robb, G.F. and Warlow, C.P. (1992) Physiotherapy intervention late after stroke and mobility. *British Medical Journal*, 304: 609–13.

Waldron, D., O'Boyle, C.A., Kearney, M. et al. (1999) Quality of life measurement in advanced cancer: assessing the individual. *Journal of Clinical Oncology*, 17: 3603–11.

Walker, A., Maher, J., Coulthard, M. et al. (2001) *Living in Britain. Results from the General Household Survey 2001*. London: The Stationery Office.

Walker, C.E. and Kaufman, K. (1984) State–Trait Anxiety Inventory for Children, in D.J. Keyser and R.C. Sweetland (eds) *Test Critiques*, Vol. I. Kansas City, MO: Test Corporation of America.

Walker, K., Macbride, A. and Vachon, M.L.S. (1977) Social support networks and the crisis of bereavement. *Social Science and Medicine*, 11: 34–41.

Walkey, F.H., Seigert, R.J., McCormick, I.A. and Taylor, A.J. (1987) Multiple replication of the factor structure of the inventory of socially supportive behaviors. *Journal of Community Psychology*, 15: 513–19.

Wallace, J.L. and Vaux, A. (1993) Social network orientation: the role of adult attachment style. *Journal of Social and Clinical Psychology*, 12: 354–65.

Wallston, K.A., Brown, G.K., Stein, M.J. and Dobbins, C.J. (1989) Comparing the long and short versions of the Arthritis Impact Measurement Scales. *Journal of Rheumatology*, 16: 1105–9.

Wallwork, J. and Caine, N. (1985) A comparison of the quality of life of cardiac transplant patients and coronary artery bypass graft patients before and after surgery. *Quality of Life and Cardiovascular Care*, 1: 317–31.

Walsh, D., McCartney, G., McCullough, S. et al. (2014) Comparing Antonovsky's sense of coherence scale across three UK post-industrial cities. *British Medical Journal*, e005792 doi:10.1136/bmjopen-2014-005792.

Walsh, J.A. (1984) Tennessee Self Concept Scale, in D.J. Keyser and R.C. Sweetland (eds) *Test Critiques*, vol. 1. Kansas City, MI: Test Corporation of America.

Walters, S.J., Munro, J.F. and Brazier, J.E. (2001) Using the SF-36 with older adults: a cross-sectional community-based study. *Age and Ageing*, 30: 337–43.

Wan, T.T.H. and Livieratos, B. (1977) A validation of the General Well-being Index: a two-stage multivariate approach. Paper presented at American Public Health Association meeting, Washington, DC.

Wang, Y-P. and Gorenstein, C. (2013) Assessment of depression in medical patients: a systematic review of the utility of a Beck Depression Inventory-II. *Clinics*, 68: 12–87.

Ward, R.A. (1977) The impact of subjective age and stigma on older persons. *Journal of Gerontology*, 32: 227–32.

Ward, R.A., Sherman, S.R. and LaGory, M. (1984) Subjective network assessments and subjective well being. *Journal of Gerontology*, 39: 93–101.

Ware, J.E. (1984) Methodological considerations in the selection of health status assessment procedures, in N.K. Wenger, M.E. Mattson, C.D. Furberg et al. (eds) *Assessment of Quality of*

Life in Clinical Trials of Cardiovascular Therapies. New York: Le Jacq.

Ware, J.E. and Karmos, A.H. (1976) *Development and Validation of Scales to Measure Perceived Health and Patient Role Propensity*, vol. 2 of a final report. Carbondale, IL: Southern Illinois University School of Medicine, publication no. PB 288–331.

Ware, J.E. and Sherbourne, C.D. (1992) The MOS 36-item short-form health status survey (SF-36): conceptual framework and item selection. *Medical Care,* 30: 473–83.

Ware, J.E. and Young, J. (1979) Issues in the conceptualization and measurement of value placed on health, in S.J. Mushkin and D.W. Dunlop (eds) *Health: What is it Worth?* New York: Pergamon Press.

Ware, J.E., Johnson, S.A., Davies-Avery, A. *et al.* (1979) *Conceptualization and Measurement of Health for Adults in the Health Insurance Study*, vol. III, *Mental Health*. Santa Monica, CA: RAND Corporation: R1987/3-HEW.

Ware, J.E., Brook, R.H., Davies-Avery, A. *et al.* (1980) *Conceptualization and Measurement of Health for Adults in the Health Insurance Study*, vol. VI, *Analysis of Relationships among Health Status Measures*. Santa Monica, CA: RAND Corporation: R1987/6-HEW.

Ware, J.E., Sherbourne, C.D. and Davies, A.R. (1992) Developing and testing the MOS 20-item Short Form Health Survey: A general population application, in A.L. Stewart and J.E. Ware (eds) *Measuring Functioning and Well-being: The Medical Outcomes Study Approach*. Durham, NC: Duke University Press.

Ware, J.E., Snow, K.K., Kosinski, M. and Gandek, B. (1993) *SF-36 Health Survey: Manual and Interpretation Guide*. Boston, MA: The Health Institute, New England Medical Center.

Ware, J.E., Kosinski, M. and Keller, S.D. (1994) *SF-36 Physical and Mental Health Summary Scales: A User's Manual*. Boston, MA: The Health Institute, New England Medical Center.

Ware, J.E., Kosinski, M. and Keller, S.D. (1995) *How to score the SF-12 Physical and Mental Health Summary Scales*, 2nd edn. Boston, MA: The Health Institute, New England Medical Center.

Ware, J.E., Kosinski, M. and Keller, S.D. (1996a) *SF-12. An Even Shorter Health Survey*. Boston, MA: Medical Outcomes Trust Bulletin, 4: 2.

Ware, J.E., Kosinski, M. and Keller, S.D. (1996b) A 12-item short-form health survey. Construction of scales and preliminary tests of reliability and validity. *Medical Care*, 34: 220–33.

Ware, J.E., Snow, K.K., Kosinski, M. and Gandek, B. (1997) *SF-36 Health Survey: Manual and Interpretation Guiide. Revised edition.* Boston, MA: The Health Institute, New England Medical Center.

Ware, J.E., Kosinski, M., Dewey, J. and Gandek, B. (2001). *How to Score and Interpret Single-item Health Status Measures: A Manual for Users of the SF-8 Health Survey.* Boston, MA: QualityMetric.

Warr, P. (1978) A study of psychological well-being. *British Journal of Psychology*, 69: 111–21.

Warr, P. (1999) Well-being and the workplace, in D. Kahnerman, E. Diener and N. Schwarz (eds) *Wellbeing: The Foundations of Hedonic Psychology*. New York: Russell Sage.

Watchel, T., Piette, J., Mor, V. *et al.* (1992) Quality of life in persons with human immunodeficiency virus infection: Measurement by the medical outcomes study instrument. *Annals of Internal Medicine*, 116: 129–37.

Watson, E. and Evans, S. (1986) An example of cross-cultural measurement of psychological symptoms in post-partum mothers. *Social Science and Medicine*, 23: 869–74.

Webb, E.J., Campbell, D.T., Schwartz, R.D. *et al.* (1966) *Unobtrusive Measures: Non-reactive Research in the Social Sciences*. Chicago, IL: Rand McNally College Publishing.

Weckowicz, T., Muir, W. and Cropley, A. (1967) A factor analysis of the Beck Inventory of Depression. *Journal of Consulting Psychology*, 31: 23–8.

Weill Cornell Medical Library (2003) A brief history of the Cornell Medical Index. New York: Weill Medical College of Cornell University, Weill Cornell Medical Library (available on line http://library.med.cornell.edu/library, accessed on 8 August 2016).

Weinberger, M., Tierney, W.M., Booher, P. and Hiner, S.L. (1990) Social support, stress and functional status in patients with osteoarthritis. *Social Science and Medicine*, 30: 503–8.

Weiss, R.S. (1973) *Loneliness: The Experience of Emotional and Social Isolation*. Cambridge, MA: MIT Press.

Welin, L., Tibblin, G., Svardsudd, K. *et al.* (1985) Prospective study of the social influences on mortality. The study of men born in 1913 and 1923. *Lancet*, 1: 915–18.

Wells, E. and Marwell, G. (1976) *Self Esteem*. Beverly Hills, CA: Sage Publications.

Wells, K.B., Hays, R.D., Burnam, M.A. *et al.* (1989a) Detection of depressive disorder for patients receiving pre-paid or fee for service care: results from the medical outcomes study. *Journal of the American Medical Association*, 262: 3298–302.

Wells, K.B., Stewart, A., Hays, R.D. *et al.* (1989b) The functioning and well-being of depressed patients: results from the medical outcomes study. *Journal of the American Medical Association*, 262: 914–19.

Wenger, G.C. (1989) Support networks in old age – constructing a typology, in M. Jefferys (ed.) *As Britain Ages*. London: Routledge.

Wenger, G.C. (1992) *Help in Old Age – Facing up to Change*. Liverpool: Liverpool University Press.

Wenger, G.C. (1994) *Support Networks of Older People: A Guide for Practitioners*. Bangor: Centre for Social Policy Research and Development, University of Wales.

Wenger, G.C. (1995) *Practitioner Assessment of Network Type (PANT). Training and Resource Pack*. Brighton: Pavilion Press.

Wenger, G.C. and Shahtahmasebi, S. (1991) Survivors: support network variation and sources of help in rural communities. *Journal of Cross-Cultural Gerontology*, 6: 41–82.

Wenger, N.K., Mattson, M.E., Furberg, C.D. *et al.* (eds) (1984) *Assessment of Quality of Life in Clinical Trials of Cardiovascular Therapies*. New York, Le Jacq.

Wentowski, G. (1982) Reciprocity and the coping strategies of older people: cultural dimensions of network building. *Gerontologist*, 21: 600–9.

Wettergren, L., Björkholm, M., Axdorph, U. *et al.* (2003) Individual quality of life in long-term survivors of Hodgkin's lymphoma – a comparative study. *Quality of Life Research*, 12: 545–54.

White, D.K., Wilson, J.C. and Ketsor, J.J. (2011) Measures of adult general functional status. *Arthritis Care and Research*, 63, S11: S297–307.

WHOQOL Group (1993) *Measuring quality of life: the development of the World Health Organization Quality of Life Instrument (WHOQOL)*. Geneva: World Health Organization.

WHOQOL Group (1994) *The development of the WHO quality of life assessment instrument (the WHOQOL)*, in J. Orley and W. Kuyken (eds) *Quality of Life Assessment: International Perspectives*. Heidelberg: Springer-Verlag.

WHOQOL Group (1995) The World Health Organization quality of life assessment (WHOQOL): position paper from the World Health Organization. Special Issue 'Quality of Life' in *Social Science and Medicine*, 10: 1403–9.

WHOQOL Group (1996) The World Health Organization Quality of Life (WHOQOL) Assessment Instrument, in B. Spilker (ed.) *Quality of Life and Pharmacoeconomics in Clinical Trials*, 2nd edn. Hagerstown, MD: Lippincott-Raven Publishers.

WHOQOL Group (1998a) The World Health Organization Quality of Life Assessment (WHOQOL): development and general psychometric properties. *Social Science and Medicine*, 46: 1569–85.

WHOQOL Group (1998b) Development of the World Health Organization WHOQOL-BREF Quality of Life Assessment. *Psychological Medicine*, 28: 551–8.

Wiest, W.M. (1965) A qualitative extension of Heider's theory of cognitive balance applied to interpersonal perception and self esteem. *Psychological Monographs: General and Applied*, 79: 1–20.

Wiggins, R.D., Netuvelli, G., Hyde, M. *et al.* (2008) The evaluation of a self-enumerated scale of quality of life (CASP-19) in the context of research on ageing: a combination of exploratory and confirmatory approaches. *Social Indicators Research*, 89: 61–77.

Wilkin, D. (1987) Conceptual problems in dependency research. *Social Science and Medicine*, 24: 867–73.

Wilkin, D. and Jolley, D.J. (1979) *Behavioural Problems among Old People in Geriatric Wards, Psychogeriatric Wards and Residential Homes, 1976-78*. Research Report no. 1, Research Section, Psychiatric Unit, University Hospital of South Manchester.

Wilkin, D. and Thompson, C. (1989) *User's Guide to Dependency Measures for Elderly People*. Sheffield Social Services Monographs: Research in Practice. University of Sheffield, Joint Unit for Social Services Research.

Wilkin, D., Hallam, L. and Doggett, M. (1992) *Measures of Need and Outcome for Primary Care*. New York: Oxford Medical Publications.

Wilkinson, M.J.B. and Barczak, P. (1988) Psychiatric screening in general practice: Comparisons of the General Health Questionnaire and the Hospital Anxiety and Depression Scale. *Journal of the Royal College of General Practitioners*, 38: 311–13.

Wilkinson, P.R., Wolfe, C.D., Warburton, F.G. *et al.* (1997) Longer term quality of life and outcome in stroke patients: is the Barthel Index alone an adequate measure of outcome? *Quality in Health Care*, 6: 125–30.

Williams, A. (1985) The value of QALYS. *Health and Social Services Journal*, 95: 3–5.

Williams, J.B.W. and Kobak, K.A. (2008) Development and reliability of a structured interview guide for the Montgomery–Åsberg Depression Rating Scale (SIGMA). *British Journal of Psychiatry*, 192: 52–8.

Williams, J.M.G. (1984) *The Psychology of Depression*. Beckenham: Croom Helm.

Williams, P. (1987) Depressive thinking in general practice patients, in P. Freeling, L.J. Downey and J.C. Malkin (eds) *The Presentation of Depression: Current Approaches*. Royal College of General Practitioners, Occasional Paper, 36: 17–20.

Williams, R.G.A., Johnston, M., Willis, M. *et al.* (1976) Disability: a model and measurement technique. *British Journal of Preventive and Social Medicine*, 30: 71–8.

Williams, S.J. and Bury, M.J. (1989) Impairment, disability and handicap in chronic respiratory illness. *Social Science and Medicine*, 29: 609–16.

Wills, T.A. and Filer, M. (2006) Interpersonal Support Evaluation List (ISEL) – college version: validation and application in a Greek Sample, *International Journal of Social Psychiatry*, 52: 552–60.

Wilson-Barnett, J. (1981) Assessment of recovery: with special reference to a study with post-operative cardiac patients. *Journal of Advanced Nursing*, 6: 435–45.

Winefield, H.R., Gill, T.K., Taylor, A.W. and Pilkington, R.M. (2012) Psychological well-being and psychological distress: is it necessary to measure both? *Psychology of Well-Being: Theory, Research and Practice*, 2: 3.

Wing, J.K. (1991) Measuring and classifying clinical disorders: learning from the PSE, in P.E. Bebbington (ed.) *Social Psychiatry: Theory, Methodology and Practice*. London: Transaction Publishers.

Wing, J.K., Cooper, J.E. and Sartorius, N. (1974) *The Measurement and Classification of Psychiatric Symptoms: An Instruction Manual for the PSE and CATEGO Program*. Cambridge: Cambridge University Press.

Witham, M.D., Fulton, R. L., Wilson, L. *et al.* (2008) Validation of an individualized quality of life measure in older day hospital patients. *Health and Quality of Life Outcomes*, 6: 27.

Wolfe, F. Michaud, K. and Pincus, T. (2004) Development and validation of the Health Assessment Questionnaire II: a revised version of the health assessment questionnaire. *Arthritis and Rheumatism*, 50: 3296–305.

Wollstadt, L.J., Glasser, M. and Nutter, T. (1997) Variations in functional status among different groups of elderly people. *Family Medicine*, 29: 394–9.

Wood, V., Wylie, M.L. and Scheafor, B. (1969) An analysis of a short self-report measure of life satisfaction: correlation with rater judgements. *Journal of Gerontology*, 24: 465–9.

Wood-Dauphinee, S. and Williams, J.I. (1991) The Spitzer Quality of Life Index: Its performance as a measure, in D. Osoba (ed.) *Effect of Cancer on Quality of Life*. Boston, MA: CRC Press.

Woods, N.F., Lentz, M., Mitchel, E. and Oakley, L.D. (1994) Depressed mood and self-esteem in young Asian, black and white women in America. *Health Care and Women International*, 15: 243–62.

World Health Organization (1947) *Constitution of the World Health Organization*. Geneva: World Health Organization.

World Health Organization (1948a) *Preamble to the Constitution of the World Health Organization as adopted by the International Health Conference, New York 19–22 June 1946*. Geneva: World Health Organization.

World Health Organization (1948b) *Official Records of the World Health Organization*, no. 2, p. 100. Geneva: World Health Organization.

World Health Organization (1958) *The First Ten Years of the World Health Organization*. Geneva: World Health Organization.

World Health Organization (1979) *Handbook for Reporting Results of Cancer Treatments*. WHO Offset Publication No. 48. Geneva: World Health Organization.

World Health Organization (1980) *International Classification of Impairments, Disabilities and Handicaps*. Geneva: World Health Organization.

World Health Organization (1985) *Targets for Health for All by the Year 2000*. Copenhagen: World Health Organization. Regional Office for Europe.

World Health Organization (1998) *ICIDH-2. International Classification of Impairments, Activities and Participation. A Manual of Dimensions of Disablement and Functioning*, Geneva: World Health Organization.

World Health Organization (2001) *International Classification of Functioning, Disability and Health*. Geneva: World Health Organization.

World Health Organization (2002) *The World Health Report 2002: Reducing Risks, Promoting Healthy Life*. Geneva: World Health Organization.

World Health Organization (2004) *International Classification of Diseases* (10th revision), vols I–III (2nd edn). Geneva: World Health Organization.

Wylie, C.M. and White, B.K. (1964) A measure of disability. *Archives of Environmental Health*, 8: 834–9.

Wylie, M.L. (1970) Life satisfaction as a program impact criterion. *Journal of Gerontology*, 25: 36–40.

Wylie, R.C. (1974) *The Self Concept*. Lincoln, NE: University of Nebraska Press.

Yang, K. and Victor, C. (2011) Age and loneliness in 25 European nations. *Ageing and Society*, 31: 1368–8.

Yates, J.W., Chalmer, B. and McKegney, F.P. (1980) Evaluation of patients with advanced cancer using the Karnofsky Performance Status. *Cancer*, 45: 2220–4.

Yen, I.H. and Kaplan, G.A. (1999) Poverty area residence and changes in depression and perceived health status: evidence from the Alameda County Study. *International Journal of Epidemiology*, 28: 90–4.

Yesavage, J.A., Brink, T.L., Rose, T.L. *et al.* (1983) Development and validation of a geriatric depression screening scale – a preliminary report. *Journal of Psychiatric Research*, 17: 37–49.

Yohannes, Y., Roomi, J., Waters, K. and Connolly, M. (1998) A comparison of the Barthel index and Nottingham extended activities of daily living scale in the assessment of disability in chronic air-flow limitation in old age. *Age and Ageing*, 27: 369–74.

Young, F.B., Lees, K.R. and Weir, C.J. (2003) Strengthening acute stroke trials through optimal use of disability end points. *Stroke*, 34: 2676–80.

Zegers Prado, B., Rojas-Barahona, C. and Förster Marín, C. (2009) Validity and reliability of the Neugarten, Havighurst & Tobin's Life Satisfaction Index (LSI-A), in a sample of adults and older adults in Chile. *Terapia Psicológica*, 27: 15–26.

Zigmond, A.S. and Snaith, R.P. (1983) The Hospital Anxiety and Depression Scale. *Acta Psychiatrica Scandinavica*, 67: 361–70.

Ziller, R.C. (1974) Self-other orientations and quality of life. *Social Indicators Research*, 1: 301–27.

Ziller, R.C., Hagey, J., Smith, M.D. *et al.* (1969) Self-esteem: a social construct. *Journal of Consulting and Clinical Psychology*, 33: 84–95.

Zimmerman, M., Chelminski, I. and Posternak, M. (2004) A review of studies of the Montgomery-Asberg Depression Rating Scale in controls: implications for the definition of remission in treatment studies of depression. *International Clinical Pharmacology*, 19: 1–7.

Zissi, A., Barry, M.M. and Cochrane, R. (1998) A mediational model of quality of life for individuals with severe mental health problems. *Psychological Medicine*, 28: 1221–30.

Zubrod, C.G., Schneiderman, M., Frei, E. *et al.* (1960) Appraisal of methods for the study of chemotherapy of cancer in man: Comparative therapeutic trial of nitrogen mustard and triethylene thiophosphoramide. *Journal of Chronic Diseases*, 11: 7–33.

Zung, W.W.K. (1965) A self-rating depression scale. *Archives of General Psychiatry*, 12: 63–70.

Zung, W.W.K. (1967) Depression in the normal aged. *Psychosomatics*, 8: 287–92.

Zung, W.W.K. (1972) The Depression Status Inventory: An adjunct to the self-rating depression scale. *Journal of Clinical Psychology*, 28: 539–43.

Zung, W.W.K. (1986) Zung Self-Rating Depression Scale and Depression Status Inventory, in N. Sartorius and T.A. Ban (eds) *Assessment of Depression*. Heidelberg: Springer-Verlag.

Zung, W.W.K., Richards, C.B. and Short, M.J. (1965) Self rating depression scale in an out-patient clinic: further validation of the ZDS. *Archives of General Psychiatry*, 13: 508–15.

INDEX

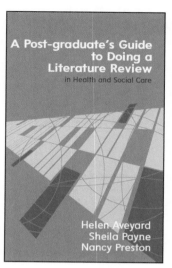

A Postgraduate's Guide to Doing a Literature Review in Health and Social Care

Helen Aveyard, Sheila Payne and Nancy Preston

9780335263684 (Paperback)
February 2016

eBook also available

This text is a comprehensive, highly readable guide to how to undertake a literature review in health and social care, tailored specifically for postgraduate study. Providing clarity and a step by step approach to doing a literature review from start to finish it will enable you to:

- Identify which type of review is appropriate for your study
- Select the literature that you need to include in your review
- Search for, appraise and analyse relevant literature
- Write up your review

The book explores the common features of a broad range of types of literature review, which serve different functions – including the literature review that is a pre-requisite prior to a larger empirical study, and the literature review that is a study in its own right. With real-life examples of written research and succinct summaries at the end of each chapter, this is the ideal text for students wanting to get the very most from their study.

www.openup.co.uk

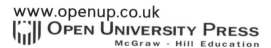

OPEN UNIVERSITY PRESS
McGraw - Hill Education

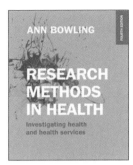

RESEARCH METHODS IN HEALTH 4/e
INVESTIGATING HEALTH AND HEALTH SERVICES

Ann Bowling

June 2014
9780335262748 – Paperback

eBook also available

This bestselling book provides an accessible introduction to the concepts and practicalities of research methods in health and health services. This new edition has been extensively re-worked and expanded and now includes expanded coverage of:

- Qualitative methods
- Social research
- Evaluation methodology
- Mixed methods
- Secondary data analysis
- Literature reviewing and critical appraisal
- Evidence based practice

Covering all core methodologies in detail the book looks at the following kinds of health research:

- health needs
- morbidity and mortality trends and rates
- costing health services
- sampling for survey research
- cross-sectional and longitudinal survey design
- experimental methods and techniques of group assignment
- questionnaire design
- interviewing techniques
- coding and analysis of quantitative data
- methods and analysis of qualitative observational studies
- unstructured interviewing

The book is grounded in the author's career as a researcher on health and health service issues, and the valuable experience this has provided in meeting the challenges of research on people and organisations in real life settings.

This book is an essential companion for students and researchers of health and health services, health clinicians and policy-makers with responsibility for applying research findings and judging the soundness of research.

www.openup.co.uk

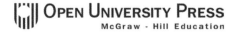

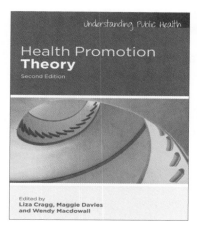

HEALTH PROMOTION THEORY
Second Edition

Liza Cragg, Maggie Davies and Wendy Macdowall

9780335263202 (Paperback)
October 2013

eBook also available

Part of the *Understanding Public Health* series, this book offers students and practitioners an accessible exploration of the origins and development of health promotion. It highlights the philosophical, ethical and political debates that influence health promotion today while also explaining the theories, frameworks and methodologies that help us understand public health problems and develop effective health promotion responses.

Key features:

- Offers more in-depth coverage of key determinants of health and how these interact with health promotion
- Revised structure to allow more depth of coverage of health promotion theory
- Updated material and case examples that reflect contemporary health promotion challenges

www.openup.co.uk

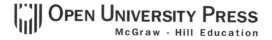

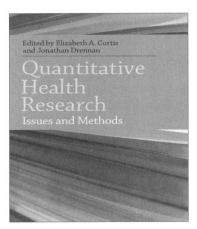

QUANTITATIVE HEALTH RESEARCH
Issues and Methods

Elizabeth A. Curtis and Jonathan Drennan

9780335245734 (Paperback)
August 2013

eBook also available

This book is a detailed and comprehensive guide to undertaking quantitative health research at postgraduate and professional level. It takes you through the entire research process, from designing the project to presenting the results and will help you execute high quality quantitative research that improves and informs clinical practice.

Key features:

- Ethical considerations of research
- Designing and planning quantitative research projects
- Data measurement and collection

www.openup.co.uk

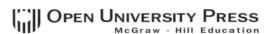

OPEN UNIVERSITY PRESS
McGraw - Hill Education

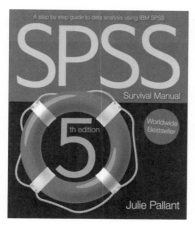

SPSS SURVIVAL MANUAL
Fifth Edition

Julie Pallant

9780335262588 (Paperback)
August 2013

eBook also available

In her bestselling guide, now covering up to version 21 of the SPSS software, Julie Pallant guides you through the entire research process, helping you choose the right data analysis technique for your project. From the formulation of research questions, to the design of the study and analysis of data, to reporting the results, Julie discusses basic and advanced statistical techniques. She outlines each technique clearly, with step by step procedures for performing the analysis, a detailed guide to interpreting data output and an example of how to present the results in a report.

Key features:

- Fully revised and updated to accommodate changes to IBM SPSS version 21 procedures, screens and output
- Additional recommended readings and websites have been added
- Supported by a website with sample data and guidelines on report writing

www.openup.co.uk
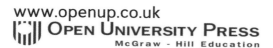
OPEN UNIVERSITY PRESS
McGraw - Hill Education

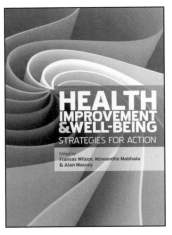

Health Improvement and Well-being
Strategies for Action

Frances Wilson, Mzwandile Andi
Mabhala and Alan Massey

9780335244959 (Paperback)
October 2014

eBook also available

This book aims to widen the perspective of health professionals to
encompass the concept of well-being across the lifespan. It has been written
to introduce students to the theory and practical application of health
improvement and well-being in the context of public health, providing
global as well as domestic perspectives on key concepts, in particular:

- Social and health inequalities
- Social justice
- Political influences
- Commissioning, funding and delivery of services

Each chapter defines and provides an outline of theoretical perspectives
relevant to each topic, allowing the reader to critically evaluate the
accepted wisdom in each field. Case studies illustrate local and global
perspectives and questions throughout the book encourage students to think
and reflect on the key points of each chapter and apply theory to practice.

This book is key reading for experienced and senior public health
professionals as well as masters level students taking modules in public
health, health improvement or health promotion.

www.openup.co.uk

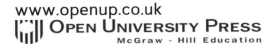

OPEN UNIVERSITY PRESS
McGraw - Hill Education